BASIC HEALTH PLANNING METHODS

Allen D. Spiegel, Ph.D.
Herbert Harvey Hyman, Ph.D.

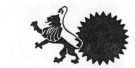

Aspen Systems Corporation
Germantown, Maryland
1978

Library of Congress Cataloging in Publication Data

Spiegel, Allen D.
Basic health planning methods.

Bibliography: p. 473.
Includes index.

1. Health planning.   I. Hyman, Herbert
Harvey, joint author.   II. Title.
RA393.867   362.1   78-10780
ISBN 0-89443-077-7

Library of Congress Catalog Card Number: 78-10780
ISBN: 0-89443-077-7
Printed in the United States of America
3 4 5

Table of Contents

Preface

Phrases such as *cottage industry, fragmented, topsy-turvy,* and *red tape* have all been used, along with other negative adjectives, to describe the health care industry. In terms of dollars spent and numbers of workers employed, the health care industry merits the serious attention of planners in general and health planners in particular. This has been reflected in recent federal legislative mandates that have emphasized maintaining the quality of health care while containing the cost.

Our purpose in writing this book is to present a large number of health planning methods and techniques that are linked to the relevant steps within a systems-oriented health planning process. Although we have concentrated on basic methods and techniques of health planning, we certainly have not included all methodologies. We have selected a variety of methods and techniques and suggest that health planners utilize this book as a jumping off point rather than as a stationary commencement point. This book should serve as a basic tool for practitioners, students, and teachers.

An introductory chapter sets the stage and emphasizes the potential impact of health planning within the health care delivery system. Each of the next six chapters is devoted to one of the steps that we have identified in a rational health planning process:

Identifying the Problem: Methods for Need Assessment and Resources Analysis
Inventorying Health Resources
Generating and Considering Alternative Courses of Action
Priority Determination
Promoting Implementation
Evaluation

In Appendix A we have included an example of the planning process as applied to family planning. We chose this example to illustrate that the steps used may differ and the words for each step may differ, but the overall process is similar for most health planning efforts.

A bibliography is also included that is a bit different. This bibliography is intended to indicate the need for health planners to keep up with the literature and to realize that changes are taking place constantly that will affect the methods and techniques utilized in the process of health planning. Therefore, we have selected about 160 items that are taken, for the most part, from journals published within the past two years. In addition, the references at the end of each chapter provide more resource material.

This book should be useful to practitioners, educators, and students and fill the void for a practical handbook on health planning methods and techniques. Practitioners such as health systems agencies staff members, hospital planners, professional standards review organization staff, governmental public health and mental health administrators, professional association committee members, and the growing number of consumers involved in decision making should be able to pick and choose methods and techniques to fit the appropriate situation. Educators have noted that they needed a text to use with students enrolled in educational programs that related to health planning. Obviously, we hope that schools teaching health planning will make use of this book, but we also hope that schools of medicine, nursing, social work, and allied health professions will consider the importance of integrating instruction about health planning methods and techniques into relevant parts of their curriculums. Students, of course, can use this book as a source and add it to their professional library for future use on their jobs.

Generally, we see our book as a stimulator and motivator. Material in the book is intended to generate ideas and to encourage adaptations. This book is not a panacea; rather, we hope that it serves to call attention to the "art and science" of health planning.

Allen D. Spiegel
Herbert Harvey Hyman
November 1978

Chapter 1

Basic Health Planning Methods: An Introduction

WHY THIS BOOK?

In an article on planning, N. Krumholz[1] noted the essential aspect of a health planner's job in relation to competence and politics:

> The power to influence decisions is directly related to professional competence. Politicians, high-ranking bureaucrats and other important actors in the public decision-making process are not interested in rhetoric. . . . Nor are they interested in planners' political "feel" of an issue. Most of them have a far better grasp of such matters than any planner. What frequently does interest them is informed recommendations directed at tangible objectives, backed by careful analysis and sound data, and presented in a manner that is meaningful to them.

Thus, the call goes out for technical competence by health planners. To echo this point, a study by W. J. Waters[2] of 42 state comprehensive health planning agencies (CHPs) documents the disparity between concepts of health planning and actual practices. Exhibit 1-1 notes the completion rate of ten key planning tasks by 42 CHPs. Only three of the ten tasks were completed by more than 50 percent of the CHPs. A question can be raised as to the value of specific action recommendations (completed by 73 percent of the CHPs) when only 19 percent ranked alternative interventions, only 26 percent established health targets, and only 36 percent agreed on a health system definition. Waters concludes from his study:

- There was a significant disparity between the practice of comprehensive health planning at the state level and the concept of

1

Exhibit 1-1 Completion of Key Planning Tasks by 42 State CHP Agencies

Key Planning Tasks	Percentage	
	Completed	Not Completed
Selected an agreed upon health system definition	36	64
Established a modus operandi for preparing a state health plan	72	28
Selected planning horizons, i.e., terminal periods	74	26
Chose problem priorities	50	50
Set and ranked health goals	41	59
Established health targets, i.e., quantified, time-related goals	26	74
Thoroughly analyzed alternative interventions	29	71
Ranked alternative interventions	19	81
Formally made specific actions recommendations	73	27
Selected criteria and procedures for intervention evaluation	43	57

Source: Reprinted with permission from the *American Journal of Health*, vol. 66, p. 139. Copyright 1976 by the American Public Health Association, 1015 Eighteenth Street, N.W. Washington, D.C. 20036.

comprehensive health planning as it evolved over time in the literature.

- State CHP agencies apparently were not engaged in technical analyses to any appreciable extent.
- Activities of the state CHP agencies appeared to lack the degree of explicitness that should be associated with planning operations.
- The majority of state CHP agencies were not setting planning priorities; i.e., not problem, end, or means priorities.
- State CHP agencies appeared to be viewing the health system in only partial terms. Further, they seemed to have only limited interests in those partial systems or subsystems.
- State CHP agencies were taking a nonintegrated approach to their planning activities.

To translate the conclusions of his study into practical application, Waters proposed a number of actions to close the gap between theory and reality:

• Greater emphasis should be placed on planning methods per se in the training of health planners.
• Increased attention should be given to the technical aspects of health planning in the allocation of health planning research funds.
• There needs to be a clearer statement of the functional priorities of health planning agencies.
• The necessity and importance of state level health planning should be reaffirmed.
• A limited number of statewide health planning demonstration projects would be beneficial.
• Health planners should give greater emphasis to preventive inputs and health status outcomes in their planning activities.

Clearly, Waters' study demonstrated the need for material about basic health planning methods that could be utilized by students as well as practitioners.

In a 1977 article in *Hospitals*, R. N. Whiting[3] commented on the continuing debate about whether or not health planning was working. In speaking to the role of the Health Systems Agencies (HSAs), he stated:

Probably the larger issue facing hospitals in their relationships with HSAs is whether the agencies will simply represent another hurdle to be dealt with or whether a more productive interaction can be developed.

Whiting also commented on the question of the HSA staff capabilities in health planning, noting the lack of formal training and actual experience in health planning. In relation to Whiting's comment about another hurdle for hospitals to jump, it should be mentioned that, historically, the hospitals have fared extremely well in jumping hurdles established by legislation and/or regulations.

These comments have been echoed by others and all lead to the conclusion that a book detailing basic health planning methods is timely. Nevertheless, a book on basic health planning methods should not be regarded as a panacea for the deficiencies mentioned above. Health planners should be aware of the precarious position that they are placed in every time they undertake any activity. A. Wildavsky[4] summed up this position neatly in his article, "If Planning is Everything, Maybe it's Nothing," explicitly describing the schizophrenic nature of the planner's job:

> Where planning does not measure up to expectations, which is almost everywhere, planners are handy targets. They have been too ambitious or they have not been ambitious enough. They have perverted their calling by entering into politics or they have been insensitive to the political dimensions of their task. They ignore national cultural mores at their peril or they capitulate to blind forces of irrationality. They pay too much attention to the relationship between one sector of the economy and another while ignoring analysis of individual projects, or they spend so much time on specific matters that they are unable to deal with movements of the economy as a whole. Planners can no longer define a role for themselves. From old American cities to British new towns, from the richest countries to the poorest, planners have difficulty in explaining who they are and what they should be expected to do. If they are supposed to doctor sick societies, the patient never seems to get well. Why can't the planners ever seem to do the right thing?

PLANNING OVERVIEW

Planning can have quite different meanings, each correct according to what it seeks to describe. In a sense, the style of planning has to be determined by the participants. It also must establish itself on a point along the continuum that runs from the purely rational through the feasible to the irrational.

E. C. Banfield[5] presents a common definition of the term planning: "a plan ... is a decision with regard to a course of action ... (a) a sequence of acts which are mutually related as means and therefore are viewed as a unit; it is the unit which is the plan." By narrowing the broad definition of planning, later use of the concept in examining problems that planners face can be facilitated.

Often social scientists attempt to clarify the meaning of a broad and/or abstract concept through use of an ideal type or model. Several models have been proposed for the planning process, and two major and quite opposite interpretations of planning can be cited. One model implies the rational and comprehensive examination of all alternatives as a basis for future action. By way of contrast, the other interpretation portrays a process of ordering future programs and policies which is both noncomprehensive and incomplete but stresses feasibility.

Charles E. Lindblom[6] presents an elaborate discussion of the contrasting extremes in planning. Lindblom proposed two models, one indicating characteristics of "rational" planning and the other showing a noncomprehensive, or "muddling through," approach.

Lindblom's characteristics of the "rational" model include the following:

- Planning proceeding from distinct values and objectives.
- Comprehensive means-ends analysis.
- Recommended alternatives of proven merit.
- Complete analysis of all variables.
- Significant reliance on theory.

In contrast, the "muddling through" approach is illustrated by the following characteristics:

- Intertwined empirical and value analysis.
- Nondistinct ends and means.
- Consensus as a measure of components.
- Limited analysis of variables (resulting in neglected alternatives and uncertain results).
- A reduced role of theory.

Banfield also sees two extremes in planning. His abridgement of the planning process in a rational model includes: (1) the decision maker lists all alternatives, (2) he identifies the results that would ensue, and (3) he settles on the action that is most favorable. Like Lindblom, Banfield has an alternative planning type that is in contrast to the rational ideal. Thus, his noncomprehensive model is described as "more or less systematic in the canvass of alternatives and probable consequences," although Banfield and Lindblom probably had different ideas in mind and Banfield would most likely object to one designating his latter approach as similar to "muddling through." Moving from a rational model to one constrained by a pluralistic complex society, R. Morris and R. Binstock's[7] feasible approach can be considered. They define feasible planning as an orderly process of evaluating the alternative ways in which goals might be achieved, in view of the opposing forces with which the actors must contend to realize their objectives.

LIMITING CONDITIONS IN PLANNING

A number of limiting conditions, serving to decrease the rationality in planning, have been noted by several commentators. Examination of some of the major limiting conditions can be grouped under three headings:

- value determination re goals and objectives, clarification and conflict;
- data and information accumulation; and
- formal and informal organizational conditions.

Value Determination re Goals and Objectives

A basic premise of the rational approach is that planning will proceed from distinct values and objectives. Yet, it seems obvious, as Lindblom notes, "social objectives do not always have the same relative values." The ambiguous meanings of such terms as goals and objectives compound the problem. These concepts may be easily distinguished, for they are often used interchangeably. R. C. Young[8] distinguishes goals as abstract, ideal, and shared by large numbers of people; objectives are specific desired ends "capable of both attainment and measurement."

Morris and Binstock tackle this issue by calling for terms to reflect the content of goals and subgoals or means and submeans to characterize the linkage between them. Thus, they develop a series of distinctions such as preamble goals, policy goals, and planning goals. A preamble goal would apply to the end most people in the planner's society would accept as normative. A policy goal would bring the goal into a decision to do something specific. A planning goal would apply to actually planning for the specific end.

These distinctions raise an old dispute—are ends or means most important in planning? This dispute can be closely related to the role of value problems in planning. Although it may be an oversimplification, different value problems are encountered in the setting of goals than in the setting of objectives or alternative methods to reach objectives. A goal to abolish slums reflects community consensus to attack the problem at a high level. At this level, value problems for the planner are often solved by decisions beyond his control. Goals can be set by public demands, official guidelines, legal constraints, or by resources available to the planner. Objectives, by way of contrast, raise difficult value problems. What are the merits of rehabilitating the houses on City Square?

Planners must use different methods to determine and clarify goals or ends than they would for objectives or means. For the former, the emphasis is often on clarification. For the latter, determination and clarification are likely to be in competition, and value conflicts must be resolved. The problem of values may be beyond ultimate solution. Both goals and objectives may shift in terms of values assigned to them. Yet, despite the ambiguity that remains, the problems raised by goals and values can be viewed as setting a possible foundation for a pragmatic planning approach.

Data and Information Accumulation

William Peterson[9] outlines the main issue that confronts planners when they seek to gather and evaluate the information necessary for "rational" or comprehensive planning:

> Indeed, our ignorance in many areas is so great that if we demanded an adequate base for planning, in many cases we could hardly begin to plan. What information exists, moreover, is seldom available in a coordinated, up-to-date, usable form to the agencies that need it.

Thus, the planner is faced with a problem of planning on the basis of only part of the facts, or not planning at all:

> The horns of this moral dilemma are sharp for a democratic empiricist. If administrators act on the basis of incomplete knowledge, they may do serious harm to those affected by their policies. But if they fail to act, the state of our knowledge will remain inadequate. For, typically the facts we need are precisely those in a human rather than a technical context, what John Dewey termed "social facts."

Peterson can be interpreted as saying that we learn by doing. Issues are clarified, and techniques are refined only through application. Perhaps this provides an insight into the dilemma of accumulating data and overcoming value objections to alternative means and objectives. Failure to devise and apply techniques for ordering factual data leads to decreased rationality in planning. As a corollary, administrators and planners cite the lack of techniques and devices for gathering facts as a reason why increased rationality in planning is impossible. This rationale approaches a self-fulfilling prophecy. Starting with an incomplete or false definition of the situation, the assumption is made that no method exists of gathering significant amounts of information. Then, by acting on this false assessment, results are assured that fill the initial description. Namely, that failure to investigate informational sources and devise tools for solving the data problem does hinder rationality in planning. A pragmatic approach to planning would attempt to discover methods of ordering required data.

Formal and Informal Organizational Conditions

Banfield notes, "in the real world, rationality means 'alternatives' and 'consequences' are considered as fully as the decision maker, given the time and other resouces available to him, can afford to consider them." This statement suggests a third major limiting condition on planning determined by organizational factors.

The degree of rationality in planning is likely to be influenced by the same formal and informal variables that are generally cited as instrumental in all bureaucratic situations. Even if values were clear and goals distinct and a technique for ordering information were available, planning might not end up approaching rationality. Factors such as Banfield mentions are indeed significant obstacles to the planning process.

Formal considerations as staff, availability of equipment and space, time to devote to the planning project, whether the agency is single-purpose or multipurpose, and similar items might be mentioned. Likewise, factors such as who initiates the planning (outside versus agency initiation), the scope and impact desired, and the responsibility or nonresponsibility for duties besides planning must be considered. Informal considerations such as leadership, political support, interest group support, and the attitudes of those doing the planning are influential in relation to the environmental climate of planning.

Clearly, to increase planning rationality calls for considerable outlays in staff, money, time, and authority. Informal requirements might not be as clear. Banfield provides an introduction to this point by noting "organizations have a decided preference for present rather than future effects." In similar fashion, Lindblom warns of the danger of "likemindedness," noting that he would introduce fresh and innovative views to planning if possible. Robert Merton[10], writing on the "Role of the Intellectual in Public Bureaucracy," notes that organizational position, rather than academic inquiry, is a determining factor in shaping an intellectual's view toward public service. Merton would also like to integrate the intellectual outside public service into a position where his insights might be of value. Although the point need not be belabored, it does seem that informal considerations may be quite significant in determining whether an effort at comprehensiveness will be attempted.

A conceptual basis for planning that attempts to be both pragmatic and rational is, in itself, difficult to outline. Yet, the planning of public programs is of major importance in our society with its rash of comprehensive planning efforts stimulated by the federal government, all aiming to achieve the best possible programs for the population.

A. Gurin and R. Perlman[11] sum it up:

> Ambiguity about the clarity of ends and means, as well as the heritage of vested interests, value commitments, predetermined limitations in the scope of choice available and widely distributed veto powers of one kind or another—all these factors have led organizational analysts to pose alternatives to a simple means-ends model . . . their general feature (the alternatives) is to look upon planning as a system of interaction and adaptation whose outcome is not completely calculable.

MAJOR TRENDS IN HEALTH PLANNING

With the passage of time and the stimulus from major federal legislation, health planning has undergone changes, and trends have emerged. Starting with the Hill-Burton Act in the mid-1940s and including legislation on facilities planning, community mental health and retardation, regional medical programs, comprehensive health planning, Section 1122 of the Social Security Amendments of 1972, and the National Health Planning and Resources Development Act of 1974 (PL 93-641), health planning has manifested seven trends:

1. A movement toward involvement of a wide range of consumers in health planning decision making has evolved. Current mandates call for majority roles for consumers.
2. Regional planning has emerged and continues to be part of the scope of health plans.
3. Comprehensive planning moved from a major emphasis on facilities and regional plans toward a broader domain, including services and total health care.

4. Financing of health care shifted from private expenditures by single agencies, nonprofit organizations, and commercial third party payers to a greater participation by the federal government for medical care costs.
5. There has been a movement to provide health planning agencies with adequate funding to employ staff and to engage in competent health planning.
6. A trend indicates efforts to achieve greater coordination and integration of health services and facilities.
7. Movement from the dominance of the private voluntary sector in health planning shows a trend toward a partnership with all levels of government, but especially with the involvement of the federal government.

These seven trends are illustrated in Exhibit 1-2 and can be seen easily by following the lines across each of the trends.

TYPES OF HEALTH PLANNING

Various types of health planning take place, and the planners utilize assorted methods for each type. No single method appears to be best suited for any particular type of planning. This does not mean that certain obvious methods tend to be indicated for a planning activity, but that the variations must be related to the other variables involved—such as geography, sociocultural factors, and political mandates. For example, coordination planning implies the use of committees, task forces, or other consensus-type methods. The following are some common types of health planning with examples:

● *Problem Solving Planning*   This involves the identification of a problem and the resolution of the problem. Planning for these problems approximates the use of the scientific method; most health professionals are familiar with it. However, the act of labeling something a "problem" can be the outcome of an ethical or moral value choice such as calling illegitimate births or premarital cohabitation a problem. An example from recent events was the outbreak of an unknown disease that resulted in high mortality: Legionnaires Disease. The organism had to be identified through the problem solving method. Incidentally, to illustrate the point about labeling, the American Legion requested that the American Medical Association come up with a more scientific name for the disease.

Exhibit 1-2 Historical Trends and National Legislation

TREND FACTORS	HILL-BURTON	FACILITIES PLANNING	CMHC ACT	RMP	CHP	"112"	"93-641"
CITIZEN INVOLVEMENT	PROVIDER-ELITE CONSUMER	SLIGHT INCREASED CONSUMER INVOLVEMENT	PROVIDER-ELITE-GRASS ROOTS CONSUMER	ELITE PROVIDER "CONSUMER GRASS ROOTS"	WIDE RANGE OF CONSUMER PROVIDER INVOLVEMENT	"B": BROAD CONSUMER INVOLVEMENT "A": ELITE CONSUMER PROVIDER	BROAD CONSUMER INVOLVEMENT
TOWARD REGIONAL PLANNING	REGIONAL PLANNING	REGIONAL PLANNING	SUBREGIONAL PLANNING	REGIONAL PLANNING	REGIONAL PLANNING	PROJECT PLANNING	REGIONAL/STATE PLANNING
COMPREHENSIVE PLANNING	EMPHASIS ON FACILITIES PLANNING	FACILITIES PLANNING	FACILITIES/ SERVICES/ MANPOWER PLANNING	BROAD MANDATE AD HOC PLANNING	BROAD MANDATE PROJECT FUNCTIONAL PLANNING	SUB-REGIONAL PLANNING	VERY COMPRE-HENSIVE SERVICES, FACILITIES
TOWARD FEDERAL FINANCIAL INPUTS/CONTROLS	INCREASED FEDERAL INPUT OF FINANCES AND CONTROL	FEDERAL FINAN-CIAL INPUT: NO CONTROL	STRONG FEDERAL FINANCIAL INPUT & CONTROL	STRONG FEDERAL CONTROLS/ FINANCIAL	VACILLATING FEDERAL CONTROLS FINANCIAL	INDIRECT FEDERAL CONTROLS-FEDER-AL FINANCIAL INCREASED	STRONG FEDERAL FUNDS/CONTROL
ADEQUATE PLANNING STAFFS	ADEQUATE PROFESSIONAL STAFF	COMPETENT STAFF OF LIMITED SIZE	COMPETENT STAFF OF LIMITED SIZE	ADEQUATE PROFESSIONAL STAFF	PROFESSIONAL STAFF OF LIMITED SIZE	ADEQUATE PROFESSIONAL STAFF	VERY ADEQUATE COMPETENT STAFF
MORE COORDINA-TION/INTEGRA-TION OF HEALTH SERVICES	NO COORDINATION-INTEGRATION OF HEALTH SERVICES	LIMITED COORDIN-ATION. NO INTEGRATION OF SERVICES	INCREASED COORDINATION INTEGRATION OF M.H. SERVICES	LIMITED COORDIN-ATION. NO INTEGRATION OF RMP PROJECTS	COORDINATION STRAINED. NO INTEGRATION	SOME COORDINATION. LIMITED INTEGRATION	INCREASED COOR-DINATION INTEGRATION OF SERVICES FACILITIES
TOWARD PRIVATE GOVERNMENT PARTNERSHIP	PRIVATE DOMINA-TION. SOME GOVERNMENT INFLUENCE	PRIVATE DOMINA-TION-NO FEDERAL INFLUENCE	PUBLIC PLANNING/ PRIVATE IMPLE-MENTATION BALANCED PARTNERSHIP	LITTLE GOVERNMENT INFLUENCE	LIMITED LOCAL BUT STRONG FEDERAL GOVERNMENT INFLUENCE	INCREASED GOVERNMENT INFLUENCE AT ALL LEVELS	BALANCED FEDER-AL PRIVATE PART-NERSHIP

Source: Health Planning and Public Accountability Seminar Workbook (Germantown, Md.: Aspen Systems Corp., 1976), p. 22. Reprinted with permission.

● *Program Planning*   This planning sets a course of action for a circumscribed health problem. Usually, the program has been predetermined elsewhere, and the health planner actually is doing the implementation planning. Influenza vaccination programs are of this type wherein the federal government sets the direction, and the states and localities plan for the actual vaccination activity itself.

● *Coordination of Efforts and Activities Planning*   Here, health planning aims to increase the availability, efficiency, productivity, effectiveness, and other aspects of various activities and programs. This involves a mutual adjustment process and maybe even occasional amalgamation or closing of services and facilities. Critics have pointed out that coordination planning tends to restrict the larger field of endeavor and possibly emphasizes the maintainence of the status quo without harm or the least harm to any of the participants in the planning process. Hospital and facility planning, wherein the various organizations meet to coordinate efforts, is a common illustration.

● *Planning for the Allocation of Resources*   This planning looks for the optimal outcome from among the alternatives to achieve the desired goals within the limited amount of resources available. Planners have to divide the budget, the manpower, and the facilities to meet existing needs and demands. Rational approaches do not always win out in this type of planning because of other factors such as power and influence. Questions such as, "Does the squeaking wheel get the oil?" or "How do we get the best bang for the buck?" permeate this type of planning. For example, automobile deaths can be reduced by wearing seat belts, installing air bags, educating drivers, enforcing laws, or redesigning highways. Consumers, manufacturers, police, and researchers all express their views, and the planners allocate funds to certain activities based on that input.

● *Creation of a Plan*   This type of planning develops a blueprint for action, including recommendations and supporting data. It is common for a commission or special task force to be created to prepare the plan. Facility projections for hospitals are typical created plans. They usually allow for changes over the years in phases.

● *Design of Standard Operating Procedures*   Planners come forth with sets of standards of practice or criteria for operation and evaluation. This can be planning mandated by legislation or created voluntarily by the parties concerned. Consensus among those involved is usually required. Guidelines for inpatient care were mandated by law and resulted in Professional Standards Review Organizations (PSROs). Voluntary standards have been established for continuing medical education by various medical specialty associations.

As the health planner becomes involved in different types of planning, the methods that work will tend to be used most often. However, the planner must be alert to the situations that require (or would certainly be more acceptable if it were so) the process to involve a broader representation rather than an internal planning group. If one has to implement, it would be better to secure agreement and participation in the planning process by those parties who have to do the task.

A WORD ABOUT METHODS AND TECHNIQUES

This book details various methods and techniques for health planners to use in their work situations. Most of the methods are considered basic to the trade. However, health planners are encouraged to add, delete, adapt, modify, revise, or in some other way change the methods to suit their own particular situation. Basically, consider this book the starting point and not the end-all for health planners. It is obvious that new methods will continue to emerge and that older techniques will become more sophisticated as time goes on. Most important, health planners should realize that the methods are tools to direct planning into the scientific mold.

Although this book divides health planning into six steps, other methods exist that have fewer or more divisions. However, the similarity of the methods is apparent as one examines the process and notes that the words are closely related regardless of the number of steps. Not only are the words related, but the actual planning process also appears to cover the same territory regardless of the number of steps (see Appendix A). Therefore, in considering the different planning methods, the planner is cautioned to examine the process and determine whether anything has been added to the method with which the planner is already comfortable.

Methods in this book are described in each of the six chapters and pertain in that specific chapter to that particular phase of the planning process. This should not constrict planners from using different methods in varying phases of the planning process. For example, the Delphi method can be used in setting priorities, in data assessment, in thinking up alternatives, and in evaluation. The technique is used a little differently each time, but the fundamentals of the technique remain the same. As the methods are described, do not limit your thinking to their use in only the examples, but be aware of where else such a method could be used or adapted.

Health planning is not as neatly ordered as in the six parts cited in this book. Such organization makes for a logical flow of ideas, but planning does not always occur logically. Planners might start anywhere in the planning process, especially when their efforts are initiated by a crisis or a report. Evaluation might yield data that cause a health planner to begin an investigation. Nevertheless, the total process will eventually occur, even in abbreviated form, to cover all phases required for a reasonable conclusion.

PROBLEMS WITH HEALTH PLANNING TOOLS

Although a goodly number of health planning tools are included in this book, the techiques have not been exhausted. Regardless of the method or technique that health planners wish to use, the problem of objective quantification and specificity of activity is difficult to achieve. For the more sophisticated space age technology the problem can be even more rigorous and could dissuade planners from attempting to employ those techniques. Highly technical engineering and mathematical planning tools lose some force in their application to human systems and human behavior, which is the core of the health care delivery model.

Another vital consideration related to health planning tools concerns the question of political or policy decisions. No matter how sophisticated the health planning tools, the decision as to where it is the health planner wants to go has to be reached first. Tools can help to plan and to evaluate effectiveness, but they cannot set the goal. Thus, health planners must exert considerable effort to establish objectives that are sound. Computer experts use the acroynm GIGO ("garbage in, garbage out") to express the importance of setting objectives. If health planners start with unsteady premises, the outcome will be shaky.

WHY PLANNING FAILS

Health planning may fail for a variety of reasons, but most of the failures can be related to common sense tenets that are often overlooked. In seeking reasons, the management literature gives insights that are pertinent to the health care system. For example the health care industry frequently has been called a "cottage industry," imply-ing a fragmented, unordered system. Therefore, the application of ex-pert businessmen relating to change and planning ought to be en-lightening.

Machiavelli, the alleged master of intrigue, noted, "There is nothing more difficult to take in hand, more perilous to conduct, or more uncer-tain in its success, than to take the lead in the introduction of a new order of things." K. A. Ringbakk[12] surveyed more than 350 American and European firms and came up with ten reasons for failure of plan-ning:

1. Corporate planning is not integrated into the total management system.
2. The different dimensions of planning have not been understood.
3. Management at all levels is not engaged in planning activities.
4. Responsibility for planning is vested solely in planning depart-ment.
5. Too much is attempted at once.
6. Management expects the plan to come true as planned.
7. Management fails to operate by the plan.
8. Extrapolation and financial projections are confused with plan-ning.
9. Inadequate information inputs are used.
10. Too much emphasis is placed on only one aspect of planning.

Certainly, "corporate" and "management" can be replaced by words relevant to the health care delivery system, and the rationale will still hold true in most instances.

When planning changes, G. Watson and E. M. Glaser[13] urge man-agement to consider the following steps:

1. Make clear the needs for change, or provide a climate in which others feel free to identify such needs.
2. Permit, encourage, and secure relevant group participation in clarifying and expanding the concept of these needs.
3. State the objectives to be achieved.
4. Establish broad guidelines for achieving the objectives.
5. Leave the details of change planning to the parts of the organiza-tion that will be affected by the change and/or must implement the plan.
6. Indicate the benefits or rewards to individuals and to the group expected as a result of successful change.
7. Materialize the benfits or rewards; i.e., keep promises.

Again, these steps do not appear to be too far afield of the health planner who has to affect change in the health care delivery system.

In an article in *Executive* magazine, W. J. Reddin[14] identified seven techniques to overcome resistance to change:

1. Diagnosis of the situation should be made first by those affected by the change.
2. Mutual objective setting should be undertaken by those instituting change and by those affected by it.
3. Group emphasis wherein the group rather than the individual makes decisions and generates ideas enhances the planning of change.
4. Maximum information about objectives, nature, methods, benefits and drawbacks should be made clear to all concerned.
5. Discussion of implementation should include agreement on the rate and method of implementation as well as the first steps and sequence of steps.
6. Use of ceremony-ritual can be used to indicate the progression from one system to another and to underline the importance of individual and institutional loyalty to the system.
7. Resistance interpretation of those who are resisting change and resolving the differences are a key part of the organizational change plan.

These three approaches, appearing in management journals, all have direct links to the health planning process. Planners need to be alert to the reasons for failure and make strong efforts to avoid the pitfalls. If large business corporations can take these steps, then surely the health care industry can do likewise.

THE IMPORTANCE OF OBJECTIVES

Specification of objectives is of vital importance in any health planning activity. The more precise the objective can be made, the more directive the health planner can be. All the steps in the planning process flow from the objective and are directly related all along the continuum.

As important as the setting of objectives is, this appears to be a major bone of contention in many planning efforts. Too often objectives are fuzzy and ill conceived, and the planning that ensues also becomes fuzzy and ill conceived. To be acceptable and valid, objectives should meet the following criteria:[15]

- The organization or institution should have the authority to undertake the objectives.
- Objectives should be within the capabilities of the agency in terms of organization, personnel, equipment, facilities, and techniques.
- The objectives should fall within budget restrictions.
- Objectives should fit into the available timetable.
- Objectives should be legal and consistent with the ethical and moral values of the community affected.
- Objectives should be practical and must be implementable.
- Objectives must be acceptable to those who are responsible for carrying them out.
- Minimum negative side effects should result from the achievement of the objectives.
- Objectives should be measurable in concrete terms.

Precise terms that can be used in preparing objectives should result in more effective health planning. Objectives that exactly identify the anticipated behavior as well as indicate a standard or criterion of acceptable performance will enhance the overall planning process. For example, many objectives use the word "understand" in a sentence such as, "The patient shall understand why he has to take the penicillin." Does understand mean that the patient can remember certain rules? When the patient understands, does he take the penicillin regularly? Does understand mean that the patient can identify the chemical reactions? Obviously, "understand" is a vague word open to various interpretations. This problem with preciseness takes place despite the fact that those planning the activity might have a logical and well-defined meaning, although not necessarily expressed in the written objective. Confusion results among the planners as well as the intended target audience when the objectives are not written using the terms that are more descriptive and less open to misinterpretation. Terms that describe and define behavior can be compared with terms that are vague in the following listing:[16]

Less Precise Terms (Many Interpretations)	More Precise Terms (Fewer Interpretations)
To know	To identify
To understand	To discuss
To understand *fully*	To list
To realize	To diagram
To appreciate	To compare and contrast
To be aware	To recall and state

To value

To be familiar with

To comprehend

To tolerate

To believe

To feel

To classify

To differentiate

To evaluate

To select

To summarize

To predict

By using precise words in the statement of objectives, the health planner can direct the activities that have to be undertaken into clearly defined channels. This will exclude the collection of extraneous data as well as delimit the amount of energy spent spinning wheels.

Examples of objectives that combine behavioral action with a standard are given below:

- Patients will be able to list correctly the six links of the infectious disease process after attending the class on health education.
- Given ethnic, sex, age, socioeconomic, and geographic data concerning the venereal disease problem, the health planner will be able to draw conclusions and state them effectively in epidemiological terms.
- Health planners will be able to compare, in writing, the relative worth of two or more similar health programs in terms of cost, availability, reliability, and validity after taking a course in evaluation.
- Patients will indicate appreciation of the hospital by talking in a supportive manner about the organization and its activities.
- Staff members will demonstrate their knowledge about nutrition by choosing foods that comprise a well-balanced diet in the cafeteria.
- Patients will place a tissue or handkerchief over their mouths when sneezing or coughing.

Note that the sample objectives deal with knowledge, attitudes, and behavior. Planners can use more precise words to express the objective in terms that lend themselves to direct evaluation. If this can be accomplished, the entire planning process can be focused without diverting time and effort to activities not germane to the project.

R. F. Mager's book on preparing instructional objectives fixed a format for developing objectives that included a performance, a criterion, and noted extenuating conditions.[17] Each objective should identify the behavior anticipated, the acceptable standard of performance and spell out the conditions under which the behavior takes place. Exhibit 1-3 contains ten objectives and is a test of the ability to determine whether each objective states a demonstratable performance, a criter-

Exhibit 1-3 Quiz on Objectives

Quickie Quiz on Objectives

To the degree of specification described for performance, criterion and conditions, an objective will spell out the intention of the planner.

Objectives should specify three characteristics:

0 Performance or behavior to be demonstrated.
0 Criteria or standards of acceptable performance.
0 Conditions under which the performance takes place.

Are each of these characteristics present in each of the objectives below? Answer YES or NO for each characteristic.

	Perf.	Crit.	Cond.
a. Health planners must be able to understand Polsby's theory for community participation. A written essay will demonstrate understanding.	___	___	___
b. Planning students should complete a 50 item multiple choice examination on planning methods and techniques within one hour without any reference materials. The lowest acceptable grade will be 35 correct answers.	___	___	___
c. Given a list of data sources and a list of data needs, health planners should be able to match all 25 data needs with the correct data sources.	___	___	___
d. Following instruction in a computer center, the planner must demonstrate the ability to prepare computer cards for a specific project. All equipment in the center can be used.	___	___	___
e. During the clinical exam, and without reference to notes, the medical student must be able to write a description of the steps involved in making a diagnosis.	___	___	___
f. Hospital administrators must know <u>well</u> the five cardinal rules of personnel administration.	___	___	___
g. Head nurses must be able to fill out a standard accident report form for the hospital after hearing an oral report.	___	___	___
h. List the important characteristics of voluntary and public hospitals.	___	___	___
i. Develop logical approaches to the evaluation of health care services in a poverty area.	___	___	___
j. List three common points of view for the failure of health planning efforts that are not supported by available research. Reference materials can be used.	___	___	___

ion, and identifies conditions. Answer yes or no for each part for each objective. Answers are given at the bottom of the page.

A rather extended listing of verbs that could be utilized in stating objectives has been compiled in a book by N. E. Gronlund[18] and is noted in Exhibit 1-4. Although this listing was prepared for an educa-

Exhibit 1-4 Illustrative Verbs

For Stating General Instructional Objectives

Analyze	Compute	Interpret	Perform	Translate
Apply	Create	Know	Recognize	Understand
Appreciate	Demonstrate	Listen	Speak	Use
Comprehend	Evaluate	Locate	Think	Write

For Stating Specific Learning Outcomes

"Creative" Behaviors

Alter	Paraphrase	Reconstruct	Rephrase	Rewrite
Ask	Predict	Regroup	Restate	Simplify
Change	Question	Rename	Restructure	Synthesize
Design	Rearrange	Reorganize	Retell	Systematize
Generalize	Recombine	Reorder	Revise	Vary
Modify				

Complex, Logical, Judgmental Behaviors

Analyze	Conclude	Deduce	Formulate	Plan
Appraise	Contrast	Defend	Generate	Structure
Combine	Criticize	Evaluate	Induce	Substitute
Compare	Decide	Explain	Infer	

General Discriminative Behaviors

Choose	Detect	Identify	Match	Place
Collect	Differentiate	Indicate	Omit	Point
Define	Discriminate	Isolate	Order	Select
Describe	Distinguish	List	Pick	Separate

Social Behaviors

Accept	Communicate	Discuss	Invite	Praise
Agree	Compliment	Excuse	Join	React
Aid	Contribute	Forgive	Laugh	Smile
Allow	Cooperate	Greet	Meet	Talk
Answer	Dance	Help	Participate	Thank
Argue	Disagree	Interact	Permit	Volunteer

Source: Reprinted with permission from Calvin K. Claus, "Verbs and Imperative Sentences as a Basis for Stating Performance Goals." Paper read at the February 10, 1968 meeting of the National Council on Measurement in Education, held in Chicago, Illinois.

tional situation, the application to health planning should be obvious. Even if the list merely serves to jog the memory, it will be worthwhile.

This type of approach to objectives is a vital part of the health planning process. Attention paid to the development of precise objectives that specify performance, criterion, and conditions will not be time wasted. The total outcome of the planning can be affected by the clarity of the objectives.

REFERENCES

1. N. Krumholz et al., "The Cleveland Policy Planning Report," *Journal of the American Institute of Planners* 41, no. 5 (September 1975): 298.

2. W.J. Waters, "State Level Comprehensive Health Planning: A Retrospect," *American Journal of Public Health* 66, no. 2 (February 1976): 139.

3. R.N. Whiting, "The Debate Continues: Is Health Planning Working?" *Hospitals* 51 (April 1977): 47.

4. A. Wildavsky, "If Planning Is Everything, Maybe It's Nothing," *Policy Sciences* 4 (April 1973): 127.

5. E.C. Banfield, "Ends and Means in Planning," *Concepts and Issues in Administrative Behavior*, edited by S. Mailick and E. Van Ness (Englewood Cliffs, N.J.: Prentice Hall, 1962), pp. 70-80.

6. C.E. Lindblom, "The Science of Muddling Through," *Public Administrative Review* 19 (Spring 1959): 79.

7. R. Morris and R. Binstock, *Feasible Planning for Change* (New York: Columbia University Press, 1966), pp. 1-27.

8. R.C. Young, "Goals and Goal Setting," *Journal of the American Institute of Planners* 32 (March 1966): 76.

9. W. Peterson, "On Some Meanings of Planning," *Journal of the American Institute of Planners* 32 (May 1966): 83.

10. R. Merton, "Role of the Intellectual in Public Bureaucracy," *Social Forces* 23 (May 1945): 405.

11. A. Gurin and R. Perlman, *Current Conceptions of Planning and Their Implications for Public Welfare*. Conference Proceedings. (Waltham, Mass.: Brandeis University, Heller School, 1966), p. 16.

12. K.A. Ringbakk, "Why Planning Fails," *European Business* 29 (September 1966): 15.

13. G. Watson and E.M. Glaser, "What We Have Learned About Planning for Change," *Management Review* 54, no. 11 (November 1965): 34.

14. W.J. Reddin, "How To Change Things," *Executive Magazine* 11 (June 1969): 22.

15. D.F. Bergwall, P.N. Reeves and N.B. Woodside, *Introduction to Health Planning* (Washington, D.C.: Information Resources Press, 1974), p. 80.

16. J.T. Fodor and G.T. Dalis, *Health Instruction, Theory and Application* (Philadelphia: Lea & Febiger, 1966), p. 57.

17. R.F. Mager, *Preparing Instructional Objectives*, 2nd Ed. (Palo Alto, Calif.: Fearon Publishers, 1975), pp. 56-57.

18. N.E. Gronlund, *Stating Behavioral Objectives for Classroom Instruction* (New York: Macmillan Company, 1970), pp. 53-56.

Chapter 2

Identifying the Problem: Methods for Needs Assessment and Resources Analysis

This chapter will focus on a crucial step in the planning process, the methods available for identifying problems in the health care field. Federal legislation has led to the development of health systems agencies and to increasing attention toward identifying methodologies for determining problems related to the health field in quantitative and measurable terms. Previously, most health plans posed problem identification in qualitative terms, so it was difficult to determine whether progress was being made in reducing the severity of the problems. The growth of the federal allocation of funds in the gross national medical budget has required greater accountability in the expenditure of these funds. Congress is increasingly concerned with whether the funds have been spent in a legal manner and with how effective the funds have been in alleviating the illnesses of people. To respond to this interest requires the posing of problems in quantitative and measurable terms.

Congress is also interested in determining how the general health status of the people of the United States has fared over time. Over the decades, there has been demonstrable improvement in many of the medical indicators used to plot trends of the nation's health. The assumption in the 1960s was that by increasing the resources available to the population the use of those resources would lead to further improvements in the indicators used to measure the health of the nation. It became disconcerting to both congressional and medical analysts that the generosity of Congress has not been rewarded by a commensurate change in the medical indicators. Mortality rates, the most important of those indicators, remained fairly static in the 1960s. Consequently, the focus shifted to an emphasis on outcome, or population status, indicators. These are concerned with what happens to specific components of the population with specific health problems, such as the diabetic conditions of women aged 29 to 38, or the tonsillectomies of children aged 6 to 10, and so forth. By concentrating on specific population cohorts with known disease conditions or higher than usual mortality rates, it would be possible to pinpoint the use of resources in a cost-effective manner. This shift from equating improvement in the health of the nation through increasing expenditures on resources to measuring it by identifying the specific medical needs of population cohorts has been spelled out in PL 93-641, the National Health Planning and Resources Development Act of 1974.

In this chapter two sets of methods will be described, those that relate to the needs assessment of specific populations and those that indicate the resources needed to deal with these problems. Public Law 93-641 requires the secretary of the Department of Health, Education, and Welfare (HEW) to assist in providing technical assistance to the health systems agencies by identifying a range of methods that are applicable to assess the needs of specific segments of the population and the resource requirements for meeting their needs. To implement this congressional directive, the Bureau of Health Planning and Resources Development (charged with the implementation of PL 93-641) has provided a number of consultant contracts to bring together the accumulated knowledge related to methods for identifying the health problems and needs of the nation. In addition, the National Health Planning Information Center has been created to spread this knowledge to the health systems agencies and others who would normally benefit from its availability. The center has also contracted out to a more limited number of health experts in the field to write papers on the state of the art of known health planning methods. Methods cited in this chapter are drawn from information that has been available through the reports of the bureau's consultant findings and the published monographs and extensive bibliographic reference library and search process of the center. In addition, methods cited in the leading medical and health journals have been elicited. These searches have produced a large number of needs assessment and resource development methods. To make this knowledge relevant to the user, it is essential to organize it in a coherent and readily usable fashion.

The first section of the chapter will deal with matters that affect all methods. These are issues related to validity, reliability, precision, and accuracy. This section will also differentiate between methods that determine "need" and those that focus on "demand." The second section will identify and describe the variety of methods available for the determination of needs assessment. Illustrations of the most important of the methods will be offered where they are not too detailed and are readily available. The strengths and limitations of varying methodologies will also be noted so the readers can render judgments on the usefulness of any particular method. Methods that are most appropriate for regional planning and for institutional planning, where relevant and available, will also be noted. It should be noted that most methods tend to focus on regional rather than institutional planning. Section three will repeat the process of section two for those methods available for determining the demand for services. Section four will present a list of available resources for gaining more detailed information about health statistics, methods, and general health knowledge.

Basically, the aim of the various methods to be discussed later in this chapter is to differentiate populations and individuals with respect to their health status before they show signs of illness. Any methods used to measure health status should be "sensitive" enough to identify small changes in the population or individuals. Thus, sensitivity becomes an important attribute in the choice of methods used.

A second attribute relates to validity. This is usually defined as the ability of the method to measure a general or specific health status of the population, such as morbidity or mortality. Thus, if a method established "poverty" as a proxy health status indicator, the question is whether that indicator can actually measure the need for health services. Poverty might be very well correlated with the degree of general morbidity or mortality compared with other income or social class groups, but it may also be a measure of poor housing, limited education, or lack of opportunity for self-improvement. Poverty might be a better indicator for mental health than for health. The point is that the methods should not utilize data to identify health status indicators that may be ambiguous of what they are measuring.

A third attribute relates to reliability. By this is usually meant the consistency or dependability of the measuring device. It is related to the variety of data required by the method to be used. This, in turn, relates to the type of questions asked in a household survey, their wording, and the order in which they are placed in the instrument. Reliability deals with the interpretation the interviewer gives to the answers received and the consistency of those interpretations among the interviewers. Likewise, the respondents should have a consistent understanding of the questions being asked. Otherwise, we may have a case where the status indicator is valid, but its reliability is in question. This simply means that different answers will be given in response to the instrument by the same or similar population. Thus, it becomes essential that the validity and reliability of the indicators and instruments are achieved to ensure the predictive capacity of the method to measure health status.

The fourth attribute refers to the accuracy of the method. Accuracy depends on the validity and reliability of the model. If either is incorrect, the accuracy of the indicators will also be in error. If data for several of the measures used to comprise a health status index are not available or are inconsistent in their availability (available for one age group but not another, for one geographic area and not another, or based on different aggregations), the final index measure will be inaccurate. Likewise, if the same population gives widely different answers to the same question at different points of time (even though nothing in their situation would warrant the different responses), the accuracy of the index will be in jeopardy.[1,2]

In addition to these generally accepted attributes of health status measures, M. K. Chen identifies several others that he considers important. These relate to the precision of measurement, the ease of collection and availability of data, and the relative ease of mathematical computations to arrive at the status indices or measures.[3] An index must be sufficiently precise that differences in subgroupings within a population or changes in the status of a population over time can be readily detected. A measure might be accurate, yet stated in such general terms or in ranges that it is not possible to determine minor differences within a population. For example, a state might have a generally low mortality rate due to heart conditions compared with the United States mean. However, unless the index is precise enough to detect differences among the population cohorts that comprise the service area, it might not be able to identify one significant subgroup in the state with a high mortality rate.

For health status indices to be used on a routine basis, the data must be readily available and collected in an efficient, cost-effective manner. One of the major obstacles to carrying out household surveys is the high cost per interview. Very few hospitals, health system agencies, or health departments can afford such methodology. Thus, although a survey might be undertaken periodically, its value becomes diluted if the information is not collected on a routine basis, whether one year, two years, or more. A method for determining a population's health status must be simple and relatively inexpensive. The development of the State Cooperative Health Statistics Program partially financed and coordinated by the National Center for Health Statistics, HEW, is a step in this direction.

Finally, the index should use mathematics that are relatively simple for health department and health planning officials to manipulate. Many planners do not have a sophisticated background either in mathematics or in statistics. They were attracted to the planning field because of their interest in changing situations. Improvement to many of the planners means new services and programs, not more highly developed statistics and sophisticated use of formulas. Thus, the index should require fairly simple mathematical formulas that can be easily computed by most planning officials.

Chen sums up the present in developing health indices by stating: "If I have painted a rather gloomy picture of health measurement endeavor, it is because the picture is gloomy."[4] Although he believes the achievement of such a health status index may not take place before the 21st century, he is generally optimistic that through incremental stages and the increased interest of investigators of health measurement this happy occurence will eventually take place. Nonetheless, these attributes must usually be implicitly or explicitly taken into account when using various methods to measure health status.

Need/Demand

Need is generally defined as "a perceived or medically defined state of illness."[5] Another way of defining need is that it is a specific condition that limits a person as an individual or a family member in meeting his full potential.[6] A child who bruises his hands such that he cannot grip a baseball bat has a definable need that prevents his involvement in one of the primary activities of his age group. A housewife with a cast on a leg is limited in getting about and taking full care of her home and family responsibilities. A person with elevated blood pressure also has a definable need, even though at any one moment it is not debilitating enough to limit daily activity. All these fall into definable types of potential medical needs.

When the need becomes severe enough that the person seeks some form of professional medical assistance, that need is then defined as a demand. The child whose mother treats his hand bruises with home remedies does not translate his hurt hands into a demand for medical services, nor does the person with an elevated blood pressure if he/she fails to seek medical treatment for the condition. Consequently, the need for medical services greatly exceeds the effective demand the population might make upon the medical system for care. On the other hand, there could be a number of people who demand medical services but might not receive them for any number of reasons. People cannot afford the service. An individual cannot get to the service at a time and place convenient to him or her. The service is simply not available. Religious beliefs prevent the use of certain type of medically needed services.

This relationship between need and demand is at the heart of planning in the health field. Health analysts are interested in knowing the nature of the medical need in a health service area, or a state, or a region. Who has what type of needs? How are these needs met: in the home, by ancillary medical staff, by medical physicians, by hospitals, and so forth? On the other hand, they are concerned about such issues as the person's accessibility to services, their availability when needed, the cost of such services, the quality offered, the continuity of care when more than one service is needed, and the acceptability of the services to the patients. All these are known as characteristics of the health care system. They determine the degree to which the services are used by people who both have a need and translate that need into a demand for service. It is only in recent years that the connection between need and demand has received much attention. In the past, it was simply assumed that the providers of medical services knew what the demand on their resources was by the number of people who called. There is now a strong awareness that many more people need services than are getting them, and that many who attempt to obtain such services are not able to receive them.

In the sections that follow, a number of methods will be described that have been used or developed to determine both need and demand. These will be described in turn with their advantages and disadvantages noted. Since it is not always possible to know all the circumstances under which a particular method will be used, no attempt will be made to determine which are the best methods for a particular situation.

NEED ASSESSMENT METHODS

G. J. Warheit and others[7] have identified six approaches to needs assessment. Each of these will be discussed in turn.

Key Informant Approach

The key informant approach is a research method of obtaining data on the needs of the community, or specific populations within a community, based on the knowledge and experiences of key persons likely to be familiar with the community being assessed. Steps in this approach are as follows:

1. A group of people interested in the survey determine what their objectives are. These should be as specifically stated as possible.

2. This committee should determine the types of key informants most familiar with the problem. These might be physicians; directors of functional health agencies who monitor the problem, such as a heart association, mental health association, or so forth; or general community leaders likely to know the conditions of the people in their area.
3. A roster of key informants should then be identified and selected for later contact.
4. A brief questionnaire should be constructed to elicit answers to all the aspects of the problem being studied. A questionnaire permits comparability when answers are given by different informants.
5. Questionnaires should be administered to the key informants. These can be done by (a) person-to-person interview, (b) mailed questionnaire, or (c) telephone interview, or some combination of all three. Of these three methods, the person-to-person interview is best because it permits other aspects to be brought out by the informant that were not identified in the questionnaire.
6. Data from the questionnaires are tabulated and analyzed. Findings are then presented to the committee and other interested persons for decision-making.
7. A final report is written based on the group's consensus of the high priority needs.

This approach has several advantages.

1. It is easy to conduct and costs little to carry out.
2. It elicits a broad range of information from knowledgeable persons, so many different facets of the needs of the community are generated.
3. In the process of obtaining knowledge, it also provides the important secondary benefit of priming the key informants to later involvement in planning and carrying out programs to meet the needs of the community.

The primary disadvantage is that the key informants are not likely to have all the knowledge of people in need of health or mental health services in the community to make appropriate decisions. This may be especially true of people who tend to avoid using health services except as a last resort. Warheit refers to these as the invisible people. Thus, the personal bias of the key informants could inadvertently omit references to various groups of people who simply do not come to their everyday attention.

Community Forum Approach

Steps to carry out the community forum approach are as follows:

1. The committee defines its goals and objectives and develops a work program for carrying out the process.
2. Questions are agreed upon.
3. One or more locations for open public community meetings are identified and secured.
4. A publicity program is developed using word-of-mouth, leaflets, mass media, and local newspapers to acquaint the target community with the meeting and its objectives. The aim is to attract as wide a cross section of the community as possible.
5. At the meeting, the moderator has a list of key questions from which responses by those attending are elicited. The meeting may be broken down into smaller groups to ensure audience participation if a large number attend. Or a series of small meetings could be held over time to ensure that persons unable to attend one can appear at another. The community forum should be flexible enough to permit participants to raise issues or discuss needs not identified by the structured key questions developed by the committee. It could be that some of these unstructured responses represent high priority needs of the community.
6. Responses are tabulated by resource persons, who collect the information from the one or more community forums. The analysts should be aware of the potential difference in needs on the part of various segments of the community.
7. A final report with high priority needs identified is developed and shared with those attending the forums.

There are three advantages to this approach.

1. Community forums are relatively easy to arrange and are not too costly compared with other approaches.
2. They encourage a wide range of community expression of need, unlike the "key informant" approach, which can be biased by the limited number of groups met.
3. They enable the sponsoring group to identify previously unidentified community persons interested in planning and developing programs to meet the needs uncovered in the forum.

Disadvantages are more numerous.

1. It may be difficult to ensure that a representative group of people from the community attends. Too often, those with the greatest interest participate to the exclusion of a number of other groups whose needs, consequently, do not receive the attention they deserve.
2. Open forum meetings are vulnerable to individuals or groups with special points of view or grievances taking over the meeting. This can lead to the committee's failure to obtain responses to its key questions as well as upsetting community residents who came to the meeting with other interests.
3. The nature of the meeting and discussion can give participants unrealistically high expectations of the benefits that might come out of a discussion of their needs. Unless checked, this could lead to rejection of later programs that fail to meet those expectations.
4. Data collected at the forums will likely be highly impressionistic and consequently not readily amenable to statistical manipulation. It is also quite possible such data are not representative of the needs of all groups in the community.

Rates-Under-Treatment Approach

The rates-under-treatment (RUT) approach has been used for many years to identify the needs of a community for health or mental health services based on its use of such services. RUT is based on the assumption that those using a service are representative of those in the community needing the service, but not using it. RUT studies have been widely used for estimating need for a number of years.

Steps in the process are the following:

1. Basic questions should be considered to help determine what is wanted, how to get it, and how to analyze and present it.
2. The basic data should include at least the following: sociodemographic characteristics of the population in need such as age, race, sex, income, etc.; presenting problem(s); type of service provided; referral sources; length and frequency of treatment; and outcome of treatment.
3. Identify where this information can be obtained. Data are generally more available from public than private sources unless a means can be devised to protect the confidentiality of the persons receiving care.
4. All the records of an agency(ies) can be used to determine need; or, if too voluminous, a sample can be used.

5. The data are then summarized into tabular form and, where appropriate, tests of significance and correlations applied.
6. Based on the analysis, a report identifying high priority needs of community populations should be developed with recommendations.

The RUT approach is a low cost method of collecting large amounts of data. Furthermore, it can provide a comprehensive overview of the services offered in the community and identify who uses the services. But it may be difficult to guarantee the type of confidentiality public and private providers require to permit use of their data. Also, it might not be possible to state with certainty that the general community population is similar to the one using the service. A number of mental health RUT studies have shown that there is a wide discrepancy between those utilizing the service compared with the number and nature of services needed by those in need of the services, but not using them.

Social Indicator Approach

The social indicator approach to needs assessment is based primarily on inferences of need drawn generally from descriptive statistics found in public records and reports. The underlying assumption of the approach is that it is possible to make useful estimates of the needs and social well-being of those in a community by analyzing statistics on selected factors which have been found to be highly correlated with persons in need. As such, these statistics are regarded, on the basis of face validity, to be indicators of need.[8]

Four factors that Warheit found to be most generally used are:

1. Spatial arrangements of people and facilities.
2. Sociodemographic characteristics (age, sex, income, etc.).
3. Social behavior and well-being of people (crime, family patterns, morbidity).
4. General social conditions within which people live (overcrowded housing, accessibility to services, etc.).

Steps needed to carry out a needs assessment using the social indicator approach are the following:

1. The group should be highly specific of the goals and objectives of its study.
2. Consideration must be given to the types of data that will best serve as indicators of need, such as housing characteristics, mortality and morbidity, crime, or education.
3. The nature of the data collected should be linked to the use to which the findings of the data will be put.
4. The unit of analysis should be determined. This is most generally at the census tract level or block groupings, a subdivision of a census tract. They have a degree of permanence and can be used as a basis for long term studies. For those in the mental health field, the National Institute of Mental Health (NIMH) has compiled a rich source of data based on the 1970 census for comparing different geographic areas using census characteristics. This body of data is referred to as the Mental Health Demographic Profile System. This system is flexible, so data from other sources such as crime, welfare, and employment can be incorporated into the geographic units of analysis to afford a more comprehensive study of the area.
5. Collect data. Data can be collected for any of the types of information noted above. These data are generally available from such sources as:

   • U.S. Bureau of Census;
   • Department of Health, Education, and Welfare, particularly the National Center for Health Statistics and the National Center for Health Services Research, NIMH;
   • National Health Planning Information Center;
   • state and local health, mental health, and welfare departments
   • court records;
   • police statistics;
   • Health Systems Agencies;
   • state Health Planning and Development Agencies; and
   • boards of education.
6. Analysis of the data can be relatively simple, using tables, charts, maps, etc., comparing various geographic units with each other. Or it can be more complex, using several characteristics at once and requiring computers.

Four advantages accrue to this approach.

1. There is a ready access to existing data, especially in the public domain.

2. Most of the data can be secured at low cost.
3. The social indicator approach is flexible in its use of data, which can be acquired from only one source or from several sources.
4. The social indicators can be readily updated and kept current with a minimum of effort.

Disadvantages include the danger that social indicators may be used incorrectly. Also, as there are efforts to correlate the characteristics of the social indicators with the general population, it should be noted that these correlations are often not accurate. The rates or averages of the social indicators "need not and often do not accurately reflect the characteristics of individuals within the areas."[9]

Survey Approach

A survey approach is based on drawing a representative sample of the community and analyzing data from that sample. If properly drawn and executed, the survey can produce the most valid and reliable findings of the health and mental health needs of the community.

Steps in the process for carrying out a survey are as follows:

1. The group must define its objectives as in the other approaches to determining community needs. At the same time, the conceptual framework must be identified and the methods explicitly stated for implementing the survey.
2. The cooperation of other interested agencies and groups must be enlisted. This ensures a wider range of relevant questions being asked, their providing the legitimacy needed to carry out the survey, and their involvement in implementing any recommendations that flow from the survey that come within their sphere of operation.
3. Data must be gathered. The same three techniques noted earlier are also relevant for the survey: person-to-person interview, mailed questionnaire, and telephone interview. Each of these techniques has its own strengths and weaknesses. The group must decide which one or combination is most pertinent for its survey by taking into account such factors as (a) the sampling procedures, (b) length of questionnaire, (c) method of collecting the data, (d) amount of time required to complete an interview, (e) acceptable nonreturn or refusal rates, (f) costs in time and dollars, and (g) validity of the findings.
4. Select the questions to be included in the questionnaire. These

should be directly related to the objective(s) of the needs assessment study. The two basic types of questionnaires are the open-ended questions, whereby respondents have freedom in answering the question as they see fit, and the closed-end or multiple choice questions in which the respondent must make one choice of the best among several possible answers to a question. Where statistical inferences are to be drawn from a reliable quantitative base, the fixed alternative question is preferable.

5. The next step is determining the sample and number of the people to be involved in answering the questions of the survey. This depends on the information needed, the data gathering technique to be used, the size of the population needed to ensure representativeness of the entire community, and the unit of analysis (an individual, a family, a neighborhood, etc.).

6. Collecting and coding the data are the next steps required. If person-to-person interviews are involved, staff must be recruited and trained. After being collected, the data are coded, i.e., transferred to predesigned formats to be analyzed. Open-ended questions are far more difficult to code because intermediary steps are usually required before the data can be converted to a quantifiable base for statistical manipulations. However, what is gained in statistical elegance is paid for by not permitting the persons being surveyed the opportunity of providing important clues to health and mental health needs that are not included among the questions and can only be elicited by the unstructured type of question. Preferably, unstructured, open-ended questions should be used to elicit the community's understanding of its own needs as a preliminary needs assessment study. Then, based on the findings of this study, the more structured, multiple choice type of question can be asked on those subjects uncovered in the first study and considered to be most relevant to the community.

7. Presenting the findings and recommendations is the final important step in the survey, as it is with the other needs assessment approaches discussed thus far. The most important factor to consider in presenting the findings is to identify the audience. Most agency administrators and the community at large are more at ease with written, descriptive material supported by easy to understand tables, charts, or graphic material. The more sophisticated, scientific audience will require an explication of the statistical methods used and the process by which the findings were developed. They are more concerned with the process; the community is more interested in the substance or final recommendations.

Advantages of the survey approach include:

1. The survey, if done correctly, can produce the most valid and reliable information regarding community health and mental health needs.
2. By going directly to a representative cross section of the community, the survey approach gets directly at what the people themselves identify as their needs. No intermediary or surrogate speaks for them whether in the form of records, key informants, or social indicators.
3. The approach is flexible and can be used to get at a wide range of community needs.
4. Its flexibility further permits it to be used in conjunction with the other approaches described above.

But the survey is generally the most costly of the approaches. Another problem is that, by going directly to the people of the community, there may be a tendency of not wanting to be interviewed at all, answering only questions with which the interviewee is comfortable, or providing inaccurate information due to memory lapses, not understanding the question, or simply trying to terminate the interview as quickly as possible. These factors, of course, can seriously affect the validity and reliability of the survey. Finally, complex surveys are generally too difficult for inexperienced groups to execute.

Service Population Approach

This approach permits a targeting in of a specific population, one that uses the services of a health or mental health agency. It elicits how people who use the service feel about it and what changes they might want with respect to it. It also provides a means for understanding the nature of problems people perceive they have, problems that activated their seeking assistance. It also gives insights into the barriers that inhibit use of the agency and its service, as well as other services they need but are not provided by the agency. The steps required to carry out this approach are similar to that of the "key informant" approach, except that the population includes the consumers rather than the providers of service.

The service population approach provides insight into a real clientele, one with specific problems using a specific service. These findings should provide a fairly realistic needs assessment of a high risk population and offer insights into how the services can be altered to render them both more accessible and more inviting than they are.

But there are disadvantages to this approach, too.

1. Fear of losing the use of the services can bias the users' answers to questions of interest to the surveyors.
2. It is dangerous to generalize from the findings of this special population to the community as a whole. Others in the community in need of such services, but not using them, might be quite different from the user population.
3. The size of the sample might be inadequate to achieve statistically valid findings. In addition, those willing to participate represent a self-selected population, making it unrepresentative of the agency's service population.

FUNCTION STATUS INDEX

J. W. Bush and others[10] have developed an index that can measure, with some sensitivity, changes in the health status of the nation. Such an index, consists of two dimensions: a function level (how a person performs his activity of daily living at a point in time) and a prognosis (changes that occur to his health and mental health at future times and result in shifts in his functional performance from one level to another—either higher or lower). He defines function status as "conformity to society's standards of physical and mental well-being, including performance of the activities usual for the social role."[11] Disturbances in the functioning of a person can be both physical and mental in origin and represent degrees of deviation from norms of well-being. Bush has been seeking to identify levels of functional performance on a scale from complete well-being to death. The problem has been to define the number of levels between these extremes on a continuum and assign valid values to the different levels. He distinguishes health status from functional status. Health status refers to changes in a person's well-being from one level to another, whereas functional status refers to a person's capacity to perform his/her social activities at some specific point in time. Three separate scales were developed related to a person's mobility, physical activity, and social activity. Exhibit 2-1 depicts a 31-level scale combining these functions with measured values assigned to each within a .00 to 1.00 continuum[12]. Exhibit 2-2 shows these levels and assigned values.[13]

Exhibit 2-1 Scales and Definitions for the Classification of Function Levels*

Scale	Step	Definition
		Mobility Scale
5	Traveled freely	Used public transportation or drove alone. For below six age group, traveled as usual for age.
4	Traveled with difficulty	(a) Went outside alone, but had trouble getting around community freely, or (b) required assistance to use public transportation or automobile.
3	In house	(a) All day, because of illness or condition, or (b) needed human assistance to go outside.
2	In hospital	Not only general hospital, but also nursing home, extended care facility, sanitarium, or similar institution.
1	In special unit	For some part of the day in a restricted area of the hospital such as intensive care, operating room, recovery room, isolation ward, or similar unit.
0	Death	
		Physical Activity Scale
4	Walked freely	With no limitations of any kind.
3	Walked with limitations	(a) With cane, crutches, or mechanical aid; or (b) limited in lifting, stooping or using inclines or stairs; or (c) limited in speed or distance by general physical condition.
2	Moved independently in wheelchair	Propelled self alone in wheelchair.
1	In wheelchair	For most or all of the day.
0	Death	
		Social Activity Scale
5	Performing major and other activities	Major means specifically- play for below 6, school for 6-17, and work or maintain household for adults. Other means all activities not classified as major, such as athletics, clubs, shopping, church, hobbies, civic projects, or games as appropriate for age.
4	Performed major but limited in other activities	Played, went to school, worked, or kept house, but limited in other activities as defined above.
3	Performed major activities with limitations	Limited in the amount or kind of major activity performed, for instance, needed special rest periods, special school, or special working aids.
2	Did not perform major activity but performed self-care activities	Did not play, go to school, work or keep house, but dressed, bathed, and fed self.

Exhibit 2-1 Continued

| 1 | Required assistance with self-care activities | Required human help with one or more of the following – dressing, bathing, or eating--and did not perform major or other activities. For below six age group, means assistance not usually required for age. |
| 0 | Death | |

*References to sources of scale items available from the authors.

Source: J.W. Bush, M.N. Chen and D.L. Patrick, *Social Indicators for Health Planning and Policy Analysis* (Springfield, Va.: National Technical Information Service, May 1974), p. 26.

Algebraically, the function status index is expressed as follows:

$$F = j\ \frac{N_j F_j}{N},$$

where $0 \leq F \leq 1$ and

N = total number of persons in a population,
N_j = number of persons in function level j,
F_j = measured weight or social preference for function level j, and
j = index for the function level—0, 1, 2, ... 30.

Exhibit 2-3 is an illustration of the use of this formula index based on the 31-level scale. It shows 95 percent of the population functioning at the highest level of performance, 30. The other three percent of the index is composed of those with various degrees of deviation from this highest level of functioning.

Advantages of the Index

Bush identifies a number of advantages for the function status index. Among these are the following:

1. It is a concise index of the health/mental health well-being of a community.
2. It is sensitive to the variations of individuals with different degrees of functional capacity.
3. The data are easily observable and can be used without knowledge of medical terms or diagnoses, or without being dependent on a person's memory.
4. Each person is exclusively assigned to only one level.

Exhibit 2-2 Function Level Classification and Measured Values*

Level Number	Mobility (Step)	Physical Activity (Step)	Social Activity (Step)	Measured Values
L 30	Traveled freely (5)	Walked freely (4)	Performed major and other activities (no symptom/problem complex) (5)	1.000
L 29	Traveled freely (5)	Walked freely (4)	Performed major and other activities (symptom/problem complex present) (5)	.804
L 28	Traveled freely (5)	Walked freely (4)	Performed major but limited in other activities (4)	.689
L 27	Traveled freely (5)	Walked freely (4)	Performed major activity with limitations (3)	.694
L 26	Traveled freely (5)	Walked freely (4)	Did not perform major but performed self-care activities (2)	.646
L 25	Traveled with difficulty (4)	Walked freely (4)	Performed major but limited in other activities (4)	.516
L 24	Traveled with difficulty (4)	Walked freely (4)	Performed major activity with limitations	.536
L 23	Traveled with difficulty (4)	Walked freely (4)	Did not perform major but performed self-care activities	.495
L 22	Traveled with difficulty (4)	Walked with limitations (3)	Performed major but limited in other activities (4)	.519
L 21	Traveled with difficulty (4)	Walked with limitations (3)	Performed major activity with limitations (3)	.522
L 20	Traveled with difficulty (4)	Walked with limitations (3)	Did not perform major but performed self-care activities (2)	.463
L 19	Traveled with difficulty (4)	Moved independently in wheelchair (2)	Performed major activity with limitation (3)	.503
L 18	Traveled with difficulty (4)	Moved independently in wheelchair (2)	Did not perform major but performed self-care activities (2)	.458
L 17	In house (3)	Walked freely (4)	Did not perform major but performed self-care activities (2)	.594

Exhibit 2-2 Continued

Level Number	Mobility (Step)	Physical Activity (Step)	Social Activity (Step)	Measured Values
L 16	In house (3)	Walked freely (4)	Required assistance with self-care activities (1)	.505
L 15	In house (3)	Walked with limitations (3)	Did not perform major but performed self-care activities (2)	.519
L 14	In house (3)	Walked with limitations (3)	Required assistance with self-care activities (1)	.436
L 13	In house (3)	Moved independently in wheelchair (2)	Did not perform major but performed self-care activities (2)	.491
L 12	In house (3)	Moved independently in wheelchair (2)	Required assistance with self-care activities (1)	.444
L 11	In house (3)	In bed or chair (1)	Did not perform major but performed self-care activities (2)	.334
L 10	In house (3)	In bed or chair (1)	Required assistance with self-care activities (1)	.436
L 9	In hospital (2)	Walked freely (4)	Did not perform major but performed self-care activities (2)	.528
L 8	In hospital (2)	Walked freely (4)	Required assistance with self-care activities (1)	.440
L 7	In hospital (2)	Walked with limitations (2)	Did not perform major but performed self-care activities (2)	.440
L 6	In hospital (2)	Walked with limitations (3)	Required assistance with self-care activities (1)	.388
L 5	In hospital (2)	Moved independently in wheelchair (2)	Did not perform major but performed self-care activities (2)	.445
L 4	In hospital (2)	Moved independently in wheelchair (2)	Required assistance with self-care activities (1)	.387
L 3	In hospital (2)	In bed or chair (1)	Did not perform major but performed self-care activities (2)	.428

Exhibit 2-2 Continued

Level Number	Mobility (Step)	Physical Activity (Step)	Social Activity (Step)	Measured Values
L 2	In hospital (2)	In bed or chair (1)	Required assistance with self-care activities (1)	.343
L 1	In special unit (1)	In bed or chair (1)	Required assistance with self-care activities (1)	.267
L 0	Death (0)			

*Rules for exclusion of other combinations of scale levels available from authors.

Source: J.W. Bush, M.N. Chen and D.L. Patrick, *Social Indicators for Health Planning and Policy Analysis* (Springfield, Va.: National Technical Information Service, May 1974), p. 27.

Exhibit 2-3 Illustrative Distribution of Persons Among Different Function Levels and Computation of the Function Status Index

Index of Function Level (j)	Number of Persons (N_j)	Function Level Values (F_j)	($F_j N_j$)
30	95,000	1.00	95,000
27	3,000	.69	2,070
17	1,000	.59	590
10	700	.44	308
2	300	.34	102
Total	100,000 ($=N$)		98,070 ($=F_j N_j$)

$$F = \frac{F_j N_j}{N} = \frac{98,070}{100,000} = .98$$

Source: J.W. Bush, M.N. Chen and D.L. Patrick, *Social Indicators for Health Planning and Policy Analysis* (Springfield, Va.: National Technical Information Service, May 1974), p. 28.

5. It is flexible as it permits cross-sectional comparisons among populations, disaggregation for comparison among populations within the community by nature of functioning or specific causes of dysfunction such as diabetes, schizophrenia, etc., and the construction of longitudinal studies of the community over time.

There are some problems with the scale. Without incorporating health status into the functioning of an individual, it fails to account for changes in a person's physical well-being or prognosis that will affect his functioning over time. Furthermore, it may take years before changes in health status are reflected in the overall function status index. Improvements in one level of the function index may be cancelled out by lower levels of functioning in other levels.

Because of this major deficiency in the function status index (FSI), Bush and his associates developed the "value-adjusted life expectancy" measure to account for the progress of individuals. It is based on four functional levels:

A—well,
B—nonbed disability,
C—bed disability,
D—death.

Based on a 90-year period of potential life within 10-year age intervals, Bush was able to compute the "equilibrium function level expectancies" for the 90 years to .724 in a well state, .050 with nonbed disability, .021 with bed disability, and .205 as years of death since the longevity expectation is about 72 years. Thus, a person can be expected to live in a well state for 65.2 years during his/her lifetime (.724 × 90 years), with nonbed disability for 4.5 years (.50 × 90), and with 1.9 years of bed disability (.021 × 90). In addition, a person will have died prematurely 18.4 years before reaching his/her potential of 90 years of age.

By multiplying the values of the function level expectancies (Y^*j) by measures of the FSI scale (F_j), the value-adjusted life expectancy (Q^*) is obtained:

$$Q^* = F_j Y^* j.$$

An illustration of this formula for a community is given in Exhibit 2-4. The value-adjusted life expectancy is similar to the expected dysfunction-free years of life. It can be used to compare population groups of all ages within a community or the health status of the same population over time. As such it can serve as a health indicator.

Exhibit 2-4 Illustrative Computation of Value-Adjusted Life Expectancy

L_j		Y^*j	F_j	Y^*jF_j
L_A	Well	65.2	1.00	65.2
L_B	Nonbed disability	4.5	.59	2.7
L_C	Bed disability	1.9	.34	.6

Value-adjusted life expectancy (Q^*) = 68.5 (years)

Source: J.W. Bush, M.N. Chen and D.L. Patrick, *Social Indicators for Health Planning and Policy Analysis* (Springfield, Va.: National Technical Information Service, May 1974), p. 29.

There are several advantages of Q^*:

1. It "combines morbidity with mortality in a single number that is independent of both age and medical diagnoses."[14]
2. It is an excellent indicator to measure the health status of total populations.
3. It can easily be replicated and thus serve as a longitudinal comparison of the health status of a population over time.

The disadvantages are as follows:

1. Causal inferences cannot be drawn from intervention procedures used to improve the health status of a population, unless a controlled experiment is designed.
2. Although it represents a major advance on earlier health status indicators, it is still in its experimental and testing stage.

INDEX FOR PROGRAM PRIORITY

Whereas Bush designed an index to provide a general indication of how the health status is faring, Chen developed a special-purpose index to meet the needs of specific problems or population groupings in a larger area.[15] Chen's G index is a modification of Miller's Q index.[16]

Both indices are based on the notion that a general reference group or population has an optimal degree of health that takes into account the capacity of modern medical technology and knowledge to treat those diseases and illnesses amenable to improvement. Any target population that has a negative deviation from this optimal reference group is thus capable of showing improvement, if equal medical care were available. Consequently, the objective of the G index is to identify the level of health of a particular group in comparison with another reference group. The G index modifies the Q index by including morbidity data. The basic formula for G is*

$$
\begin{aligned}
\text{G Index} &= (M_t/M_r)\ (D_1 + D_2) \\
&= (n_t/N_t)\ (n_r/N_r)\ (D_1 + D_2) \\
&= (n_t N_r/n_r\ N_t)\ (D_1 + D_2).
\end{aligned}
$$

To arrive at the G index, a number of prior calculations must be made. Exhibit 2-5 explains the calculations and illustrates the use of Chen's formula to compute the statistics using fictitious values. When the G values are compared with each other in this illustration, they show that Disease B is 105 times as serious as Disease C and about twice as serious as Disease A.

Advantages of this index include:

1. The G index uses data that are readily available and fairly reliable.
2. It provides a fairly accurate method for comparing the relative seriousness of diseases within a target population.
3. It is fairly simple to calculate the ratios involved in the formula.

However, disadvantages must be noted. While Chen points out a way to validate the index, it has not been validated yet. Also, the index cannot be used alone to interpret the needs of the target population. Those using it must also have other data related to indicators of quality of life, such as housing, employment status, availability of health services, etc., if one is to have a framework within which to interpret the real meaning of the index.

FUNCTION LIMITATION SCALE

M. Berdit and J. W. Williamson[17] have developed a function limitation scale to measure the outcome of medical intervention on patients treated at ambulatory clinics. The object of the scale is to test the quality of care of the physicians by measuring the outcome of treat-

Exhibit 2-5 Values of G Index for Three Hypothetical Diseases

Quantity	Disease A	Disease B	Disease C
n_r	1,000.00	2,000.00	5,500.00
N_r	200,000,000.00	200,000,000.00	200,000,000.00
n_t	700.00	1,500.00	70.00
N_t	400,000.00	400,000.00	400,000.00
M_r/100,000	.50	1.00	2.75
M_t/100,000	175.00	375.00	17.50
E_r	20.00	35.00	10.00
E_t	30.00	30.00	55.00
W_r	20,000.00	70,000.00	55,000.00
W_t	21,000.00	45,000.00	3,850.00
H_r	20,000.00	45,000.00	9,000.00
H_t	18,000.00	39,000.00	4,812,000.00
C_r	75,000.00	150,000.00	13,000.00
C_t	80,000.00	100,000.00	8,955,000.00
T_r	123.29	260.27	36.53
T_t	122.37	198.17	21,361.64
W'_t	40.00	140.00	7.70
T'_t	.25	.52	.07
D_1	20,960.00	44,860.00	3,842.30
D_2	122.12	197.65	21,361.57
G	7,378,742.00	16,896,618.75	160,388.26
Priority...	46.00	105.35	1.00

Key:

n_r = total deaths from specific class of disease in reference population

N_r = size of reference population

n_t = total deaths from specific class of disease in target population

N_t = size of target population

M_r = crude disease-specific mortality for the reference population

M_t = crude disease-specific mortality for the target population

E_r = average life expectancy at average age of death from specific class of disease in reference population

E_t = average life expectancy at average age of death from specific class of disease in target population

W_r = total years lost from disease-specific mortality in reference population

W_t = total years lost from disease-specific mortality in target population

H_r = total hospital days from specific disease for reference population

H_t = total hospital days from specific disease for target population

Exhibit 2-5 Continued

C_r = total clinic visits for specific disease in reference population
C_t = total clinic visits for specific disease in target population
T_r = total years lost from disease-specific morbidity in reference population
T_t = total years lost from disease-specific morbidity in target population
W'_t = *expected* years lost from disease-specific mortality in target population if disease impact on target and reference populations were the same
T'_t = *expected* years lost from disease-specific morbidity in target population if disease impact on target and reference populations were the same
D_1 = difference between observed and expected years lost from disease-specific mortality in target population
D_2 = difference between observed and expected years lost from disease-specific morbidity in target population

Source: Reprinted with permission from *Health Status Indexes*, edited by Robert L. Berg. Copyright 1973 by the Hospital Research and Educational Trust, 840 North Lake Shore Drive, Chicago, Illinois 60611.

ment as perceived by the patient and comparing it with standards developed by physicians. As such, the scale has both policy and practice implications when used at the microlevel of analysis for measuring the day-to-day activity of a clinic.

This scale is based on a six-point ordinal continuum of patient functioning, ranging from one's capacity to be fully active at one end to death at the other end (Exhibit 2-6). Basically, a paramedical "health accountant" telephones patients and asks them several questions to arrive at an evaluation of their level of functioning.

Does the patient function at his usual activities? If he does, does he nevertheless need medical care on a regular basis to control his condition? Does he find that his condition is beginning to impinge on his ability to carry out his usual activities? If he cannot carry out his full range of usual activities, can he carry out some of them? Is he ambulatory or is he entirely dependent on others to care for him?[18]

Exhibit 2-6 Function Limitation Scale

Function Limitation	Definition
0. Fully active—asymptomatic, no care needed	No impairment. Participants fully in "usual activities."* No symptoms. No more than average health risk.
1. Fully active—asymptomatic, medical care needed	Minimal impairment. Participates fully in usual activities."* No symptoms, but has detectable signs of illness of which he may be unaware. Usually requires diagnostic and therapeutic care. Higher than average health risk.
2. Fully active—symptomatic	Aware of impairment. Symptoms minor to severe. Participates in 80%–100% of "usual activities"* but may experience reduced comfort and productivity.
3. Restricted active	Participates partially (less than 80%) or not at all in "usual activities."* Can care for self.
4. Dependent	Cannot participate in usual activities or care for self. Dependency may be partial (help needed in self-care) or total (as in comatose state).
5. Dead	Total, irreversible loss of function.

*"Usual activities" are defined as those appropriate to the patient's life stage. The criteria for ranking in the active and in the restricted levels at the various stages are as follows:

Life Stage	Fully Active (Levels 0–2)	Restricted Active (Level 3)
Schoolchild	Attends school over 80% of the time. Plays as much as other children. Engages in out-of-school activities consistent with age and personality.	Misses school at least 20% of the time. Cannot play as much as other children. Change in out-of-school activities not explained by maturational phase.
Adult in productive years	Carries on housework, job, community work at least at 80% of normal rate. Works at least four days a week.	Works less than four days a week. Needs significant help with housework. Has had to curtail community work.
Adult in retirement	Participates in activity generally engaged in (from work to reading) during past year and is satisfied with activity level.	Has had to cut down on previous activity of past year (whether or not because of problem under study), or is continuing activity but is not satisfied with activity level.

Source: Reprinted with permission from *Health Status Indexes*, edited by Robert L. Berg. Copyright 1973 by the Hospital Research and Educational Trust, 840 North Lake Shore Drive, Chicago, Illinois 60611.

The scale is fairly inexpensive to use, and it does not require high cost and skilled staff to implement. Furthermore, such a method provides a ready outcome measure of how a clinic is operating. Since the scale involves the patient's own perception of health, it can take into account both his physical and mental health. A physician's account would yield data related only to the patient's physical condition.

But the scale has not been tested for its validity or reliability. Also, it requires physician acceptance and cooperation. If physicians do not accept it, they will not use it to guide their practice. Finally, because paramedicals are used to collect data, they must be trained to ensure a uniform understanding, reporting, and evaluation of the data to be scored properly on the scale.

Exhibit 2-6 illustrates the function limitation scale.

DELPHI FORECASTING

Delphi is a method for forecasting social and organizational futures, which was predominantly used, until recently, in the area of technological forecasts. Determining the needs and organizational structure of hospitals and other medical facilities and services is one of the uses of Delphi.

Basically, Delphi is a technique for obtaining consensus from a panel of experts on the probability that future events will occur. Panel members do not interact with each other, but through an intermediary. This permits the experts to present their best estimates without being biased by the presence of strong-willed persons of high status or prestige, as in a face-to-face situation. Panelists do not know each other's identity during the proceedings, though they are generally experts in the medical field. The process takes three to four rounds before the differences among the panelists can be narrowed to form a consensus about the future. In each round, the respective panelist's descriptions and predictions of the future are circulated among the other panelists, leading to comparison and contrasts among them. In time, through refinement and clarification of each panelist's position, a consensus is reached.

Panelists should have heterogeneous backgrounds to ensure that a range of values is offered to the subjects under discussion. Each panelist must be an expert in his/her own right to avoid a situation where someone else's point of view is summarily accepted without question. The illustration of how the responses are collected and formatted is shown by the need of a hospital to have a range of options for future use of its facilities and services.[19]

Exhibit 2-7 shows, for example, that 60 percent of the panelists agreed that the probability of there being a change in hospital sponsorship in the next ten years is only 10 percent. In sum, the panelists see little change occurring. However, with respect to greater regulation of hospitals in the next ten years, 80 percent of the panelists believe in a 90 percent probability of that occurring. The investigators who carried out this Delphi study define a consensus as 75 percent of the panelists coming to an agreement on one of the three probabilities occurring in ten years, very high probability—90 percent, unsure of the direction of change—50 percent, and very low probability—10 percent.

Advantages of Delphi forecasting include:

1. In a situation where the complexity of a subject or the availability of quantitative data is lacking, the Delphi method is a positive approach to identifying either the needs of populations for medical care or those of medical systems.
2. It is a relatively inexpensive method.
3. It enables a range of options to be elicited from which experts are in a position to come to a possible consensus. In this way, the power of a vocal few who may overwhelm a gathering of persons and shut out the eliciting of options from the more timid persons is reduced.
4. Forecasts of future needs can be monitored so, as they arise, future iterations of the Delphi forecasts can be made to correct distorted predictions.

But there are some disadvantages, too:

1. A poor selection of panelists can lead to bias occurring.
2. Panel fatigue, usually coming in the third round, often leads to premature closure or agreement when, in fact, the panelists do not agree. Experts in the Delphi method can determine whether such fatigue has occurred by examining the amount of change in responses between round two and three or three and four.
3. Delphi can be used for purposes for which it was not intended, such as assuming that the results were based upon available data and are statistically significant.
4. Because the assessments are subjective in nature, they are neither valid nor reliable. A different group of panelists could well develop a different set of findings.

Exhibit 2-7 Medical Service Organizational Patterns and Their Effect on Hospitals*

Futures	Percent of panelists indicating likelihood of occurrence in next 10 years of:		
	90%	50%	10%
Hospitals in Respect to Sponsorship			
(a) Little or no change	20	20	60
(b) More profit-oriented ownership	0	35	65
(c) Government run hospitals will convert to private nonprofit status	15	45	40
(d) Hospitals will assume status of quasi-public utilities	45	50	5
(e) Federation of hospitals into central sponsorship/ownership	20	45	35
Hospitals in Respect to Public Accountability			
(f) Little or no change	5	5	90
(g) More voluntary public responsiveness in terms of types of services, financial accounting, expansion, etc.	35	55	10
(h) More representation of the underserved public on hospital boards	55	45	0
(i) Public disclosure of hospital income, expenses and plans	95	5	0
(j) Officially authorized agency review of performance in fiscal management and of service quality	55	45	0
(k) Greater commission-type regulation of services, expansion, and rates	80	20	0
Hospitals in Respect to Relationship with Other Hospitals			
(l) Little or no change	5	20	75
(m) Continued voluntary development of shared services not involving patient contact	35	55	10
(n) Greater voluntary coordination, cooperation and functional specialization among hospitals regarding all services, research, and education	65	30	5
(o) Stronger management alliances	55	35	10
(p) Formation of consortia of hospitals which will jointly assume financial risk	35	40	25
(q) Physical consolidations and complete organizational merger	15	40	45
Hospitals in Respect to Medical Staff Organization			
(r) Physicians will be required to admit all of their cases to one hospital rather than several	0	35	65
(s) Hospitals will continue to have their own medical staff and will continue to be closed to non-staff physicians	50	25	25
(t) Hospitals will no longer have their own medical staff, physicians will become members of a common staff which is sponsored by a federated organization such as a health care corporation	10	20	70
(u) Staff privileges among hospitals will be interchangeable	20	40	40
(v) Hospitals will contract with medical care foundation for medical staff	5	55	40
(w) One medical staff for two or more hospitals	45	40	15
(x) Greater physician participation in hospital affairs, including direct operating responsibilities	40	45	15
(y) Doctors will be closer to their principal hospital, having an interlocking incentive and penalty system linked to the hospital	10	80	10
(z) Medical staff will be more oriented into health teams coordinated with neighborhood clinics in addition to hospitals	30	50	20

*This exhibit shows the proportion of panelists, rounded to the nearest five percent, who estimated with .90, .50, and .10 probability, respectively, that the conditions para-

DEMAND ASSESSMENT METHODS

In this section, five major demand methods will be discussed as well as several variants for special needs of health care facilities or services. Although there are a number of others that could have been selected, these represent the ones most widely in use. In addition, they all have the advantage of ease of use in their mathematical formulation as well as the availability of data and the ease of data access.

The Formula Approach

This is the Hill-Burton approach used by most states to determine future need for medical facilities, particularly beds. It is based on projecting future utilization by summing the use rate by some estimated projected population.

$$\frac{\text{current patient-days}}{\text{current population}} = \text{use rate}$$

$$\frac{(\text{use rate}) (\text{projected population})}{365} = \text{average daily census}$$

$$\frac{\text{average daily census}}{\text{desired occupancy rate}} = \text{projected beds required}$$

---

phrased by each statement will occur in the next five to ten years. Rectangles and squares are used to graphically indicate the degree of consensus for each statement. Consensus is defined as 75 percent or more of the panel having reached agreement on one or two probability choices. If that proportion of the panel agreed on two probability choices (i.e., .10 and .50 or .50 and .90), "general consensus" was achieved. If the 75 percent proportion converged on a single probability choice (i.e., .10 or .50 or .90), "strong consensus" was evidenced. General consensus is indicated by rectangles, and strong consensus by larger squares. A smaller square within a rectangle denotes a future circumstance in which 50 percent or more but not 75 percent of the panel converged on one probability estimate. Results reported here are undifferentiated by respondent background. Each panel member's assessment was equally weighted. Since the panel used in this study was made up of persons with widely divergent expertises and approaches to medical care, the futures upon which consensus was reached would seem to have general significance.

Source: Reprinted with permission from D.B. Starkweather, et al. "Delphi Forecasting of Health Care Organization," *Medical Care*, 12: 37 (1975). Copyright 1975 by J.B. Lippincott Company, East Washington Square, Philadelphia, Pennsylvania 19105.

Example:

$$\frac{400,000 \text{ patient-days}}{1,600,000 \text{ people}} = .25 \text{ use rate}$$

If the projected population for the health systems agency (HSA) region were 2 million people by 1985, the future utilization would be found by multiplying this figure by the use rate, .25:

$$(.25) \ (2,000,000) = 500,000 \text{ patient-days.}$$

Average daily census is computed then by dividing the expected total number of annual patient days by 365, the number of days in a year:

$$\frac{500,000}{365} = 1,370 \text{ average daily census (1370).}$$

The final step is to divide the average daily census (1,370) by the desired occupancy rate. This figure is usually considered between 80 percent and 85 percent, depending on the state and the component parts of a hospital's facilities that comprise the average daily census.

$$\frac{1370}{80} = 1712.5, \text{ or } 1,713 \text{ beds required by 1985.}$$

Through alterations in various parts of the basic series of steps noted above, it is possible to make adjustments to take into account such factors as changes in the use rate, the differential utilization of the major components of a hospital (medical/surgical, obstetric, and pediatric), age/sex differences of those using the hospital such as child-bearing women between the ages of 15 and 44, and differences in the origin of the patient (those living within the boundaries of the HSA compared with those coming from outside its area). For example, to account for an increased use rate projected for 1985 of .005/annually based on an increased aging population, a modification in the formula would be made as follows:

Future/use rate = current use rate (1978) ×
                        [1 + (rate of change) ×
                        (number of years in the projection)]
           = .25 × [1 + (.005) × (8 years)]
           = .25 × (1 + .04)
           = .25 × 1.04 = .26

Future utilization $= 2,000,000 \times .26$
$\qquad\qquad\qquad = 520,000$ patient days
Average daily census $= \dfrac{520,000}{-365} = 1,425$
Beds needed by 1985 $= \dfrac{1,425}{.80}$

This anticipated increase in use rate results in a need for 68 additional beds required for the year 1985.

Advantages of the formula approach are:

1. Data to compute the formula are readily available and generally reliable.
2. The formula is fairly simple to use.
3. Through adjustments in the formula, it can take into account some basic factors of the population and its use of hospital facilities to arrive at a more realistic assessment of bed need in the HSA region.
4. It is most reliable and valid when used in a region with a relatively stable population.

There are four disadvantages, though:

1. The formula does not take into account alternatives to bed use that may be altering the need for beds in the future such as health maintenance organizations, minisurgery, and emphasis on preventive care.
2. Although the formula might be able to account for some population variables such as children or women in the child-bearing years, it cannot account for important factors such as diagnosis, family circumstances, or insurance availability to meet hospital costs, which cumulatively affect the use rate and the need for beds.
3. It fails to discriminate between proper and improper utilization of the hospital facility. Recent surveys have shown that anywhere from 10 percent to 60 percent of the admitted patients to hospitals and nursing facilities are inappropriately placed for the type of service needed.
4. The formula also does not take into account persons in the population who are not using the facility even though they have a legitimate and proper need for its services.

The Stochastic Method

This method translates utilization of a medical facility into bed needs and is based on probability theory.[20] It assumes that admissions and discharges of patients into a facility is a random choice. By averaging the percentage of persons who enter and leave the facility during the year it is possible to match these random occurrences against a normal distribution of Poisson curve. Queuing theory can then be used to determine the pattern of patient admissions by comparing these with the Poisson and normal distribution curves. By applying the standard deviation of the average census, the number of times that average daily census will be surpassed during the year can be predicted. It therefore becomes a decision of how often a hospital is willing to accept a higher than average daily census for it to determine how many beds it needs. Thus, unlike the formula method, which is based on population change, this method is based on fluctuations in hospital census.

Steps in the use of this method are as follows:

1. After examining the actual census level of a medical facility, a frequency distribution is drawn up. This will show the number of times each year a census level is reached. The pattern will probably resemble a bell-shaped curve.
2. This is compared with that which would have been predicted by Poisson and normal distribution.
3. The standard deviation of the average census is then determined.
4. The facility's decision makers determine which among the various levels are acceptable in meeting the future needs of its patient population. Thus, if the average daily census is 10,000, the standard deviation is considered to be 100 (under the Poisson/normal distribution, standard deviation is the square root of the mean), so the number of beds needed can be chosen. To meet the demand on all but nine days a year, 10.196 beds would be required. (10,000 divided by 1.96 × 100). Or if one wants to guarantee that there will be enough beds 99 percent of the time, then 10,233 beds (2 standard deviation) would be necessary.[21]

Advantages of the stochastic method are that it is fairly accurate for assessing the need for beds in a single institution and it provides flexibility in setting different levels of bed need. Further, the method tends to reduce the number of hospital beds needed. The larger the hospital, the higher the occupancy rate; the smaller the hospital, the more excessive capacity is needed to produce a specified level of care.

However, there are several disadvantages. Because this method does not assume the interchangeability of one set of beds (pediatric for surgical for example) or that one set of beds in one hospital is interchangeable with those in another, it cannot be used to generate bed need for an entire HSA region. The method also does not take into account alternative forms of care that can reduce or increase the need for beds, such as health maintenance organizations or the use of health prevention services. It should be noted that it cannot be assumed that past utilization, which varies by some statistical distribution, will continue to hold true in the future. Finally, this method is based on a normal curve distribution. Consequently, unless one can assume that such a distribution is present, then it is of questionable validity.

Exhibit 2-8 illustrates the results of applying the stochastic method.

Clinical Appraisal of Existing Utilization

This method is basically used to determine the appropriateness of use of existing medical facilities. It is based on a combination of the survey approach and evaluations based on expert opinion. It rests on the assumption that if all those persons in need of service, whether receiving care or not, are identified, then it is possible to determine the appropriate level of care required by them and thus maximize the use of medical facilities and services.[22, 23]

Steps required to carry out this method are as follows:

1. Define the population in need in the HSA region by its demographic characteristics (age, sex, race, income, etc.).
   a. Inpatient population is identified by means of those already in medical facilities. Those in need of service and not obtaining it are identified by contacting all those professionals in the community likely to come in contact with potential patients: visiting nurses, physician office practices, local social service agencies, senior citizens, clergy and church groups, local pharmacists, mail carriers, and a mail survey supported by the local medical society.
   b. This list is examined and duplicates eliminated.
2. Survey teams comprised of a physician and a nurse are developed.
3. Survey teams should agree in advance on the definitions of level of care. They should all be involved in common orientation sessions to ensure common understanding and acceptance of the surveys and the procedures to be followed.
4. The patients' records should be surveyed; and the nurse, using a

Exhibit 2-8 Distribution of Daily Census, Pediatrics

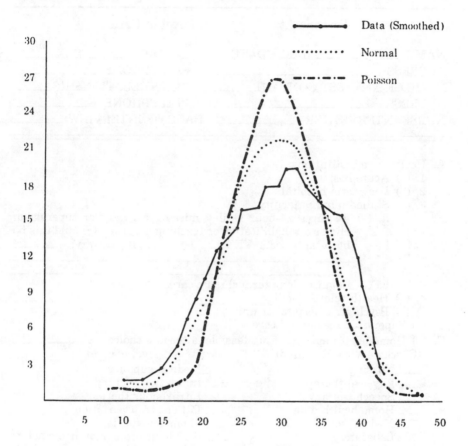

Source: Richard DuFour, "Planning for Acute Inpatient Services—A Probabilistic Model for Relating the Determination of Bed Requirements to the Level of Services to be Provided." Paper presented at Symposium on Methods, sponsored by BHPRD, HEW, February 3-5, 1975, p. 7.

standard form (Exhibit 2-9), makes her recommendation on the type of care the patients require. The physician reviews the nurse's forms without her judgments and makes an independent decision. The two then meet to discuss and come to an agreement of the level of care required. Home visits are made initially by a nurse; and then, if the persons are agreeable, the physician is invited. It was found that those at home were more comfortable with nurses than physicians.

Exhibit 2-9 Level of Care Evaluation

Persons At (   ) Level of Care

NAME _____ BIRTHDATE _____ AGE _____ SEX _____
ADDRESS _____ TELEPHONE _____
NAME OF NEAREST CONTACT _____ RELATIONSHIP _____
ADDRESS _____ TELEPHONE _____
NURSE INTERVIEWER _____ DATE OF INTERVIEW _____

A. Health care institutions
   1. ( ) Acute hospital
   2. ( ) Long term hospital
   3. ( ) Skilled nursing facility
      a. ( ) Requires 24-hour skilled nursing care and/or supervision and/or a rehabilitation or teaching program. (Should this be hospital-based?) YES ____ NO ____ . If yes, why? _____
_____
_____

      b. ( ) Requires long term chronic care.
   4. ( ) Health related facility
   5. ( ) Psychiatric hospital or unit
B. ( ) Supervised residential care
C. ( ) Home health agency. If not feasible, alternate choice _____
   (Check Services Required)   (Write out level of care)

____ Nursing	____ Medical supplies
____ Physical therapy	____ Inhalation therapy
____ Speech therapy	____ Intravenous therapy
____ Home health aide	____ Patient transportation
____ Medical social work	____ Meals-on-wheels
____ Laboratory	____ 8-10 hour companion-homemaker
____ Medical equipment	____ Other (specify) _____

_____

D. ( ) Other (specify) _____
E. ( ) None of the above

2. AMBULATION
   ( ) Unlimited $\bar{c}$ or $\bar{s}$ mechanical aid
   ( ) Outdoors $\bar{c}$ personal ass't or super.
   ( ) Indoors, semiambulant $\bar{c}$ personal assistance and/or supervision
   ( ) Wheelchair $\bar{c}$ aid in transfer
   ( ) Bed to chair $\bar{c}$ aid in transfer
   ( ) Bedfast, can turn self
   ( ) Bedfast, must be turned
   ( ) Other _____
         specify

Exhibit 2-9 Continued

3. CONTINENCE
( ) Completely continent
( ) Incontinent, urine, occ.
( ) Incontinent, urine, always
( ) Indwelling catheter, condom dr.
( ) Incontinent, feces, occ.
( ) Incontinent, feces, always
( ) Completely incontinent
( ) Colostomy—not regulated
( ) Colostomy—regulated

4. PERSONAL CARE ASSISTANCE

Bathing	Dressing	Toileting	Feeding	
				No help needed
				Minimal help/supervision
				Moderate help/supervision
				Complete help/supervision

5. OTHER PROBLEMS (Elaborate if needed)
( ) Vision _____
( ) Hearing _____
( ) Decubiti _____
( ) Prostheses _____
( ) Speech _____
( ) Language barrier _____

6. MENTAL STATUS — was mental status for those in supervised homes for adults verified c̄ staff? ___ YES ___ NO

( ) Alert, oriented, no discernable memory loss.
( ) Requires supervision in open environment for mild confusion, for example the administration of medications.
( ) Requires supervision in open environment for management of behavior because of moderate or severe confusion.
( ) Requires care in a closed psychiatric setting.

7. MEDICATIONS (Name Only)
(ORAL)
( ) None ..... _____ _____ ....Able to self-adm.
( ) Few ...... _____ _____ ..... s̄ supervision
( ) Moderate _____ _____ .....Pt. needs reminding
( ) Many .... _____ _____ .....Needs drug supervision

Exhibit 2-9 Continued

(PARENTERAL)   ____ Requires adm. &
( ) None .....   _____ _____   skilled observation
( ) Few   ...... _____ _____
( ) Moderate ..   _____ _____
( ) Many ....   _____ _____

8. EQUIPMENT AND TREATMENTS REQUIRED:
   List special equipment and treatments required. Include dressings, irrigations, tube feedings, inhalation therapy, intravenous therapy, etc.

9. OTHER PATIENT CARE REQUIREMENTS
   ( ) Special diet
   ( ) Lab work and/or x-ray and/or EKG as needed
   ( ) Physical therapy
   ( ) Speech evaluation and/or therapy
   ( ) OT evaluation and/or therapy
   ( ) Social work
   ( ) Dental care
   ( ) Specialized consultation _____
                          (specify)
   ( ) Periodic podiatry
   ( ) Reality orientation
   ( ) Diversional activities
   ( ) _____

10. DAY CARE — Could the patient benefit from a day care program ____YES ____NO ____CANNOT JUDGE

Source: T.F. Lantry et al., *Methods for Determining and Projecting Needs and Demands for Acute Inpatient Care Services* (Washington, D.C.: Arthur Young & Company, 1975), pp. 60-63.

5. The individual records are then tabulated to determine the "real" need and the level of that need in the HSA region. This should result in a measure of misutilization and nonutilization of services.
6. Periodic surveys are required to determine what changes, if any, are occurring in the appropriate use of medical services.

Advantages of this method include:

1. It permits the identification of real needs for medical and mental health services in the HSA region.
2. It has very good validity as it is based on the needs of the people interviewed about their own physical and mental health.
3. It identifies the ideal levels of care that should be offered to inpatients or potential patients according to their needs.

But the method does not recommend what levels of utilization of services are required to meet the needs uncovered, and it makes no forecast of what the utilization will be in the future. The method also fails to deal with one important group of persons, those living outside the region and obtaining service within the region. Finally, it does not investigate the causes of illnesses from the sociodemographic factors affecting demand.

Index of Institutional Commitment and Relevance

This is a method for evaluating how many resources are being used by a specific service population in a metropolitan area. Rather than attempt to define the total service area being served by an urban hospital, this method attempts to determine the utilization of the medical facility by the patients from a specific geographic area, in this case census tracts. It assumes that a hospital located in a community would play a larger leadership role, if not the principal one, if it had a way of knowing how much it was already committing to a specific geographic territory and how relevant that commitment has been to the people of the area. This in turn would generate an assessment of unmet need in the area through dialogue with community leaders and HSA planners for developing a community health plan.

Two indices are required: an index of commitment and an index of relevance.[24] The index of institutional commitment is defined by the proportion of a hospital's resources devoted to serving the medical needs of a specific community. For example, 300 annual admissions to hospital X out of 9,000 overall come from a given census tract. The index of commitment is 300/9,000, or .033. In addition, 5,000 out of the 40,000 outpatient visits also are derived from that same census tract, or a .125 index of commitment.

The index of relevance refers to the degree the people from a given census tract utilize the hospital. Thus, if the census tract produces 3,000 inpatients to all hospitals, then X hospital with 300 inpatients has an index of relevance of 300/3,000, or .10. Likewise, if 15,000 outpatient visits are made to all hospitals, its outpatient index of relevance is .33 (5,000/15,000). It is also possible to determine the dollar value of X hospital's resources to the area. Thus, from $12 million annually, its budget for inpatient services, it provides $396,000 (3 percent of its budget) worth of services to the census tract. In addition, out of its $800,000 outpatient budget, it provides $100,000 worth of services. In sum, almost a half million dollars of medical services are provided to the area. In planning for future needs for the community, these levels of commitment and relevance are useful bases upon which to develop future services to the community.

There are three advantages to this index:

1. It gives to the medical facility an accurate indication of the total support it renders the community.
2. It provides to the consumers of medical service in that community their degree of dependence and need of X hospital. It also enables the community to gauge the hospital's level of commitment to their needs.
3. It offers a tool for examining the nature and demographic characteristics of the portion of the community who uses the hospital. Is it only the residents from one small area that use the hospital and not others? Are these the more affluent or the low income residents of the area? Questions like these can be used to determine future direction for medical services.

But two disadvantages exist. In a large metropolitan area, it is difficult to collect the demographic data needed to survey who uses the hospital from the census tract. Most data will have to be generated by the records of the hospital itself. Patient origin studies are usually not geographically specific enough to assist in identifying where all the patients from a given census tract go to obtain their medical care. Also, data for outpatient and emergency services are generally not standardized, as are inpatient data. This will make comparing one hospital with another difficult and severely limit the use the community makes of various hospital services.

Regression Methods

Regression analysis is a technique that incorporates a series of independent variables into an equation to extrapolate future values of a dependent variable.[25-27] It is mainly used for estimating the need for beds of highly specific services, such as obstetrics or pediatrics. This method requires the identification of variables that are comparable with the demand for the service. For example, having medical insurance and the number and age of child-bearing women may be associated with maternity beds.[28] The method is based on several assumptions:

1. The number of patient days is some function of the level of a set of causal factors (e.g. price, demographic and social characteristics).
2. There is some stability over time among the relationships used as components of the causal factors.

3. The variables used represent a substitute or surrogate measure of demand.
4. The variables used in the analysis will also be the important ones in the future.

The Method

The simplest regression model is that of multiple linear regression:

$$Y = a + bX,$$

where

X = the independent variable(s),
Y = the variable being predicted (e.g., patient days), and a and b = constants describing y and the slope intercept of that function.

A form of regression most likely to be used for analysis is the following:

$$Y = a + b_1x_1 + b_2x_2 + \ldots b_nx_n,$$

where Y (paticnt days or visits) is predicted on the basis of a constant a plus the effects of each variable x weighted by a coefficient b. The degree to which the factors included explain the level of patient days Y is expressed by the squared coefficient of multiple correlation (i.e., the coefficient of determination), R^2. The value of R^2 can range from zero, meaning that the variables do not account for any Y, to one, which is interpreted to mean that the xs completely explain Y. Analysis is then included regarding the level of confidence with which the prediction is made.

The regression method should have fairly good validity because of the many variables used to predict Y. It should be noted, though, that it is most useful with stable populations with a short range time frame. There are several disadvantages, however:

1. The analysis appears to have a causal relationship between the dependent and independent variables. In fact, the independent variables in the equation have a correlational relationship to the dependent variable based on a past pattern of demand.

2. Because many variables are normally included in the analysis, the analysis can become quite complex and require the use of a computer.
3. To ensure the validity of the method, the data selected should have a strong direct or proxy relationship to the dependent variable.
4. The prediction of the analysis may be distorted by nonquantifiable factors such as medical technology or the referral patterns of physicians.
5. There is a danger the population being planned for might not be clearly defined, thereby misrepresenting the actual population and resulting in an inaccurate prediction of demand.
6. The method cannot be used in rapidly changing situations. This is particularly true of urban/suburban populations.

SOURCES OF DATA

Data sources are proliferating at a rapid pace. Although much of the data required to identify needs and undertake analysis of different population cohorts are available at the regional and state levels, they are often absent at the small area level. However, regardless of the availability and usages to be made of the data, unless they are readily accessible and the sources known from which they can be sought, the data serve no purpose. The relevance of the methods for determining need and demand is basically dependent on data that are both reliable and accurate. To assist those who depend on the regular use of data, the major sources for different types of data are listed in chart form. This list is by no means complete, but it provides most of the major sources of data at the national, state, and local levels.[29]

One of the important sources of data is the 1970 U.S. Census, particularly the second and fourth count summary tapes. This provides data on general population, socioeconomic status, ethnic composition, household composition and family structure, type of housing (urbanization), condition of housing, and community instability. It is highly useful for undertaking social area analysis and comparing different subareas within a health service area or a mental health catchment area. It is also used to make comparisons by selecting relevant characteristics for use as indicators. The Biometry Division of the National Institute of Mental Health has made extensive use of the census data to develop methods for identifying potential high risk populations. Exhibit 2-10 lists the most commonly used of the census characteristics.

Exhibit 2-10   Selected Statistics for (Designated Area) and Comparison Areas Based on 1970 Census Second and Fourth County Summary Tapes

General Population Data

Total population
Number of males (in households)
Number of females (in households)
Population in group quarters
Population white
Population black

Socioeconomic Status

Economic status
    Income of families and unrelated individuals: median income of families and unrelated individuals
    Families in poverty: percent of all families below poverty level

Social status
    Low occupational status, males: percent of employed males 16 and over who are operatives, service workers, and laborers, including farm laborers
    High occupational status, males: percent of employed males 16 and over who are professionals, technical and kindred workers, and managers except farm

Educational status
    School years completed: median school years completed by persons 25 and over

Ethnic Composition

Black: percent of household population black
Other nonwhite: percent of household population nonwhite and nonblack
Foreign origin: percent of population who are foreign born or native born of foreign or mixed parentage

Household Composition and Family Structure

Husband-wife households: percent of all households with husband-wife families
Age of household heads: median age of household heads

Exhibit 2-10 Continued

Youth dependency ratio: persons under 18 per 100 persons 18-64 in household population

Aged dependency ratio: persons 65 and over per 100 persons 18-64 in household population

Type of Housing (Urbanization)

Single dwelling units: percent of all year-round housing units that are single detached (excluding mobile homes and trailers)

High rise apartments: percent of all year-round housing units that are in structures of seven or more stories

Condition of Housing

Overcrowding: percent of persons in households in housing units with 1.01 or more persons per room

Standard housing: percent of occupied housing units with direct access and complete plumbing and kitchen facilities for exclusive use

Community Instability

Recent movers: percent of population who moved into present residence 1969-1970.

Source: Health Planning and Public Accountability Seminar Workbook (Germantown, Md.: Aspen Systems Corporation, 1976), pp. 219-220. Reprinted with permission.

Other sources and types of data related to health care are the following.

Sources of Data

Population at Risk
    Census profile   U.S. Bureau of the Census
    Population estimates   U.S. Bureau of Census
                             Federal-State Cooperative Program for Local Population Estimates
                             Local agencies
                             State health departments
                             Universities
                             Local planning agencies

Sources of Data (Continued)

Health Status
  Vital statistics

Mortality data	Death certificates
	U.S. Bureau of Vital Statistics
Death rates	Death certificates
Perinatal and infant mortality	Birth certificates
Natality	Birth certificates
	National Center for Health Statistics
Marriage and divorce	National Center for Health Statistics
	State Vital Statistics Office
Morbidity	National Center for Health Statistics
	Disease registries
	Local surveys
Disability	Industry records
	Mental retardation registries
	Disability claims
	Welfare programs for the blind or partially disabled
	School records
	Home health agency records
	Local surveys
	Uniform Hospital Abstracts
	State and local mental health authorities
	Employment commissions
	Visiting Nurses Association
	State administrators of vocational rehabilitation
	American Board of Physical Medicine and Rehabilitation
	National Center for Health Statistics

Inpatient Facilities and Services

Characteristics of facilities	Hospitals

	National Center for Health Statistics
	American Hospital Association
	Joint Commission on Accreditation of Hospitals
	Licensure boards
	Local transportation departments
	Professional organizations
	Chambers of Commerce
Capacity of facilities	Hospitals
	State hospital association
	Hill-Burton Agency
	American Hospital Association
	National Center for Health Statistics
	Cost review commissions
Staffing of facilities	State directory of physicians
	Department of Health, Education, and Welfare, *Area Resource File*
	American Medical Association
	Hospital annual budgets or reports
	State hospital cost review commissions
	Department of Health, Education, and Welfare
	Bureau of Health Resources Development
	Bureau of Health Manpower Education
	National Center for Health Statistics
	Institute of Medicine report on manpower
Services and utilization	Boards of health
	Hospital associations
	American Hospital Association Guide
	Area Resource File
	Hospital Statistics
	Hospital records
	Hill-Burton Agency
	Special studies

Mental health	Psychiatric hospitals Mental health agency Department of Health, Education, and Welfare National Institute of Mental Health
Status and disposition of patients	Individual hospitals that utilize the hospital abstract system or aggregated data from reports or commissions
Payment for services	Social Security Administration Social and Rehabilitation Service Blue Cross-Blue Shield, *Source Book of Health Insurance Data* State and local governments Hospitals Social service agencies Government finance agencies
Quality of care	National Center for Health Statistics, length of stay statistics Professional Activity Study, Medical Audit Program Hospitals Commission on Professional and Hospital Activities Professional Standards Review Organizations (where established) Discharge abstract systems (ambulatory and hospital) Individual facilities Hospital commissions
Ambulatory Care Patient	Providers who utilize the uniform minimum basic data set for ambulatory medical care records Health Resources Administration National Ambulatory Medical Care Survey
Provider	Providers who utilize the uniform minimum basic data set for ambulatory medical care records Health Resources Administration

	National Ambulatory Medical Care Survey
Encounter	Providers who utilize the uniform minimum basic data set for ambulatory medical care records
	Health Resources Administration
	National Ambulatory Medical Care Survey
Outpatient services	Admission records of facilities
	State and local health departments
Mental health	Statewide mental health information systems
	Mental health records
	Local health department
	Immunization program records
Manpower	American Medical Association
	Licensure boards
	American Board of Medical Specialists
	American Dental Association
	Department of Health, Education, and Welfare
	Licensed Optometrists in (state)
	Registered Pharmacists in (state)
	American Medical Association Physician Masterfile
	National League for Nursing
	American Nurses' Association
	Area Resource File
	State Register of Licensed Dental Hygienists

Finally, there are important supportive data that provide a framework of other services and the environment, which influence health care services, health status, and trends with respect to these.

Sources of Data By Type and Source—Examples

Demography

Population	
Race	
Age	
Sex	U.S. Census Bureau
Mobility status	
Distribution of subgroups in population	

Socioeconomic

Per capita income	
Median family income	U.S. Census Bureau
Occupational status	
Value of housing	
Educational level	
Number of one-parent families	
Household size	
Number engaged in agriculture, industry, service, etc.	
Overcrowding index	
Unemployment rate	State Department of Labor
Number of families receiving Aid to Dependent Children	
Number of persons receiving public assistance	Local or state department of social welfare or social service
Number of persons receiving Medicaid	
Number of persons receiving food stamps	
Number of persons receiving Medicare	Social Security Administration
Number and percént of juvenile court referrals per 1,000 under 18 years of age	Local courts

Geographic Data

Size and geographic features of areas
Location of health and other facilities
Public transportation available and routes

Major roadways
Traffic patterns to health care
Natural barriers
Special features, i.e., reservations, parks
Ratio of developed/undeveloped land area
Percent of land use, i.e., residential,
    business, agricultural

Local planning commissions, Chambers of Commerce, road maps, public transportation administrations, geography texts

Environment

Condition of housing	Local government
	Household survey
Rubble, refuse	Household survey
Heavy industry	
Water system and supply	
Sewage, garbage disposal, sanitation system	Planning Commission
Average air pollution count	

Health Status Indicators

Total number live births	Birth certificates at state or local office of vital statistics
Fertility rate	
Number of illegitimate births	
Number of abortions	
Infant death rate	
Perinatal death rate	Death certificates at state or local office of vital statistics
Neonatal death rate	
Maternal death rate	
Crude death rate	
Standard mortality ratio	
Proportional mortality ratio	
Age-specific death rates by cause and residence	
Incidence of specific diseases	
Rate of occurrence of communicable disease	School records Household survey
Functional disability categorical (involuntary restriction	Industry absentee records

of activities: disability days annually
per 1,000 population)
    Incidence or prevalence of impair-
    ment
Accident rate   Local police department

Health Facilities

Acute, short term, and psychiatric hos-
    pitals   Local health planning
    number and type   agency
    location
    number of beds by service
    construction planned
Long term care facilities
    number and type   Administrator
    location
    admissions policy
    number of beds
Emergency rooms and specialty clinics
    number and type   Local health planning
    location   agency
    admissions policy   Administrator
    services provided
Department of Health
    number served   Commissioner or director
    services provided
    locations
Department of Social Services—Health
Related Services
    number served   Commissioner or director
    services provided
    locations
Department of Mental Health
    number served   Commissioner or director
    services provided
    locations
Proprietary health-related services
    number served
    services provided
    locations   Administrator
Voluntary social agencies providing
    health and mental health services

number served	
services provided	Administrator
locations	
Mental health clinics	
number served	
services provided	Administrator
locations	
Rehabilitation agencies	
number served	
services provided	Administrator
locations	
Public school health programs	
number served	
services provided	Superintendent of Schools
locations	
Industrial health care facilities—union	
and management	
number served	
services provided	Public Relations Depart-
locations	ment

Among those most familiar with the use of health data, a growing list of acronyms has grown up as a shorthand method for talking about various health services information systems. The most familiar are identified in Exhibit 2-11.

CONSIDERATIONS REGARDING DATA SOURCES

Although some data sources have already been considered in the sections on need and demand assessment methods, Exhibit 2-12 lists a few additional ones. For each of the sources some advantages and disadvantages are cited.

Representative interviews is a method similar to the key informant one. Health planners choose people they believe to be representative and interview them to collect data.

Opinion polls and surveys are familiar to most planners and to the public. Data might be available from polls and surveys that have been conducted by others and reported elsewhere. Planners should check to see if such already collected information is useful before conducting their own poll or survey.

Vital statistics are usually available in large numbers. Here, the problem is to select the data that can be applied to the specific problem.

Exhibit 2-11 Key to Often-Used Abbreviations in Health Services Information Systems

AHA	American Hospital Association	Primary source of information on hospitals
AMA	American Medical Association	Primary source of information on physicians
FMC	Foundation for Medical Care	Organization of fee-for-service physicians to provide comprehensive health care plan & peer review
HAS	Hospital Administrative Services	Standard cost-accounting system sponsored by AHA
HCFA	Health Care Financing Administration	Primary source of information on Medicare, health financing, costs & expenditures
HIAA	Health Insurance Association of America	Primary source of information on health insurance coverage
HIP	Health Insurance Plan of Greater New York	One of early health insurance plans involving group practice
HMO	Health Maintenance Organization	Organization providing comprehensive health services to an enrolled population on a prepaid basis
HUP	Hospital Utilization Project	Hospital discharge abstract system in Western Pennsylvania
ICDA-9-CM	International Classification of Diseases, Adapted, 9th Revision	Official U.S. version of WHO's classification of disease
MAP	Medical Audit Program	PAS-related system for data collection & peer review of hospital inpatient utilization
NAMCS	National Ambulatory Medical Care Survey	New NCHS continuing survey of visits to office-based physicians
NCHS	National Center for Health Statistics	Principal government agency responsible for collecting & disseminating health information
NCHSR	National Center for Health Services Research	New name for National Center for Health Services Research & Development (government agency involved in developing health information systems
NDTI	National Disease and Therapeutic Index	Continuing survey of office-based practice supported by ethical drug industry
NHDS	National Hospital Discharge Survey	Continuing NCHS sample survey of hospital discharges
NHPIC	National Health Planning Information Center, Health Resouces Administration, PHS, DHEW	Provides an information service, library, search, abstracting, and bibliographies related to all aspects of health planning

Exhibit 2-11 Continued

NHS	National Health Survey	Major NCHS program comprising Health Interview Survey (HIS), Health and Nutritional Examination Survey (HANES), & Health Resources Survey (HRS)
NTIS	National Technical Information Service, Department of Commerce	Provides technical reports, bibliographies, and searches of governmental documents sponsored by the federal, state, and local government, including health
PAS	Professional Activity Study	Largest hospital discharge abstract system in U.S.
PSRO	Professional Standards Review Organization	New, federally authorized organization of professionals charged with reviewing quality & appropriateness of medical services to recipients of public funds.
QAP	Quality Assurance Program	Peer review method sponsored by AHA
QUEST	Quality, Utilization, Effectiveness, Statistically Tabulated	Hospital discharge abstract system in Northeast Ohio
SEARCH	Rhode Island Health Services Research, Inc.	One of the new consortiums of public & private health services agencies sponsoring a comprehensive health information system
UHDDS	Uniform Hospital Discharge Data Set	Official set of 14 uniformly defined data elements for hospital discharge abstracts

Source: Health Planning and Public Accountability Seminar Workbook (Germantown, Md.: Aspen Systems Corporation, 1976). Reprinted with permission.

An expert interview is a rapid source of data since the health planner has only to seek out the right expert and secure answers to questions. A few experts can supply the major data. In this age of sophisticated technology, the question that must be considered is whether the planner has chosen the right expert.

Position papers provide data from concerned parties who are asked to submit written statements containing their information and rationale. Those invited may include experts and the lay public and any concerned organization or individual. Obviously, the planner then has to decide whose position paper presents a valid viewpoint.

Public hearings are similar to the community forum approach noted under needs assessment methods.

Citizen committees could be task forces, ad hoc groups, or other gatherings appointed to secure data and prepare an opinion and recommendations. Health planners usually provide staff people to assist the committees. As a source of data, the citizen committee varies in direct ratio to the input of the citizens.

Research studies and investigative reports both generate data in volume. Both are usually expensive and time consuming. Again, planners should check to ensure that prior work does not exist before launching their own research or investigation.

Computer literature searches provide a tremendous source of data if they are available to the health planner. Health planners should know that these searches are available from the National Library of Medicine and other resources and can be had for free or a nominal charge since the work has already been done and copying is all that is required.

In reviewing Exhibit 2-12, note that the list is not complete and that more pluses and minuses could be added. However, the illustration indicates that health planners must consider various aspects of the sources of data.

OBSTACLES TO THE RECEIVING OF TECHNICAL INFORMATION

Much of the information utilized in health planning is of a technical nature. Obviously, not all health planners will be expert about each phase of the project. There will have to be a reliance on others for sources of technical data and for evaluating information gathered. Several difficulties related to the technical nature of the information include the following:[30]

- Technical and scientific information deals in probabilities—not certainties with a margin of error. Physicians and other scientists cannot say that something will never happen. There is always a chance that some unforseen event will occur. Although a vaccine might be 99 percent effective, the 1 percent probability can take place, even if unlikely.
- Outstanding personalities involved in the data-gathering efforts can divert attention from the issue. A world-famous surgeon develops a new surgical technique to reduce coronary artery disease. People flock from all over to seek the surgery. The mere presence of the personality involved could overshadow any efforts to garner technical data about the true value of the technique.
- Technical differences of opinion among experts have mixed effects, but mainly they are negative effects. Where experts disagree,

Exhibit 2-12 Considerations Regarding Data Sources

Source	Advantages	Disadvantages
Representative interviews	grass roots feeling variety of viewpoints	bias, prejudice locating representative source
Opinion polls	covers more people comparative data usually closed end questions	expensive expertise needed limited questions
Surveys	sample population accurate collection	cost, manpower, expertise respondents' attitudes
Vital statistics	long term data comparative data usually accurate	limited to hard data local barriers to collection and utilization currentness questionable
Expert interviews	quick	right expert?
Position papers	quick	bias?
Public hearings	grass roots participation legitimation	repetitive controlled?
Citizen committees	concerned parties participate	time-consuming
Research studies	authoritative	expensive, time-consuming
Investigative reports	data generated in volume	expense, time political?
Literature search— MEDLARS computers	volume data	not all journals in system

Source: Health Planning and Public Accountability Seminar Workbook (Germantown, Md.: Aspen Systems Corporation, 1976), p. 216. Reprinted with permission.

people seem to feel that it is best to wait and see. Data generated by opposing experts all weigh the same.
- Sensationalism related to the area under investigation produces mixed effects. An issue is inflated by sensationalism and may attract pseudo experts and a great deal of visibility. However, can the information be evaluated rationally? A number of the dieting regimens achieve this sensationalism, and there is little that can be done to wash away the élan and find the truth.
- Unproven hypotheses based on experience, myths, or other derivations might be treated as valid when, in fact, there is some doubt. Testimonials from "cured" patients fall into this grouping, and the placebo effect is discounted. Some folk remedies and cures can also

be considered here. How to displace strong emotional beliefs with scientific evidence is a serious problem.

THE VALUE OF STATISTICS

Common maxims often note that "statistics don't lie, but liars use statistics." Health planners should be aware of the pitfalls regarding the use of statistics. A former commissioner of labor statistics, upon his retirement from that post, stated,[31] "I obtained more mileage from stale and mediocre ideas, presumably backed with statistics, than I ever derived from fresh and brilliant ideas when I was younger." This excommissioner went on to cite several misuses of statistics ranging from the comical to the tragic. Yet, the following practical guidelines were listed for the use of statistics:

* There is a need for more and better statistics to illuminate the problems more adequately.
* Statistics should be interpreted with greater skill and discretion. Administrators should not be permitted to confuse them with complex, elusive realities or regard them as significant entities in their own right.
* Specious quantification of the unquantifiable can be as mischievous as ignoring it. Unlike the present generation of computers, the human brain can deal with qualitative issues in their own right.
* There is no substitute for the intuitive feel of a problem resulting from first-hand exposure to it.

Obviously, statistics are part of the required art form of health planning. Yet, health planners should realize that a malfunction *can* cause the computer to answer five when adding two and two.

REFERENCES

1. G.D. Brown, G. Candia and G. Gavin, *Methods for Hospital Service and the Bed Need Assessment* (University Park, Pa.: Pennsylvania State University, dated, about 1976), pp. 25-26.
2. J.E. Ware et al., *The Measurement of Health Concepts* (Springfield, Va.: National Technical Information Service, 1972), pp. 58-59.
3. M.K. Chen, "Health Status Indicators: From Here to Where?," paper presented at National Center for Health Statistics workshop, Orlando, Florida, April 1975.
4. M.K. Chen, "Health Status Indices and Health Services Planning," paper presented at meeting on Institutional Health Indicators at the University of Wisconsin, August 1975, p. 17.
5. Brown, *op. cit.*, p. 3.

6. Chen, "Basic Status Indices and Health Services Planning," *op. cit.*

7. G.J. Warheit, R.A. Bell and J.J. Schwab, *Planning for Change: Needs Assessment Approach* (Washington, D.C.: National Institute of Mental Health. Dated, about 1972), p. 47.

8. *Ibid.*

9. *Ibid.*, p. 59.

10. J.W. Bush, M.K. Chen and D.L. Patrick, *Social Indicators for Health Planning and Policy Analysis* (Springfield, Va.: National Technical Information Service, 1974).

11. *Ibid.*, p. 5.

12. *Ibid.*, p. 26.

13. *Ibid.*, p. 27.

14. *Ibid.*, p. 17.

15. M.K. Chen, "The G Index for Program Priority," *Health Status Indexes* by R.L. Berg (Chicago: Hospital Research and Educational Trust, 1973), pp. 28-34.

16. J.E. Miller, "An Indicator to Aid Management in Assigning Program Priorities," *Health Services Reports* 85 (August 1970): 725.

17. M. Berdit and J.W. Williamson, "Function Limitation Scale for Measuring Health Outcome," *Health Status Indexes* by R.L. Berg (Chicago: Hospital Research and Educational Trust, 1973), pp. 59-65.

18. *Ibid.*, p. 63.

19. D.B. Starkweather, L. Gelwicks and R. Newcomer, "Delphi Forecasting of Health Care Organization," *Inquiry* 12 (March 1975): 37.

20. R.C. Dufour, "Predicting Hospital Bed Needs," *Health Services Research* 9 (Spring 1974): 62.

21. *Ibid.*

22. R.M. Crane, "Methods Used in Determining Health Services and Facility Requirements," *Health Regulation, Certificate of Need and 1122* by H.H. Hyman (Germantown, Md.: Aspen Systems Corporation, 1977), pp. 118-121.

23. T.F. Lantry et al., *Methods for Determining and Projecting Needs and Demands for Acute Inpatient Care Services* (Washington, D.C.: Arthur Young & Company, 1975), pp. 60-63.

24. J.P. Zimmerman, "Serving Areas and Their Needs Must be Reassessed," *Hospitals* 49 (September 1975): 46.

25. Brown, *op. cit.*

26. Crane, *op. cit.*

27. Medical Service Consultants, Inc., *Criteria and Standards Monograph for Review of Obstetrics/Gynecology Inpatient Services* (Washington, D.C.: Health Resources Administration, dated, about 1977), Appendix I-8 to I-10.

28. *Ibid.*

29. HEW, Health Resouces Administration, Bureau of Health Planning and Resources, *Guide to Data for Health System Planners: Health Planning Information Series* (Washington, D.C.: U.S. Government Printing Office, 1976), pp. 345-350.

30. Library of Congress, Legislative Reference Service, *Technical Information for Congress* (Washington, D.C.: U.S. Government Printing Office, 1969), pp. 507-510.

31. A.M. Ross, "Ross Hits Statistics 'Mis-Use,' Says Officials Fool Themselves," *Washington Post*, June 30, 1968.

Chapter 3

Inventorying Health Resources

Once the problem has been identified and, perhaps, some initial data have been collected relative to the problem, then the resources in the community must be identified. The first step is to designate the boundaries of the health care delivery system so planners can see where to concentrate their efforts. Boundaries can be defined geographically or across other lines, such as community of interest or special demographic characteristics. But geographic boundaries usually prove to be the easiest to handle, and they allow for resources outside of the area to be utilized. However, J. R. Hammond[1] does note that the Health Systems Agencies (HSAs) and Professional Standards Review Organizations (PSROs) do not have congruent geographic boundaries, which might impede planning. M. H. Lepper[2] also comments on boundary lines and the people's health and cites difficulties with the area designation process.

Within the defined boundaries, resources are inventoried most frequently in terms of manpower, materials, and money. Manpower includes professional, ancillary, management, clerical, and voluntary categories. Materials include equipment, facilities, and supplies. And money can be thought of as private or public or, perhaps, in terms of barter.

MANPOWER

In planning for manpower needs, attention should be given to all types of sources as well as to the specific task that has to be accomplished. It is evident in the health care field that tasks and functions have been shifting about for some time; many new personnel are coming into the field to handle tasks that were previously thought to be solely within the domain of other professionals. For example, a physician's assistant can give injections, do physical exams, and take laboratory cultures under general supervision. Therefore, to do an appropriate inventory of manpower resources in the community there should be an adequate understanding of the tasks involved in the project and an initial concept of the type of personnel required. Obviously, this concept will change as more information is secured while doing the inventory of resources.

Professional manpower inventories include many various practitioners in the community. The yellow pages of the phone book is an easily available listing of physicians, dentists, opticians, marriage counselors, psychologists, and others. Of course, professional associations probably have directories of members, but not every professional is a member. (The American Medical Association claims to have about 50 percent of the physicians in America as members.) State registration authorities might also be able to supply a list of professionals that require state certification.

Ancillary personnel could include people with first aid certificates, former armed forces medical corpsmen, aides of all kinds, and individuals having any type of special skill that would be useful in attacking the identified problem. Inventorying this manpower group will require more specific identification of tasks related to the problem.

Management manpower will be needed as administrators of various aspects of the project. Most administrators will come from the sponsoring agency, but there may be a need for special talent. In areas with a United Fund, planners will be familiar with the loaned executive concept. (Industries loan one or more of their executives for a short time to assist the fund-raising activities of the United Fund.) Similarly, highly trained executives might be loaned to oversee aspects of the planning project.

Clerical manpower has been secured in the past from the ranks of retired persons, high school and university students, and workers given released time by their employers. Of course, a core of salaried employees is usually included in the project.

Services of volunteers are familiar to most hospital staff. "Candy stripers," "gray ladies," and the like perform many crucial tasks.

MATERIALS

In planning for materials, again all the needs might not be evident immediately. So the inventory might have to be done when more information is available about the proposed program. However, some initial idea will be guiding the preliminary inventory of resources.

Equipment needs should be obvious in the problem identified. Do you need x-ray capability? Is there a need for transport vehicles? Are portable lights required for night mobile clinics? In any event, equipment sources should be sought out and listed. Small equipment should also be considered, such as duplicating equipment, typewriters, and the like. Although some equipment can be purchased, it is possible that most can be donated or loaned, thereby leaving funds free to provide additional services.

Facilities would include hospitals, clinics, private offices, nursing homes, institutions, and other "bricks and mortar" edifices. Since these facilities are readily identifiable, there should be no difficulty pinpointing them. But planners should be alert to the fact that facilities can be utilized for purposes other than their obvious intention. For example, a bus can be converted into an ambulance carrying 10 to 12 persons for disaster drills.

Supplies would include the usual office supplies and all disposable materials. Although most projects plan for the usual paper and pencil supplies, supplies unique to the project must be considered. An inventory of potential sources should be compiled for future use.

MONEY

Money sources must be considered in the planning process. Private funds could include fees charged for services, insurance or other third party monies, or donations from foundations or commercial companies. Foundation directories exist to furnish planners with selected information about the many foundations and their interests.

Public sources for funding could come from tax monies through state and federal governmental agencies. Directories of the agencies and their contract and grant activities are an aid. Regional offices of the Department of Health, Education, and Welfare are often a useful starting point to find the right agency for a particular problem.

A barter system, exchanging services for money is an important source of funds. Perhaps an employee could be shifted to another agency that has an opening, so that salary could then be freed for use on the project.

In considering an inventory of resources of manpower, materials, and money, flexibility and innovation are key words. The problem should be identified specifically to ease the job of completing the inventory. Needs can be pinpointed and alternatives can be considered that best meet the situation. Maps showing the location of facilities and other vital locations aid in visualizing the available service elements that can be brought to bear on the problem.

But bear in mind that there is no such thing as a closed-end inventory. As the planning proceeds, more resources might be uncovered and added to the compilation.

INVENTORY DEVELOPMENT

Although a good deal of information might be readily available in existing directories or other listings, there will probably be a need to compile original data. Various individuals maintain their inventory information on cards, on sheets in a loose-leaf book, or even on a computer, depending on what method the person is most comfortable with and what is available. In any event, basic data should be retrievable quickly, be accurate, and be complete.

Following are examples of major sources of existing inventory directories:[3]

Alcoholism	*Alcoholism Treatment Facilities Directory: United States and Canada* Alcohol and Drug Problems Assn. of North America 1101 15th Street N.W., Washington, D.C. 20005
	National Clearinghouse for Alcohol Information P.O. Box 2345, Rockville, Maryland 20852
Blind	National Accreditation Council for Agencies Serving the Blind 79 Madison Avenue, New York, New York 10016
	Directory of Agencies Serving Blind Persons, U.S. American Foundation for the Blind 15 West 16th Street, New York, New York 10011
Blood banks	*Establishments and Products Licensed Under Section 351 of the Public Health Service Act* Director, Bureau of Biologics Food and Drug Administration 8800 Rockville Pike, Bethesda, Maryland 20014
Clinical and public health laboratories	(Listing of licensed facilities) Center for Disease Control Chamblee Facility, Atlanta, Georgia 30333
Community Mental Health Centers	*Directory: Federally Funded Community Mental Health Centers* National Clearinghouse for Mental Health Information 5600 Fishers Lane, Rockville, Maryland 20852

Dentists	*American Dental Directory* American Dental Association 211 E. Chicago Avenue, Chicago, Illinois 60611

Drug abuse	*National Directory of Drug Abuse Treatment*
	   Programs
	National Clearinghouse for Drug Abuse
	   Information
	5600 Fishers Lane, Rockville, Maryland 20852

Exceptional children	*Directory for Exceptional Children* Porter-Sargent Publishers, Inc. 11 Beacon Street, Boston, Massachusetts 02108

Halfway houses	*Directory: Halfway Houses for the Mentally Ill*
	   and Alcoholics
	National Clearinghouse for Mental Health
	   Information
	5600 Fishers Lane, Rockville, Maryland 20852

Health Maintenance
   Organizations
Neighborhood
   Health Centers
Migrant Health
   Programs
Maternal & Child
   Health Centers
	(Directory listings)
	Bureau of Community Health Services
	5600 Fishers Lane, Rockville, Maryland 20852

Homemaker–
   home health
   aides
	Directory
	National Council for Homemaker-Home Health
	   Aide Services, Inc.
	67 Irving Place, New York, New York 10003

Hospitals	*Guide to the Health Care Field* American Hospital Association 840 North Lake Shore Drive, Chicago, Illinois 60611

Nursing
   homes
	Directory of Accredited Long-Term Care Facilities
	Joint Commission on Accreditation of Hospitals
	645 North Michigan Avenue, Chicago,
	   Illinois 60611
	
	Directory of Nursing Home Facilities
	National Center for Health Statistics
	Center Bldg., 3700 East-West Highway
	Hyattsville, Maryland 20782
	
	Directory of Medicare/Medicaid Providers and
	   Suppliers of Services
	U.S. Government Printing Office,
	   Washington, D.C. 20402

Osteopaths	*Yearbook & Directory of Osteopathic Physicians* American Osteopathic Association 212 E. Ohio Street, Chicago, Illinois 60611
Physicians	*American Medical Directory* American Medical Association 535 N. Dearborn Street, Chicago, Illinois 60611

	U.S. Physician Reference Listing Fisher-Stevens, Inc. 120 Brighton Road, Clifton, New Jersey 07012
	Directory of Medical Specialists Marquis Who's Who, Inc. 200 E. Ohio Street, Chicago, Illinois 60611
Poison control centers	*Directory* National Clearinghouse for Poison Control Centers Bureau of Drugs, FDA 5401 Westbard Avenue, Bethesda, Maryland 20016
Psychiatric clinics	*Mental Health Directory* *U.S. Facilities and Programs for Children with Mental Illness: A Directory* National Clearinghouse for Mental Health Information 5600 Fishers Lane, Rockville, Maryland 20852
Rehabilitation	Commission on Accredition of Rehabilitation Facilities 4001 W. Devon Avenue, Chicago, Illinois 60646
Retarded	Accreditation Council for Facilities for the Mentally Retarded Joint Commission on Accreditation of Hospitals 875 N. Michigan Avenue, Chicago, Illinois 60611
	Directory of Inpatient Facilities for the Retarded National Center for Health Statistics Center Bldg., 3700 East-West Highway Hyattsville, Maryland 20782
	Clinical Programs for Mentally Retarded Children Bureau of Community Health Services 5600 Fishers Lane, Rockville, Maryland 20852
Suicide prevention	*Directory of Suicide-Prevention/Crisis Intervention Centers in the United States* American Association of Suicidology Baylor University 1200 Moursund Avenue, Houston, Texas 77025

Original Inventory Collection Via Forms

After securing all the available information from existing sources, the planner might still have to resort to the collection of original data using the telephone, mail questionnaires, or other sources. A step-by-step inventory development procedure is outlined below with specific attention to the data items needed, the making of a specific list, and the updating requirement.

Examples of forms that could be adapted for the collection of data about hospitals, nursing homes, ambulance services, manpower, and outpatient-nonpatient health resources are also given. In addition to the example of a form for outpatient/nonpatient data collection, a list is included of organizations and agencies for which this inventory method may be appropriate.[4]

Step-by-Step Inventory Development Procedures

1. Identify resources and determine information needed about each one.
   A. Select resources for compilation and for inventory list.
   B. Define resource to distinguish from other resources.
   C. Prepare list of data items to be collected about each resource.
   D. Define each data item.
   E. Name sources from which the data can be obtained.
2. Develop a list of specific resources and their services using the specific resources identified in Step 1.
   A. Compile a list of resources by name, address, phone.
   B. Check for inconsistency with those identified in Step 1.
   C. Verify the citations with other sources.
3. Obtain data enumerated in Step 1, D.
   A. Decide on storage mode for data; paper sheet, cards, computer, etc.
   B. Obtain the data.
   C. Check to see that data have been collected to meet needs.
   D. If data are not collected, design mechanism to obtain missing information such as phone interview, questionnaire, personal interview, or combination.
4. Update inventory.
   A. Select appropriate time interval for updating.
   B. Update inventory as new information becomes available from existing sources.

Guidelines for Hospital Data Collection Form (Exhibit 3-1)

1. The hospital's full, legal name.
2. Street number and name, city, county, zip code.
3. Telephone area code and number.
4. Accreditation status by Joint Commission on Accreditation of Hospitals (JCAH), certified for participation in Medicare by HEW.
5. Hospital identification number—special number for this inventory listing.

6. Date data collected.
7. Person spoken to, if any.
8. Number of patients accepted for inpatient service during 12-month reporting period, excluding newborns.
9. Average number of inpatients receiving care each day during 12-month period, excluding newborns.
10. Number of persons on the payroll as of the close of the reporting period, including full-time equivalents of part-time personnel but excluding trainees, private nurses, and volunteers. Two part-time persons equal one full time person.
11. Type of service by service provided to the majority of admissions.
12. Yes or no.
13. Type of organization responsible for the day-to-day operation and management.
14. Number of beds, by type, regularly available. Do not include newborn bassinets, holding beds for patients prior to transfer to other facilities, beds assigned to patients for a portion of their stay who have other beds available to them (e.g. labor room, postoperative recovery, postanesthesia and psychiatric holding beds).

Side two:
15. Check the services available.

Guidelines for Nursing Home Data Collection Form (Exhibit 3-2)

1. Identification number for planning inventory.
2. Full, legal name.
3. Street number and name, city, county, and zip code.
4. Name of contact person and phone number.
5. Identify type of facility.
6. Accredited status by JCAH as extended care facility (ECF), nursing care facility (NCF), or resident care facility (RCF). Date of accreditation.
7. Number of patients or residents admitted during the most recent 12-month reporting period. Calculate on monthly admission if annual data not available. Date of admission period.
8. Check services routinely provided.
9. Fill in the numbers.

Side two:
10. Check type of organization owning the facility.

Exhibit 3-1 Hospital Data Collection Form

[side one]

1 Name:_____

2 Address:_____

_____

3 Telephone:_____ 4 ☐ JCAH
☐ Medicare

Hospital ID:_____ **5**
Date:_____ **6**
Contact:_____ **7**
Annual no. of admissions:_____ **8**
Patient census:_____ **9**
Total personnel:_____ **10**

---

11 Type of service:

☐ general medical and surgical

☐ other, specify treatment area:

_____

12 Admissions restricted primarily to children:

☐ yes
☐ no

13 Operation:

☐ government, nonfederal

☐ nongovernment, not-for-profit

☐ investor-owned (for profit)

☐ government, federal

☐ osteopathic

14 Number of beds:

☐ medical/surgical
☐ coronary care
☐ all other IC beds
☐ obstetrical
☐ pediatrics
☐ communicable disease
☐ long-term care
☐ psychiatric
☐ tuberculosis
☐ rehabilitation (Date:_____)

[side two]

15 Facilities and services:
Date:_____

☐ Postoperative recovery room
☐ Intensive cardiac care unit
☐ Intensive-care unit
☐ Open-heart surgery
☐ Pharmacy with FT reg. pharm.
☐ Pharmacy with PT reg. pharm.
☐ X-ray therapy
☐ Cobalt therapy
☐ Radium therapy
☐ Diagnostic radioisotope
☐ Therapeutic radioisotope
☐ Histopathology laboratory
☐ Organ bank
☐ Blood bank
☐ Electroencephalography
☐ Other

☐ Inhalation therapy
☐ Premature nursery
☐ Self-care unit
☐ Extended care
☐ Inpt. renal dialysis
☐ Outpt. renal dialysis
☐ Burn care unit
☐ Physical therapy
☐ Occupational therapy
☐ Rehabilitation inpt.
☐ Rehabilitation outpt.
☐ Psychiatric inpt.
☐ Psychiatric outpt.
☐ Psychiatric partial hospitalization program
☐ Psychiatric emergency
☐ Hospital auxiliary

☐ Psychiatric foster and/or home care
☐ Psychiatric consultation and education
☐ Clinical psychologist
☐ Organized outpt. dept.
☐ Emergency dept.
☐ Social Work dept.
☐ Family planning
☐ Genetic counseling
☐ Abortion – inpt.
☐ Abortion – outpt.
☐ Home care dept.
☐ Dental
☐ Podiatrist
☐ Speech therapist
☐ Volunteer services

Comments:

Source: A Guide to the Development of Health Resource Inventories, No. 3 in Health Planning Information Series, 1976. Available from National Technical Information Service, Springfield, Virginia.

11. Fill in number of full-time and part-time personnel. Exclude trainees, private nurses, and volunteers.
12. Number of patients or residents housed in the facility currently.

Exhibit 3-2 Nursing Home Data Collection Form

```
1    2                          [side one]
     I.D.#                      Name:
3 Phone:                   Street:                City:
4 Contact:                 County:          State:      Zip:

Type:  5                          Services:  8

  ☐ skilled nursing facility (certified    ☐ supervision over medications which may be
    under either Medicare or Medicaid)        self-administered
  ☐ skilled nursing facility unit of a     ☐ medications and treatments administered
    hospital                                  in accordance with physician's orders
  ☐ nursing care unit of a retirement      ☐ rub and massage
    center                                  ☐ help with tub bath or shower
  ☐ sheltered or custodial care home       ☐ help with dressing
    (include homes for the aged)           ☐ help with correspondence or shopping
  ☐ other type of nursing home             ☐ help with walking or getting about
    specify:_____            ☐ help with eating
                                           ☐ room and board ONLY

  Accreditation Status:      Annual        Number and Certification of Beds:
         (JCAH)            7 number of     9 licensed bed capacity          ☐
                            admissions       number Medicare-certified beds ☐
                                             number Medicaid-certified beds ☐
  ECF  ☐                                         skilled nursing            ☐
  NCF  ☐                                         intermediate care          ☐
  RCF  ☐                    ☐               beds currently set up and staffed ☐
                                             for use
  Date:_____     Date:_____
10                              [side two]
  Ownership:                       I.D.#_____

  ☐ government                     Name_____
  ☐ proprietary
  ☐ nonprofit-church related       Miscellaneous Information
  ☐ other nonprofit

  Date:_____

  Personnel:  11
     FT                    PT
  ☐                     ☐
  ☐        physician    ☐
  ☐           RN        ☐
  ☐        LPN/LVN      ☐
             other

12     Current Patient Census

           ☐

     Date:_____
```

Source: A Guide to the Development of Health Resource Inventories, No. 3 in Health Planning Information Series, 1976. Available from National Technical Information Service, Springfield, Virginia.

Guidelines for Ambulance Providers Data Collection Form (Exhibit 3-3)

    A. Full, legal name; street number and name; city, county, state, and zip code; and area code and phone number.

Exhibit 3-3 Ambulance Providers Data Collection Form

A [side one]

PLEASE ANSWER ALL QUESTIONS AS OF (date)   THANK YOU FOR YOUR COOPERATION

1 Do you provide ambulance service
(emergency and/or non-emergency
transportation of patients)
in_____(area)_____?

__ NO (Please return card in
postage paid envelope)

__ YES (Please answer questions
2 through 5)

3 How many ambulance personnel do
you employ?

____ full-time employees (35 or
more hours per week)

____ part-time employees (less
than 35 hours per week)

---

2 How many ambulance vehicles do
you operate (by type of vehicle)?

____ conventional ambulance coaches

____ station wagons

____ hearses or hearse-ambulance
combinations

____ vans and trucks

____ other

4 What type of training do these
personnel have (indicate number in each category)?

____ EMT training

____ advanced first aid

____ basic first aid

____ other

[side two]

5 Please indicate the number of
ambulance runs made by your
service in the past year
(from ____ to ____).

____ emergency runs

____ non-emergency runs (e.g.,
scheduled transfers)

____ no service or false
alarms

6 What types of services do you
normally provide (check all
that apply)?

____ emergency transportation

____ emergency medical care

____ non-emergency transportation

____ rescue and extrication

____ other (specify)_____
_____
_____

Source: A Guide to the Development of Health Resource Inventories, No. 3 in Health
Planning Information Series, 1976. Available from National Technical Information
Service, Springfield, Virginia.

---

1. Yes or no.
2. Fill in the number of vehicles.
3. Fill in numbers.
4. Fill in numbers.

Side two:
5. Fill in total number of runs made in past year.
6. Check appropriate services.

Exhibit 3-4 Outpatient/Nonpatient Health Resources Data Collection
Form

```
                            [side one]
1 _____
   (Agency name)

   _____        _____
   (Agency address)                            (Telephone)
                                        2 _____
   _____        _____
   (Agency address cont'd.)                    (Hours of operation)
3 _____
   (Full-time personnel:  number and type)

4 _____
   (Part-time personnel:  number and type)

5 _____
   (Intake procedures, waiting list, etc.)
```

```
                            [side two]
6 Type of service provided:                    Charges, if any


   _____|_____
   _____|_____
   _____|_____
   _____|_____
   _____|_____
   _____|_____


7 Date information collected:_____Name of respondent_____
```

Source: A Guide to the Development of Health Resource Inventories, No. 3 in Health
Planning Information Series, 1976. Available from National Technical Information
Service, Springfield, Virginia.

*Guidelines for Outpatient/Nonpatient Health Resources Data Collection
Form (Exhibit 3-4)*

1. Full, legal name; street number and name; city, county, state,
   and zip code; and area code and phone number. If another address, etc., is used for administrative offices, list both.
2. Days of week agency provides services, and hours open on each
   day.
3. Indicate number and type of full-time staff. Minimum categories
   MD, DO, dentist, RN, LPN, physical therapist, psychologist, social worker, other.
4. Indicate part-time staff as above.

5. Is there a waiting list? Is written application required in advance of treatment?

Side two:
6. List all major services provided and charges for these services.
7. Name and date person contacted.

Outpatient and Nonpatient Health Resources Inventory Information Needs (Exhibits 3-5 and 3-7)

The following inventory deals only with nonresidential facilities, or with services provided to patients or clients at home or in outpatient and nonpatient settings. Services provided by institutions that exist primarily to serve inpatients, though they are being provided to outpatients (e.g., hospital emergency rooms and outpatient departments) are excluded. Listed below are examples of those facilities, organizations, and agencies for which this inventory method may be suitable.

Outpatient and Nonpatient Health Resources

Blood banks:	Blood bank service
	Community blood bank
	Regional blood center
	Transfusion facility
	Transfusion service
Clinical (medical and dental) laboratories:	Bacteriological laboratory
	Independent (clinical) laboratory
	Medical laboratory
	Public health laboratory
	Dental laboratory
Comprehensive health services programs:	
Community mental health center	(Comprehensive) (community) mental health center
Migrant health program	Migrant health project
	Migrant health service
Neighborhood health center	Community health center
Health maintenance organization	Comprehensive neighborhood health center
	Comprehensive neighborhood health service program
	Health care center
	Public health center
	Rural health center

Exhibit 3-5 Manpower Data Collection Form

```
NAME:_____
              last                  first               middle

ADDRESS:_____
            number              street name          room/suite

         _____
            city           county         state        zip code

Type:  ☐ M.D.   ☐ D.O.   ☐ D.D.S.   ☐ D.M.D.    Age:_____
                                                     (year of birth)

Federal employment status:  ☐ non-federal   ☐ federal:

                                             __ U.S. Public
                                                Health Service
                                             __ other

Primary specialty:_____

Professional activity:  ☐ active:            ☐ inactive
                           ☐ direct patient care
                           ☐ training
                           ☐ other
```

Source: A Guide to the Development of Health Resource Inventories, No. 3 in Health Planning Information Series, 1976. Available from National Technical Information Service, Springfield, Virginia.

Family planning clinics:	Birth control clinic
	Family planning service
	Maternal and child care clinic
	Planned parenthood clinic
	Vasectomy clinic
	Well-baby clinic
Home health agencies:	Community nursing service
	Home health aide service
	Visiting nurse association
Medical/dental practices:	Solo practice
	(General practice) medical group
	Group clinic
	Medical group clinic
	Medical group practice
	Multispecialty medical group
	Single-specialty medical group
Opticianry establishments:	Retail optical shop
	Optical department (of store)

Exhibit 3-6 Health Manpower Occupations Data Collection Form

```
                    _____
                        occupational category


_____    I.D.# _____
name of institution


number of graduates:_____    year:_____


enrollment:                       reporting period:_____

   first year  _____

   second year _____          accreditation status if not
                                   fully accredited:
   third year  _____

                                   _____
   fourth year _____

                                   _____
   fifth year  _____

   total       _____          _____
```

Source: A Guide to the Development of Health Resource Inventories, No. 3 in Health Planning Information Series, 1976. Available from National Technical Information Service, Springfield, Virginia.

Pharmacies:	Chain drugstore
	Chain pharmacy
	Community pharmacy
	Drug chain
	Independent pharmacy
	Noncommunity pharmacy
	Prescription pharmacy
	(Retail) drugstore
Poison control centers:	Poison information center
	Poison treatment center
Psychiatric outpatient clinics:	(Free-standing) outpatient psychiatric clinic
Rehabilitation outpatient facilities:	(Comprehensive) rehabilitation center
	Free-standing rehabilitation center
	Homebound program
	Rehabilitation program
	(Sheltered) workshop
	Speech and hearing center

Exhibit 3-7 Health Manpower Educational Institutions Data Collection Form

```
_____  I.D.#:_____
name of institution

_____
street address

_____
city          county          state          zip code

_____
telephone number
-----------------------------------------------------------

Program types (health manpower occupations trained):

☐ Chiropractor        ☐ Doctor of Osteopathy   ☐ Pharmacist

☐ Dental Hygienist    ☐ Nurse, Registered      ☐ Physical Therapist

☐ Dentist             ☐ Nurse, Practical       ☐ Podiatrist

☐ Doctor of Medicine  ☐ Optometrist            ☐ Veterinarian
```

Source: A Guide to the Development of Health Resource Inventories, No. 3 in Health Planning Information Series, 1976. Available from National Technical Information Service, Springfield, Virginia.

Suicide prevention centers:	Crisis intervention agency Suicide "hotline" Suicide prevention program
Specialty outpatient facilities, clinics, or programs:	Halfway houses Programs for treatment of addiction Renal dialysis clinic Prenatal care clinic Maternal and child health clinic Disability appraisal center
Programs or facilities for the aged or handicapped:	Transportation service Day care center Meals on wheels Homemaker service
General or specialized preventive programs:	Preventive health Immunization First aid Venereal disease

General or specialized health
and medical agencies:

Society for Crippled Children
March of Dimes
Agency serving blind or deaf
Leukemia foundation
Cerebral palsy association
American Cancer Society
Diabetes association
Mental health association
Kidney foundation
Multiple sclerosis society
Muscular distrophy association
Colostomy association

POTENTIAL RESOURCES

Efforts should be made to investigate the resources of manpower, materials, and money that might be available from other community agencies and organizations, whether governmental or private organizations (private organizations should include the nonprofit group as well as the profit making agencies). Governmental sources could be on a national, state, county, or local level, or some combination of governments such as a special district commission. Finally, even though a project is local, a federal agency might have a local office to provide assistance, such as an agricultural extension agent. Nonprofit and profit-making organizations might include associations of professional practitioners, hospital associations, nursing home associations, university departments, trade associations, commercial manufacturers, and consultant groups.

Organizations, however, vary tremendously in the names that are given to similar units. The list in Exhibit 3-8 suggests key words to look for in directories or other compilations of organizations listed as administrations, agencies, bureaus, departments, divisions, offices, sections, and the like. Surely other key words will be found as more resources are located. But as one uses these to search for resources, a listing of agencies will be compiled for aid in further health planning.

In using a key word list approach to discovering potential resources, health planners would do well to work up their own listing of words particularly germane to the project being considered. The examples given here should merely stimulate one's train of thought. Once a key word list is compiled, all researchers can direct their efforts toward locating a wide variety of possible resources.

Exhibit 3-8 Key Word List for Potential Resources

Adolescent health
Adult health
Air pollution
Alcohol abuse
Alcoholism
Birth and death records
Child abuse
Child care
Child health
Child neglect
Clinics
Colleges
Communicable disease
Communicable disorders
Community health
Dental health
Dental services
Drug abuse
Drug control
Drug treatment
Education
Emergency medical services
Employment security
Employment services
Environmental health
Environmental protection
Epidemiology
Examiners (health professions)
Family planning
Geriatric health
Health
Health facilities
Health statistics
Higher education
Home care
Hospitals

Human resources
Immunization
Infant health
Institutional care
Institutions
Licensing (health professionals)
Manpower
Maternal health
Maternal services
Medicaid
Medical assistance
Medical social services
Mental health
Mental hospitals
Mental hygiene
Narcotics treatment
Occupational health
Public assistance
Public health
Public instruction
Public welfare
Radiological health
Sanitary engineering
Sanitation
Schools
School health
Social services
Social welfare
Tuberculosis
Universities
Venereal disease
Vital statistics
Vocational rehabilitation
Welfare
Youth health

USUAL AND UNUSUAL RESOURCES OF MANPOWER, MATERIALS, AND MONEY: EXAMPLES FROM ACTUAL PROGRAM EXPERIENCES

A vital consideration in seeking out resources is a frame of reference that allows the planner to ask for anything, no matter how outlandish it may seem. The first law of request is, "The most that anyone can do is say no!"

A couple of examples will illustrate the point. One planner had difficulty meeting a report deadline due to the lack of an extra typewriter. He called a local firm featuring a new style electric typewriter, explained his problem to the manager, and asked for the loan of a machine. The manager agreed to loan him four typewriters, all with the same type face. It was easy for the planner to find three more typists and finish the report in plenty of time with the loaned typewriters.

In another case a mimeograph machine was loaned to a planner to print flyers advertising the location of health screening units. When copies of the flyers were sent to the manufacturer who had loaned the machine, the planner received a phone call from the manufacturer's representative indicating that he would send a better machine and extra equipment because he did not like the way the print appeared.

The following list of how various sources aided individual projects is but a starting point in seeking manpower, materials, or money. Experience can only prove to add to the list; one's own contacts and ideas should not be ignored.

Block associations, tenant organizations
　Volunteers cleaned the streets in sanitation effort.
Church clubs, men's and women's
　Provided clerical manpower for multiphasic screening project.
Civic associations, historical societies
　Donated funds for rodent eradication project.
Fraternities, sororities, social clubs
　Held dance marathons to raise funds for mentally retarded.
Grange, farmer's union, garden clubs
　Donated table settings for a conference of volunteers.
Health councils
　Supplied and ran off announcements and distributed the same to
　membership.
Hobby groups, photo club, old car collectors
　Took and prepared photos for newspapers.
Knights of Columbus, Pythian Temples
　Provided transportation for the elderly to the health center.

Labor unions
Donated the use of their health center for a diabetes screening program.
League of Women Voters
Supplied volunteers to work on research project on coronary care.
Lions, Kiwanis, Rotary
Donated funds to buy volunteers awards for a tuberculosis project.

Ministerial associations
Agreed to read messages from pulpit on venereal disease screening project.

Political clubs
Provided expert consultation on local community leaders and translation services.
Professional associations
Duplicated letters to members and mailed them on their own stationery.
PTAs, public and parochial
Provided manpower for community nutrition program.

Quasi-practitioners, faith healers, witch doctors
Participated in mental health screening activities.

Radio and television stations
Donated air time for public service announcements.
Religious charities
Allowed the use of their computer system for a research project.
Research, consultation, and management firms
Donated funds and loaned staff to assist in planning stages.

Schools, colleges, and universities
Graduate school class members each prepared promotional kit for tuberculosis project.

Talent agencies, model agencies, and public relations firms
Sent entertainers to blood testing program and gave popcorn giveaways.
Trade associations, merchants associations', Chambers of Commerce
Paid for and printed 250,000 advance self-sticking cards for x-ray publicity.

Voluntary health agencies, United Funds, Community Chests
Donated furniture, office space, and clerical help for health education project.
YMCA, YWCA, YMHA, YWHA
Supplied volunteers for training as civil defense first aiders.

RESOURCES GRID TO INVENTORY RESOURCES

A resources grid can be used as an aid in building an inventory of resources when one is reasonably familiar with agencies and organizations in the community. What the grid does is to order thinking around the generic sources and the organizational level. Then, the planner with a particular problem in mind, goes through the grid filling in the boxes to construct a compilation of resources that relate to the project. A further sophistication of this grid technique would allow for labeling of the resources by type of resource available. To aid in completing your grid, Exhibit 3-9 is an initial listing of international, national, and regional organizations.[5] Another source is the consumer health education directory prepared by the federal government.[6]

As an exercise, consider the grid in Exhibit 3-10. We will identify a problem and go through part of the inventory resource building. Suppose that our problem deals with the establishment of an outpatient diabetic education service in a local community. Let us list the source and the type of resource possible.

Commercial	Local representative of Ames Corporation—literature, drug samples, money.
Cultural	Local drama club—perform playlet for high risk populations at Golden Age Club.
Government	Local health department—provide professional speakers, literature.
Hospitals	Speciality service of local hospital or speciality hospital—provide continuing education for professionals.
Mass media	Local radio, television and newspapers—assign reporters to do stories on diabetes.
Professional	Local medical society—provide speakers for lay groups.
Recreational	Local parks department—provide facilities for field day for diabetics.
Religious	Catholic charities, Jewish Federation, Protestant charities—donate funds for printing of diabetic cookbooks.
Schools	Local colleges, community colleges—supply manpower for door-to-door survey.
Voluntary	Local branch of American Diabetic Association—literature, speakers, movies, training materials.

Exhibit 3-9 Professional Organizations

Other sources of information many times overlooked are professional organizations. Included in this section is a list of selected organizations, many of which maintain data and regularly publish pertinent information that may be useful to the health planner. These organizations may also have state, regional, or local chapters. It is important to note that other professional organizations exist in addition to those listed.

Ambulance Association of America	72 15th Avenue, S.W. Cedar Rapids, Iowa 52404
American Academy of Family Physicians	1740 West 92nd Street Kansas City, Missouri 64114
American Academy of Medical Administrators	6 Beacon Street Boston, Massachusetts 02108
American Academy of Ophthalmology and Otolaryngology	15 Second Street, S.W. Rochester, Minnesota 55901
American Academy of Orthopaedic Surgeons	430 N. Michigan Avenue Chicago, Illinois 60611
American Academy of Pediatrics	1801 Hinman Avenue Evanston, Illinois 60204
American Association for Hospital Planning	2284 Main Street Concord, Massachusetts 01742
American Association for Maternal and Child Health, Inc.	Box 965 Los Altos, California 94022
American Association of Homes for the Aging	347 National Press Building Washington, D.C. 20004
American Association of Medical Assistants	1 East Wacker Drive, Suite 1510 Chicago, Illinois 60601
American Association of Obstetricians and Gynecologists	Johns Hopkins Hospital Baltimore, Maryland 21205
American Association of Public Health Physicians	2401 Bluffview Drive Austin, Texas 78704
American Board of Internal Medicine	3930 Chestnut Street Philadelphia, Pennsylvania 19104
American Board of Medical Specialties	1603 Orrington Avenue, Suite 11160 Evanston, Illinois 60201
American Board of Obstetrics and Gynecology, Inc.	100 Meadow Road Buffalo, New York 14216

Exhibit 3-9 Continued

American Board of Ophthalmology	8870 Towanda Street Philadelphia, Pennsylvania 19118
American Board of Orthopaedic Surgery, Inc.	430 North Michigan Avenue Chicago, Illinois 60611
American Board of Pediatrics, Inc.	Museum of Science and Industry 57th St. and S. Lake Shore Dr. Chicago, Illinois 60637
American Board of Physical Medicine and Rehabilitation	Suite D-1A, Kahler East Rochester, Minnesota 55901
American Board of Preventive Medicine	615 North Wolfe Street Baltimore, Maryland 21205
American Board of Psychiatry and Neurology, Inc.	Box 1157 Rochester, Minnesota 55901
American Board of Radiology, Inc.	Kahler East Rochester, Minnesota 55901
American Board of Surgery, Inc.	1617 John F. Kennedy Blvd. Philadelphia, Pennsylvania 19103
American Board of Thoracic Surgery	14624 East Seven Mile Road Detroit, Michigan 48025
American Board of Urology, Inc.	Kansas University Medical Center 39th and Rainbow Kansas City, Kansas 66103
American Cancer Society, Inc.	219 East 42nd Street New York, New York 10017
American College of Emergency Physicians	241 East Saginaw Street East Lansing, Michigan 48823
American College of Obstetricians and Gynecologists	1 East Wacker Drive Chicago, Illinois 60601
American College of Physicians	4200 Pine Street Philadelphia, Pennsylvania 19104
American College of Preventive Medicine	801 Old Lancaster Road Bryn Mawr, Pennsylvania 19010
American College of Surgeons	55 East Erie Street Chicago, Illinois 60611
American Dental Association	211 East Chicago Avenue Chicago, Illinois 60611
American Geriatrics Society	10 Columbus Circle New York, New York 10019

Exhibit 3-9 Continued

American Hospital Association	840 North Lake Shore Drive Chicago, Illinois 60611
American Medical Association	535 North Dearborn Street Chicago, Illinois 60610
American Medical Record Association	875 North Michigan Avenue Suite 1850 Chicago, Illinois 60611
American National Red Cross	17th and D Sts., N.W. Washington, D.C. 20006
American Nurses' Association	2420 Pershing Road Kansas City, Missouri 64108
American Nurses' Foundation, Inc.	2420 Pershing Road Kansas City, Missouri 64108
American Nursing Home Association	1200 15th Street, N.W. Washington, D.C. 20005
American Public Health Association, Inc.	1015 18th Street, N.W. Washington, D.C. 20037
American Society of Internal Medicine	703 Market Street San Francisco, California 94103
American Society of Medical Technologists	5555 West Loop Street Houston, Texas 77401
American Society of Planning Officials	1313 East 60th Street Chicago, Illinois 60637
Association of American Medical Colleges	1 DuPont Circle, Suite 200 Washington, D.C. 20036
Association of American Physicians	Vanderbilt University School of Medicine Nashville, Tennessee 37115
Association of American Physicians and Surgeons, Inc.	2111 Enco Drive, Suite N-515 Oak Brook, Illinois 60521
Association of Mental Health Administrators	2901 Lafayette Lansing, Michigan 48906
Blue Cross Association	840 North Lake Shore Drive Chicago, Illinois 60611
Commission of Professional and Hospital Activities	1968 Greed Road Ann Arbor, Michigan 48105
Community Health Association	13936 Woodward Avenue Highland Park, Michigan 48203
Emergency Care Research Institute	913 Walnut Street Philadelphia, Pennsylvania 19107
Federation of State Medical Boards of the United States, Inc.	1612 Summit Avenue Suite 304 Fort Worth, Texas 76102

Exhibit 3-9 Continued

Hospital Research and Educational Trust	840 North Lake Shore Drive Chicago, Illinois 60611
Joint Commission of Accreditation of Hospitals	875 North Michigan Avenue Chicago, Illinois 60611
Mental Health Institute	1200 East Washington Street Mount Pleasant, Iowa 52641
National Academy of Sciences—National Research Council	2101 Constitution Avenue, N.W. Washington, D.C. 20418
National Ambulance and Medical Services Association	Box 359 Westfield, Massachusetts 01085
National Association of State Mental Health Program Directors	1001 Third Street, S.W. Washington, D.C. 20024
National Association for Mental Health, Inc.	1800 North Kent Street Arlington, Virginia 22209
National Association of Blue Shield Plans	211 East Chicago Avenue Chicago, Illinois 60611
National Board of Medical Examiners	3930 Chestnut Street Philadelphia, Pennsylvania 19104
National Council for Homemaker-Home Health Aid Services	67 Irving Street New York, New York 10003
National Council on Alcoholism, Inc.	2 Park Avenue New York, New York 10016
National Council on the the Aging	1828 L Street, N.W., Suite 504 Washington, D.C. 20036
National Federation of Licensed Practical Nurses	250 West 57th Street, Suite 323 New York, New York 10019
National Geriatrics Society	212 West Wisconsin Avenue Milwaukee, Wisconsin 53203
National League for Nursing	10 Columbus Circle New York, New York 10019
National Medical Association, Inc.	2109 E Street, N.W. Washington, D.C. 20037
National Safety Council	425 North Michigan Avenue Chicago, Illinois 60611
Pan American Health Organization/World Health Organization	525 23rd Street, N.W. Washington, D.C. 20037

Source: Health Resources Administration, DHEW, *Guide to Data for Health Systems Planners,* Health Planning Information Series #2, Pub. No. (HRA) 76-14502 (1976).

Exhibit 3-10 Resource Grid

Generic Source	Organizational Level				
	International	National	State	Local	Other
Commercial					
Cultural					
Government					
Hospitals					
Mass Media					
Professional					
Recreational					
Religious					
Schools					
Voluntary					

Source: Health Planning and Public Accountability Seminar Workbook (Germantown, Md.: Aspen Systems Corporation, 1976), p. 238. Reprinted with permission.

It is apparent that, as one goes through the grid, one can think of many other resources. Money might be sought from other pharmaceutical companies, from different government agencies, from religious organizations, or from voluntary health agencies. Equipment, facilities, and supplies might be forthcoming from almost any of the resources cited, if the request is specific enough. Manpower assistance could be sought from a governmental health department, hospitals, professional societies, religious agencies, schools, or voluntary health and welfare organizations.

The use of the grid can be further illustrated by observing a completed chart. While no specific disease or condition is being used, the completed grid shows the spectrum of agencies that could be utilized. Listed below are examples of actual organizations:

Generic	Organizational Level			
Source	International	National	State	Local
Commercial	IGF Corp.	Schering Corp.		
Cultural		National Theatre Company		New York City Opera Co.
Government	World Health Organization	HEW	Alabama State Health Dept.	Essex County Welfare Dept.
Hospitals		National Hospital for Asthmatics	Mass. Correctional Institution	Grady Memorial Hospital
Mass media		American Public Relations Assn.	S. Carolina Educational TV	WNYC AM/FM and TV
Professional	World Medical Assn.	American Dental Assn.	Minn. Nurses Assn.	Reno Podiatry Assn.
Recreational		Natl. Parks Assn.		Los Angeles Recreation Dept.
Religious	Vatican City	American Jewish Congress	R.I. Catholic Charities	N. Dakota Prostestant Federation
Schools		National Education Assn.	State Univ. of Ohio	Cincinnati City Univ.
Voluntary	Federation Dentaire	American Heart Assn.	Fla. Cancer Society	Houston Mental Health Assn.

System Resource Grids

When an entire health care delivery system is the object of an inventory of resources, the approach could be centered around the problem and the agencies available in the community. First, the agencies that have available resources are identified and listed, as shown in Exhibit 3-11, and the problems are listed on the opposite axis of the chart. Then the planner proceeds down the agencies and lists the resources available from each that impinge on a specific problem. On completion of this grid, the planner should have identified all components of the

Exhibit 3-11 Systems Resources Grid

Agency Resources	Diabetes	X-Rays	Multiphasic Screening	Rehab	Home Care
Health Dept.					
Welfare Dept.					
Police Dept.					
Hospitals					
Schools					
Fire Dept.					
Highway Dept.					
Legal Dept.					

Source: Health Planning and Public Accountability Seminar Workbook (Germantown, Md.: Aspen Systems Corporation, 1976), p. 237.

health care delivery system under study that affect the specific problem.

For example, the health department might supply the staff to do testing for diabetes but not treatment services, could arrange for mobile or fixed location chest x-rays, could put together a package of tests for multiphasic screening, but have no rehabilitation or home care services. The welfare department might provide funds for diabetics in need but not x-ray or multiphasic screening resources, or perhaps it could pay for rehabilitation and home care services.

Obviously, the list of agencies can grow longer as the grid is plotted. However, the major difference between this and a regular resource grid is its orientation. This grid is problem oriented rather than agency directed; agency resources are related to specific identified problems. The resultant grid produces a systems approach and a systems identification of resources having something to do with the identified problem. The advantage of this method is that the grid could then be used to plot decision trees and referral diagrams since most of the data are available from the boxes.

Resource Identification Worksheet

Using a resource identification worksheet (Exhibit 3-12) is a mechanism for individual creative brainstorming about resources. Resources

Exhibit 3-12 Resource Identification Worksheet

RESOURCE	Source
People:	
sponsors or supporters _____	Heart Assn, public health, industry
providers of service _____	hospitals, clinics, pharmacies
leaders _____	mayor, physicians
staff skills and time:	
medical _____	med colleges, hospitals
organizational _____	health plan agencies, Heart Assn, colleges
planning _____	health plan agencies
clerical _____	volunteers, students, unemployed
educational _____	Heart Assn, public health, schools
analytical _____	colleges, dept. of vital statistics
Equipment:	
tables, chairs, etc. _____	same as facilities
BP devices _____	discount from med supply, hospitals, public health
lab equipment _____	hospitals, public health
data processing equipment _____	city, county, colleges
typewriters, calculators, etc. _____	same as facilities
filing cabinets _____	same as facilities
Supplies and materials:	
paper, pens, etc. _____	same as facilities
pamphlets _____	NHBPEP, AHA, pharmaceutical firms
posters _____	NHBPEP, AHA, pharmaceutical firms
forms _____	other HBP control programs, hospitals, health dept.
a/v materials _____	NHBPEP, AHA, pharmaceutical firms
medication, lab supplies _____	county medical facilities
Information:	
HBP and its consequences _____	physicians, AHA, NHBPEP
community health care system _____	physicians, health planners, health dept.
status of HBP control in community _	physicians, health planners, health dept., Heart Assn
community resources _____	health plan, health dept., Heart Assn, industry, foundations
Facilities: (use and alteration) _____	business/industry, health dept., hospitals, Heart Assn
Money: (for any of the above) _____	patient fees, third-party payers, grants, government

Source: National Heart, Lung, and Blood Institute, *Handbook for Improving High Blood Pressure Control in the Community* (Washington, D.C.: U.S. Government Printing Office, 1977), p. 29.

are listed on one side of the worksheet as cues to trigger an immediate response from knowledgeable people about the possible source of that specific resource. Of course, the resource cues can be amended to provide both sides of the worksheet. Often, this type of worksheet is most effective because those filling out the responses usually are well acquainted with the source and are reasonably sure about its ability to contribute to a program.

Another method for expanding the resource worksheet concept is to take a completed worksheet and then have another person add to the existing listings. This "hitchhiking" serves as an impetus to the individual working on the additional rounds.

In any event, the worksheet should be used for "word association" types of responses in a creative atmosphere, rather than for detailed mulling. For such a routine approach, the expanded checklist method given next in this chapter could be utilized.

Two-Way Resource Checklist for a Specific Source and/or Resource

The two-way resource checklist shown in Exhibit 3-13 consists of two columns—one lists the possible resources, and the other the potential sources. To use the checklist, you check the source column and read back to the corresponding resource item or items a specific organization or individual might contribute. On the other hand, if you need a particular resource and you are looking for an organization or individual to provide it, check the resource column and read across to identify potential sources. Although some sources will be specifically identified in the quick two-way resource checklist, most will be generic to allow the user to expand on the method and adopt this technique to the unique conditions existing in any individual community.

Potential Resources in a Classification Scheme for Health System Services and Settings

A framework has been recommended by the federal government for use by health planning agencies as they analyze their proposed plans. This framework classifies health system services against health system settings, as shown in Exhibit 3-14. By recommending this classification framework, the federal government hopes to achieve consistency and uniformity in the terminology of all planning agencies. Specifically, consistent use of an analytic framework might provide similar directions to various planning agencies as they develop resources to meet deficiencies.

Exhibit 3-13 Two-Way Quick Checklist

Resource	Source	
People:		
Leaders Sponsors Supporters	Business/industry Celebrities Clergy Ethnic groups Government officials Hospitals Mass media	Medical scoieties Politicians Private practitioners Professional assns. PTAs Public health depts. Schools Social clubs Unions Voluntary health assns.

Health care
providers
	Clinics
	First aid squads
	Hospitals
	Medical society
		Neighborhood health
		  center
		Private practitioners
		Professional assns.
		Public health dept.
		Schools (medical,
		  nursing etc.)

Staff (may be consultants, committee members and providers of service):

Medical	Clinics
	Hospitals
	Industry
	Medical society
		Neighborhood health
		  center
		Private practitioners
		Professional assns.
		Public health dept.
		Schools (professional)
		Voluntary health assn.
		  (Heart, cancer, etc.)

Clerical	Business/industry Civic groups Hospital Private citizen	PTAs Public health dept. Schools Senior citizen groups Social clubs Unions Voluntary health assn. "Y"s

Analytical	Business/industry
	  (computers)
	Health planning agency
	Professional assn.
	  (statisticians)
	Public health dept.
	Schools (management,
	  computer)
	Voluntary health assn.	

Organizational or planning	Business/industry Chamber of commerce Civic groups Clergy Consumer groups Govt. officials Health planning agency	Neighborhood health center Politicians Private practitioners Professional assns. PTAs Public health dept.

Exhibit 3-13 Continued

Resource	Source	
	Hospital Medical society	Schools Social clubs Tenant organization Unions Voluntary health assn.
Educational	Clinics Consumer groups Hospital Insurance company Mass media Medical society	Private practitioners Professional assns. Public health dept. Schools Voluntary health assns.
Equipment:		
Office equipment (tables, chairs, etc.)	Business/industry Chamber of commerce Civic groups Clinics Consumer groups Hospital Neighborhood health centers	Professional assns. Public health dept. Schools Trade assns. Unions Voluntary health assns. "Y"s

Devices,
  equipment
	Armed forces (VAs)
	Business/industry
	  (mfgrs.)
	Clinics
	First aid squads
	Govt. officials
	Hospital
	Medical society
		Neighborhood health
		  center
		Private practitioners
		Professional assns.
		Public health dept.
		Schools
		Trade assns.
		Voluntary health assns.

Computer equipment	Business/industry Government officials Health planning agency Hospital	Public health dept. Schools Trade assns. (mfgrs.)
Supplies:		

Office supplies	Business/industry
	Civic groups
	Consumer groups
	Government
	Hospital
	Neighborhood health
	  center
		Professional assns.
		Public health dept.
		Schools
		Unions
		Voluntary health
		  assns.

Pamphlets,
posters, audio-
visual material
	Business/industry
	  (ad agency)
	Civic groups
	Clinics
	Consumer groups
	Government
	Hospital
	Mass media
		Medical society
		Professional assns.
		Public health dept.
		Unions (health plans)
		Voluntary health
		  assns.

Lab supplies, medication	Business/industry Government Hospital Private practitioners	Professional assns. Public health dept. Trade assns. Voluntary health assns.

Exhibit 3-13 Continued

Resource	Source	
Information:		
Status of, and how to get things done in the community health care system	Consumer groups Health planning agency Hospital Medical society Politicians	Professional assns. Public health dept. Schools Voluntary health assns.
Community resources	Business/industry Chamber of commerce Civic groups Clergy Clinics Consumer groups Ethnic groups Fraternal societies Government officials Health planning agency Hospital	Mass medial Medical society Politicians Professional assns. Public health dept. Schools Social clubs Tenants organization Trade assns. Unions Voluntary health assns. "Y"s
Facilities:		

Use	Business/industry
	Chamber of commerce
	Civic groups
	Clergy
	Government
	Hospital
		Neighborhood health
		  center
		Professional assns.
		Schools
		Social clubs
		Tenant organizations
		Unions
		Voluntary health
		  assns.
		"Y"s

Alteration	Business/industry (construction firms) Unions (labor)	
Cash:	Business/industry Civic groups Foundations Fraternal societies Government Private citizens	Professional assns. Third party payers Unions Voluntary health assns.

Source: National Heart, Lung, and Blood Institute, *Handbook for Improving High Blood Pressure Control in the Community* (Washington, D.C.: U.S. Government Printing Office, 1977), p. 29.

Exhibit 3-14 Simplified Taxonomic Classification of Health System Services and Settings

HEALTH SYSTEM SERVICES *	HEALTH SYSTEM SETTINGS *					
	HOME	MOBILE	AMBULATORY	SHORT-STAY INPATIENT	FREE-STANDING SUPPORT	COMMUNITY
COMMUNITY HEALTH PROMOTION AND PROTECTION						
PREVENTION AND DETECTION						
DIAGNOSIS AND TREATMENT						
HABILITATION AND REHABILITATION						
MAINTENANCE						
PERSONAL HEALTH CARE SUPPORT						
HEALTH SYSTEM ENABLING						

*Health system services and health system settings are defined and illustrated with examples in the pages following Exhibits 3-14 and 3-15.

Source: Health Resources Administration, *A Taxonomy of the Health System Appropriate for Plan Development*, No. 4 in Health Planning Methods and Technology Series (Washington, D.C.: U.S. Government Printing Office, 1977), p. 18.

Exhibit 3-15 Analytic Framework of Health System Services and Settings

HEALTH SYSTEM SERVICES		HOME MOBILE	AMBULATORY		SHORT-STAY INPATIENT		LONG-STAY INPATIENT		FREE STANDING SUPPORT	COMMUNITY
			Hospital	Other	Hospital	Other	Hospital	Other		
COMMUNITY HEALTH PROMOTION AND PROTECTION	Health Educ. Services									
	Mental Health Promotion Services									
	Environmental Quality Management									
	Food Protection									
	Occupational Health and Safety									
	Radiation Safety									
	Biomedical & Consumer Product Safety									
PREVEN-TION AND DETEC-TION	Individual Health Protection Services									
	Detection Services									
DIAGNOSIS AND TREATMENT	Obstetric Services									
	Surgical Services									
	Diagnostic Radiology Services									
	Therapeutic Radiology Services									
	Clinical Laboratory Services									
	Emergency Medical Services									
	Dental Health Services									
	Mental Health Services									
	General Med. Services									
HABILITATION AND REHABILITA-TION	Habilitation and Rehabilitation Services									
	Therapy Services									
MAINTEN-ANCE										
PERSONAL HEALTH CARE SUPPORT	Direct Patient Care Support Services									
	Administrative Services									
HEALTH SYSTEM ENABLING	Health Planning									
	Resources Development									
	Financing									
	Regulation									
	Research									

Health System Settings spans AMBULATORY, SHORT-STAY INPATIENT, and LONG-STAY INPATIENT columns.

Source: Health Resources Administration, *A Taxonomy of the Health System Appropriate for Plan Development,* No. 4 in Health Planning Methods and Technology Series (Washington, D.C.: U.S. Government Printing Office, 1977), p. 19.

Exhibit 3-15 expands on the services and settings noted earlier in the classification scheme. This diagram rapidly provides cues for the type of services and settings for which resources must be found to provide comprehensive services in a community. To clarify the terms used in the settings and services, definitions and examples are included. Ideas for the development of resources should become obvious as the definitions and examples are examined.

*Health System Services Definitions**

- *Community health promotion and protection services*—Services directed at the community level toward improving the personal health behavior of community residents and improving the quality of factors in the environment that affect their health.

    1. *Health education services*—Those services directed toward informing, educating, and motivating the public to adopt personal life styles and nutritional practices that will promote optimal health, avoid health risks, and make appropriate use of health care services in the community. Health education services include:
        a. transfer of health knowledge,
        b. transfer of health information, and
        c. motivation toward positive health behavior (including the modification of poor health habits).

    2. *Mental health promotion services*—Services to promote optimum mental well-being among individuals in the community, including consultation with schools, police, and other community entities.

    3. *Environmental quality management*—Those measures taken to protect the community from environmental hazards causing or contributing to disease, illness, injury, or death. Environmental hazards include air, water, and noise pollution, as well as hazards related specifically to unsafe residential and community environs. Prominent concerns of environmental quality management include:
        a. water supply treatment and waste water disposal,
        b. solid waste disposal,
        c. air pollution control,
        d. noise control,
        e. housing and residential hazards control,
        f. vector control,
        g. recreational area hazards control, and
        h. highway safety.

    4. *Food protection*—Those measures taken to assure wholesome and clean food free from unsafe bacteria and chemical con-

---

*The material in this and the next section comes from Health Resources Administration, *A Taxonomy of the Health System Appropriate for Plan Development,* No. 4 in Health Planning Methods and Technology Series (Washington, D.C.: U.S. Government Printing Office, 1977), pp. 27–43.

tamination; natural or added deleterious substances; and decomposition during production, processing, packaging, distribution, storage, preparation and service; and to assure that marketed foods comply with established nutritional quality and packaging identification guidelines. The major components of food protection are:

    a. sanitation,

    b. safety, and

    c. nutritional quality.

5. *Occupational health and safety*—Actions taken to assure the recognition, prevention, and control of occupational health hazards and illnesses, and those taken to promote the physical and mental well-being of employed persons. Occupational health and safety concerns are typically different for each of the following occupational categories:

    a. mining (including oil and gas drilling and similar extractive occupations);

    b. construction;

    c. agriculture;

    d. transportation and utilities; and

    e. manufacturing, service, and other.

6. *Radiation safety*—Actions taken to protect the community from unnecessary exposure to ionizing and nonionizing radiation from controllable industrial and nuclear sources and to minimize exposure of patients and medical personnel to clinical radiation. The major areas of concern in radiation safety include:

    a. industrial radiation

    b. medical radiation, and

    c. radioactive wastes.

7. *Biomedical and consumer product safety*—Those measures taken to ensure that drugs, cosmetics, therapeutic devices, and all types of consumer products including cleaning fluids, pesticides, and children's toys are safe and appropriate for their intended use and are clearly labeled as to the potential harm resulting from abuse or misuse. The major subcategories of biomedical and consumer product safety include:

    a. drugs and medical devices, and

    b. hazardous substances and products.

• *Prevention and detection services*—Services delivered to individuals in order to promote optimum physical and mental well-being, including protection from the development of disease and ill health. This category also includes identification of disease or ill health at the presymptomatic or unrecognized symptomatic stage to permit early intervention.

1. *Individual health protection services*—Individual education, routine examination and use of drugs, substances, or devices to protect an individual against disease and promote his optimum health. Illustrative service categories include:
   a. immunization,
   b. well-person maintenance,
   c. dental prophylaxis, and
   d. mental health consultation.
2. *Detection services*—Routine evaluation and screening of individuals without recognized symptoms to identify the persons at risk who have certain diseases or conditions. Illustrative service categories include:
   a. condition-specific screening,
   b. multiphasic screening, and
   c. contact/collateral follow-up.

- *Diagnosis and treatment services*—Services for evaluating the health status of individuals and identifying and alleviating disease and ill health or the symptoms thereof.

1. *Obstetric services*—The diagnosis and treatment of any abnormalities during pregnancy, and services for the promotion and maintenance of optimum mental and physical well-being of the individual woman and her child from the onset of labor until the end of the perinatal period. Illustrative service categories include:
   a. diagnosis and treatment of prenatal complications,
   b. labor and delivery care,
   c. postpartum care, and
   d. newborn care.
2. *Surgical services*—The diagnosis and treatment of physical diseases and conditions or their symptoms by means of operative techniques in conjunction with the administration of anesthesia when appropriate. Illustrative service categories include:
   a. surgery (including general surgery and surgical subspecialities),
   b. postoperative recovery care,
   c. postsurgical care, and
   d. anesthesiology.
3. *Diagnostic radiology services*—The detection of physical dis-

eases and other ill health conditions through the use of radiant energy. Illustrative techniques used include:

a. general roentgenography,
b. contrast radiology,
c. computerized transaxial tomography, and
d. nuclear medicine.

4. *Therapeutic radiology services*—The treatment of physical diseases or other ill health conditions through the use of radiant energy. Illustrative techniques used include megavoltage therapy, orthovoltage therapy, and interstitial radium therapy.

5. *Clinical laboratory services*—The testing of specimens from the human body to aid in the diagnosis and treatment of physical diseases and other ill health conditions. Illustrative types of clinical laboratory services include:

a. hematology,
b. chemistry,
c. histology, and
d. microbiology.

6. *Emergency medical services*—Diagnosis and treatment in response to the perceived need of an individual for immediate medical care to prevent loss of life or aggravation of physiological illness or injury. Illustrative components of emergency medical services include emergency communication, transportation, and medical treatment.

7. *Dental health services*—The diagnosis and treatment of diseases and other conditions of the teeth and oral cavity. Illustrative service categories include:

a. dental restoration,
b. periodontics, and
c. oral surgery.

8. *Mental health services*—The diagnosis and treatment of emotional and mental diseases and conditions or their symptoms through the administration of medication and specialized therapy. Illustrative services include:

a. general psychiatric services,
b. alcoholism treatment,
c. drug abuse treatment, and
d. psychological therapy.

9. *General medical services*—The diagnosis and treatment of non-emergent physical diseases and other ill health conditions or their symptoms by techniques distinct from those used in obstetrics, surgery, diagnostic and therapeutic radiology, and

clinical laboratory services. Illustrative components of general medical services include:
  a. clinical diagnosis, prescription, and medical care management;
  b. specialized diagnostic procedures (e.g., electrocardiography, electroencephalography, cardiac catheterization); and
  c. renal dialysis.

- *Habilitation and rehabilitation services* — Services to restore the ill or disabled individual to, or to assist the developmentally disabled individual to achieve the fullest physical, mental, social, vocational, and economic usefulness of which he is capable.
  1. *Medical habilitation and rehabilitation services* — The medical evaluation of the needs of the ill or disabled individual and the design, management, and evaluation of a habilitation or rehabilitation program to meet those needs.
  2. *Therapy services* — The therapeutic techniques used in implementing a program of habilitation or rehabilitation designed to meet the needs of an ill or disabled individual. Illustrative techniques include:
     a. physical therapy,
     b. occupational therapy,
     c. recreation therapy,
     d. prosthetic/orthotic services,
     e. communication therapy, and
     f. social therapy.
- *Maintenance services* — Services provided to individuals with chronic physical and mental ill health conditions to prevent deterioration in those conditions, as well as services provided to individuals in need of assistance in activities of daily living. The purpose of such services is to enable an individual to participate in the community to the fullest degree to which that individual is capable. Maintenance services do not include habilitative or rehabilitative services, since the primary purpose of the latter is to *increase* functional ability rather than maintain an existing level of function.
- *Personal health care support services* — Services that do not involve direct medical care but assist in the prevention, diagnosis, and treatment of diseases or ill health conditions or in the habilitation, rehabilitation, or maintenance of ill or disabled individuals.
  1. *Direct patient care support services* — Those services lending assistance to the prevention, diagnosis, and treatment of disease or other ill health conditions and to the restoration or habilitation of the ill or disabled. Illustrative examples include:

   a. pharmacy services;
   b. tissue services (i.e., storage, preservation and distribution of blood, body organs amenable to transplant, and skin);
   c. medical social work services; and
   d. medical records services.
2. *Administrative services* —Those services provided to assure adequate management of medical care resources as well as adequate management of the patient care environment. Illustrative examples include management and supervision of medical care resources and facility maintenance and housekeeping services.

- *Health system enabling services*—Organized activities designed to influence the means by which, and conditions under which, health system services are delivered.
  1. *Health planning*—A process that establishes desired future levels for health status and health system performance, designs and selects among alternative actions aimed at modifying the health system so future levels of both health status and health system performance conform to desired levels, and suggests steps for implementation of the recommended actions. The sequential components of health planning include:
     a. data assembly and analysis,
     b. goal determination,
     c. action recommendation, and
     d. implementation strategy.
  2. *Resources development*—Activities that focus especially on the recruitment and education of health care professionals or the construction and modernization of health care facilities. Areas of concern in resources development include: manpower, facilities, and equipment.
  3. *Financing*—The sources and methods of financing both resources development and health system services. Areas of concern include the appropriate use of such modes of financing as:
     a. third party reimbursement,
     b. public grants and direct public expenditures for service,
     c. philanthropic grants and payments for service, and
     d. construction loans and loan guarantees (bonding authority, commercial, etc.).
  4. *Regulation*—The intervention of government or accreditation associations in the health system by means of rules and regulations that typically influence, control, or set standards relative to the services provided within the health system, the settings

in which and the resources by which those services are provided, and the manner in which providers of service are reim-
bursed. Regulatory programs and concerns include:
  a. certificate of need,
  b. 1122 agreements,
  c. manpower licensure and certification,
  d. facility licensure and certification,
  e. rate regulation,
  f. insurance regulation, and
  g. JCAH and other association accreditation.
5. *Research*—Scientific investigation or inquiry. Research concerns within the health system can be classified as follows:
  a. biomedical,
  b. behavioral,
  c. technological, or
  d. organizational and services delivery.

Health System Setting Definitions

- *Home setting*—A person's usual or temporary place of residence
  (except where such place of residence is a health care institution),
  with the result that the patient does not travel to receive services.
- *Mobile setting*—A movable structure or specially equipped vehicle
  used to provide continuing or periodic health care services in a
  location selected to assure geographic accessibility to an identified
  target population, or a vehicle used to provide health care services
  during transportation of patients. Mobile settings include:
  a. ambulances,
  b. mobile screening units, and
  c. mobile health centers.
- *Ambulatory setting*—A location where organized health care services are provided to patients who travel to the site of care, receive
  a service or services, and leave the site the same day. An ambulatory setting typically has no provision for overnight patient stay.
  1. *Hospital*—Any hospital-based outpatient clinic, emergency de-
     partment, or ancillary department serving ambulatory pa-
     tients.
  2. *Other than hospital*—Any location that is not an organizational
     component of a hospital where personal health care services
     are provided on an outpatient basis. Illustrative settings ap-
     propriate to this category include:
     a. neighborhood health centers,
     b. public health centers,

c. primary care physician offices (including general and family practice physicians, internists, pediatricians, and obstetrician/gynecologists),
d. specialist physician offices,
e. dentists' offices,
f. dental clinics,
g. surgicenters,
h. renal dialysis centers,
i. mental health centers,
j. alcoholism and/or drug abuse treatment centers,
k. well-child clinics,
l. family planning clinics,
m. rehabilitation centers,
n. multiphasic screening clinics,
o. abortion clinics,
p. suicide prevention centers,
q. adult day care centers,
r. schools,
s. places of employment, and
t. residential institutions (including residential schools, colleges and universities, and prisons).

- *Short stay impatient setting*—A location where personal health care services are provided to patients who stay overnight, at least 50 percent of whom leave less than 30 days following admission.
  1. *Hospital*—An institution whose primary function is to provide inpatient diagnostic treatment or therapeutic services to patients. Short stay hospitals can be further classified as unrestricted or restricted in accordance with written policies that limit the hospital's use to persons with a specific health condition, demographic characteristic (e.g., age, sex), or affiliation. Illustrative categories include:
  a. general hospitals,
  b. children's hospitals,
  c. maternity hospitals,
  d. ophthalmologic hospitals,
  e. psychiatric hospitals, and
  f. veterans' administration hospitals.
  2. *Other than hospital*—Any location where personal health care services are provided on a short term inpatient basis and which is not considered an organizational component of a hospital. Illustrative settings appropriate to this category include: crisis intervention centers and convalescent centers.

- *Long stay inpatient setting*—A location where personal health care services are provided to patients who stay overnight, at least 50 percent of whom remain 30 consecutive days or longer.
  1. *Hospital*—An institution whose primary function is to provide inpatient diagnostic, treatment, therapeutic, or maintenance services to patients. Long stay hospitals may be further classified as unrestricted or restricted to people with particular characteristics. Illustrative categories include:
     a. general hospitals,
     b. psychiatric hospitals,
     c. orthopedic hospitals,
     d. physical rehabilitation hospitals,
     e. turberculosis hospitals, and
     f. chronic disease hospitals.
  2. *Other than hospital*—Any location where personal health care services are provided on a long term inpatient basis and which is not considered an organized component of a hospital. Illustrative settings appropriate to this category include:
     a. skilled nursing facilities (physician supervision and one RN at all times),
     b. intermediate care facilities (setting for nursing and related services),
     c. personal care homes (setting for assistance in activities of daily living), and
     d. sheltered care homes (protective environment).

- *Free-standing support setting*—A location where health services are provided that support the delivery of personal health care services without providing direct patient care. It is not a component of an organization that delivers personal health care services in another setting. Free-standing support settings include:
  a. medical laboratories,
  b. dental laboratories,
  c. pharmacies,
  d. tissue banks (including blood, organ and skin banks), and
  e. health information centers.

- *Community setting*—Settings in which community health promotion and health system enabling services, rather than personal health care services or patient related support services, are provided. Voluntary or public agencies or schools for health professions/occupations typically provide services in community settings.

Additional Types of Resources Classification

Although the federal government is recommending the classification scheme that uses services run against settings, others have used different techniques for developing categories. One divides the health care services into bed and nonbed related, with special and support services as additional categories. Another has categories for hospitals, nursing homes, other health facilities and health manpower. Still another scheme combines a geographic concept with the level of care and derives a classification system with neighborhood/local services (primary care), and subregional services (intermediate care and regional services' tertiary care). Exhibits 3-16 to 3-19 illustrate these and other classification methods.

The classification schemes depicted in the following exhibits provide a starting point when it comes to identifying and inventorying health care system resources. In most cases the identification and inventory process will be directly affected by the demands emanating from the specific problem situation. These classification methods will then be judged for their suitability to the situation and used as is or adapted to the specific need of the planning agency. In an ideal setting, the categorization provides a listing that acts as a trigger mechanism for the planner's thinking.

Mapping Resources With Overlays

At some time in the process of identifying and inventorying health care resources, the question of maps will arise. Maps do provide an easy visual familarity with the geography and the spatial relationships among the resources. For most projects, maps will be required and will be an important aid in planning.

To save time, effort, and money, the overlay method of preparing maps fits the bill. Starting with the basic geographic area with streets or main thoroughfares identified and other common characteristics pinpointed, the maps can be built up by the addition of clear plastic overlays. Separate plastic maps should be made for each of the resources required and located on the clear plastic with different symbols from the other resources (Exhibits 3-20 and 3-21). Each clear plastic map need only have the area outline drawn on it since the plastic will be placed over the basic map and thereby gain the streets, thoroughfares and other identifiable highlights. Thus, separate clear plastic maps could be prepared showing the locations of hospitals, health centers, mental institutions, schools, group practices, and so on. As a

Exhibit 3-16 Standard Categories of Health Care Services for Certificate of Need, New Jersey

---

A. Bed-Related

1. Medicine, surgery
2. Obstetrics, gynecology
3. Pediatric
4. Intensive care
5. Cardiac care
6. Psychiatric
7. Rehabilitation and long term care categories
8. Skilled nursing care
9. Intermediate care
10. Sheltered care

B. Nonbed-Related

1. Outpatient and clinic services
2. Emergency room services
3. Diagnostic radiology
4. Nuclear medicine
5. Laboratory services
6. Physical medicine
7. Dentistry
8. Vocational/disability services
9. Social services
10. Home health agency
11. Drug rehabilitation
12. Alcohol rehabilitation
13. Free-standing health screening centers

C. Special Services

1. Renal dialysis
2. Cardiac catheterization
3. Burn center
4. Neurosurgery
5. Open heart surgery
6. Organ transplant
7. Therapeutic radiation
8. Organ bank
9. Blood bank
10. Neonatal intensive care
11. Health maintenance organizations

D. Support Services

1. Accounting
2. Admitting
3. Central sterile supply
4. Dietary and cafeteria
5. Electronic data processing
6. General administration
7. Housekeeping
8. Laundry and linen
9. Operation of plant
10. Maintenance of plant
11. Medical records
12. Purchasing
13. Security

Source: Health Resources Administration, *A Taxonomy of the Health System for Plan Development,* No. 4 in Health Planning Methods and Technology Series (Washington, D.C.: U.S. Government Printing Office, 1977), Appendix A.

Exhibit 3-17 Health Resources Classification

A. Hospitals
   1. General medical and surgical
   2. Specialty

B. Nursing homes
   1. Nursing care homes
   2. Personal care homes with nursing
   3. Personal care homes without nursing
   4. Domiciliary care homes

C. Other health facilities
   1. Other inpatient care facilities
      a. Facilities for alcoholic and drug abusers
      b. Facilities for the blind and deaf
      c. Facilities for the crippled and physically handicapped
      d. Facilities for the mentally retarded
      e. Facilities for unwed mothers
      f. Juvenile correctional facilities
      g. Orphanages and homes for dependent children
      h. Homes for emotionally disturbed children
   2. Outpatient and nonpatient health resources
      a. Ambulance providers
      b. Blood banks
      c. Clinical medical and dental laboratories
      d. Comprehensive health services programs (i.e., HMOs)
      e. Family planning clinics
      f. Home health agencies
      g. Medical and dental practices, solo and group
      h. Opticianry establishments
      i. Pharmacies
      j. Poison control centers
      k. Psychiatric outpatient clinics
      l. Rehabilitation outpatient facilities
      m. Suicide prevention centers
      n. Hospital outpatient departments
      o. Emergency rooms
      p. Ancillary services
      q. Other hospital-based departments
      r. Other

Exhibit 3-17 Continued

D. Health manpower
   1. Physicians, M.D. and D.O.
   2. Dentists, D.D.S. and D.M.D.
   3. Other

E. Health manpower educational institutions

Source: Health Resources Administration, *Guide to the Development of Health Resources Inventories* (Washington, D.C.: U.S. Government Printing Office, 1976), pp. 7-8.

project arises, the maps can be prepared by adding whatever resources apply in the situation, and the final product would be a composite map showing the varied resources easily identifiable with the legend telling what each symbol stands for on the map (Exhibit 3-22).

For presentations before audiences, the overlays could be in color to make the resources stand out even more in an auditorium or conference hall. Of course, if you can duplicate in color, these could also be used for that purpose.

Another technique in mapping relates to the use of an altered map to reflect the population density. Exhibit 3-23 is the usual geopolitical map with resources indicated by dots. However, Exhibit 3-24 shows the same area plotted with the population as a base. Note the changes when a population-based map is used. What appeared in Exhibit 3-23 as a highly intensified resource system has resurfaced in Exhibit 3-24 as a fairly evenly distributed system, even in the most heavily populated area of the state. A. G. Dean[7] originally prepared the illustrations to illustrate the distribution of a salmonella outbreak. G. E. A. Dever[8] discussed the application of computer graphics to health administration decisions and illustrated the numerous usages of computers to print out display material visualizing the resources vividly.

Ideally, population based maps and other types are best drawn by computer. However, they can be drawn by hand on graph paper. The shape of each area can be altered, if necessary, to preserve the contiguous geographic boundaries in the geopolitical map.

Exhibit 3-18 A Community Health Care System Model, in *A Planning Framework,* Arthur Young and Company (Draft)

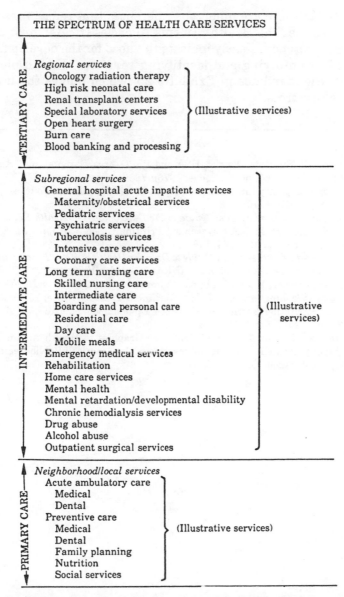

THE SPECTRUM OF HEALTH CARE SERVICES

TERTIARY CARE

Regional services
  Oncology radiation therapy
  High risk neonatal care
  Renal transplant centers
  Special laboratory services   } (Illustrative services)
  Open heart surgery
  Burn care
  Blood banking and processing

INTERMEDIATE CARE

Subregional services
  General hospital acute inpatient services
    Maternity/obstetrical services
    Pediatric services
    Psychiatric services
    Tuberculosis services
    Intensive care services
    Coronary care services
  Long term nursing care
    Skilled nursing care
    Intermediate care
    Boarding and personal care   } (Illustrative
    Residential care   services)
    Day care
    Mobile meals
  Emergency medical services
  Rehabilitation
  Home care services
  Mental health
  Mental retardation/developmental disability
  Chronic hemodialysis services
  Drug abuse
  Alcohol abuse
  Outpatient surgical services

PRIMARY CARE

Neighborhood/local services
  Acute ambulatory care
    Medical
    Dental
  Preventive care
    Medical   } (Illustrative services)
    Dental
    Family planning
    Nutrition
    Social services

Source: Health Resources Administration, *Taxonomy of the Health System Appropriate for Plan Development,* No. 4 in Health Planning and Technology Series (Washington, D.C.: U.S. Government Printing Office, 1977), p. A-5.

Resources and the National Health Planning and Resources Development Act (PL 93-641)

In PL 93-641 there are numerous references that refer to resources and activities that the Health Systems Agencies (HSAs) must undertake. These references clearly indicate the need for the development of methods of inventorying and identifying resources. Health planners can review the mandates in Exhibit 3-25, which quotes the law and defines the resources.

References

1. J. R. Hammond, "Substate District, HSA and PSPO Area Designations," *American Journal of Public Health* 66, no. 8 (August 1976): 788.
2. M. H. Lepper, "Boundary Lines and the People's Health," *American Journal of Public Health* 66, no. 8 (August 1976): 738.
3. Health Resources Administration, *Guide to the Development of Health Resources Inventories* (Washington, D.C.: U.S. Government Printing Office, 1976), pp. 61–81.
4. *Ibid.*, pp. 33, 48, 88–92, 125, 154, 158.
5. Health Resources Administration, *Guide to Data for Health Systems Planners,* Health Planning Information Series #2, Pub. No. (HRA) 76-14502 (1976).
6. Public Health Service, Health Resources Administration, *Consumer Health Education. A Directory* (Washington, D.C.: U.S. Government Printing Office, 1976).
7. A.G. Dean, "Population Based Spot Maps: An Epidemiologic Technique," *American Journal of Public Health* 66 (1976): 988.
8. G. E. A. Dever, "The Application of Computer Graphics to Health Administration Decisions," paper presented at the annual meeting of the American Public Health Association, 1977, Washington, D.C.

Exhibit 3-19 Facilities Reported in the American Hospital
Association Guide to the Health Care Field

1. Postoperative recovery room
2. Intensive cardiac care unit
3. Intensive care unit
4. Open heart surgery facilities
5. Pharmacy with full-time registered pharmacist
6. Pharmacy with part-time registered pharmacist
7. X-ray therapy
8. Cobalt therapy
9. Radium therapy
10. Diagnostic radioisotope facility
11. Therapeutic radioisotope facility
12. Histopathology laboratory
13. Organ bank
14. Blood bank
15. Electroencephalography
16. Inhalation therapy department
17. Premature nursery
18. Self-care unit
19. Extended care or long term nursing care unit
20. Inpatient renal dialysis
21. Outpatient renal dialysis
22. Burn care unit
23. Physical therapy department
24. Occupational therapy department

25. Rehabilitation inpatient unit
26. Rehabilitation outpatient unit
27. Psychiatric inpatient unit
28. Psychiatric outpatient unit
29. Psychiatric partial hospitalization program
30. Psychiatric emergency services
31. Psychiatric foster and/or home care
32. Psychiatric consultation and education services
33. Clinical psychologist services
34. Organized outpatient department
35. Emergency department
36. Social work department
37. Family planning service
38. Genetic counseling service
39. Abortion service (inpatient)
40. Abortion service (outpatient)
41. Home care department
42. Dental services
43. Podiatrist services
44. Speech therapist services
45. Hospital auxiliary
46. Volunteer services department

Source: Health Resources Administration, *A Taxonomy of the Health System Appropriate for Plan Development,* No. 4 in Health Planning and Technolgy Series (Washington, D.C.: U.S. Government Printing Office, 1977), Appendix A.

Exhibit 3-20 New York City Mental Health Areas and Facilities

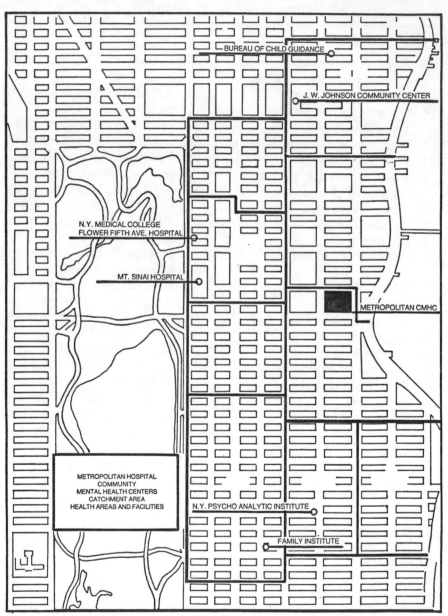

Source: National Institute of Mental Health, *Services to the Mentally Disabled of Metropolitan Community Mental Health Center Catchment Area,* Series B, No. 10 (Washington, D.C.: U.S. Government Printing Office, 1976), pp. 11-12.

Exhibit 3-21 New York City Public Transportation Routes

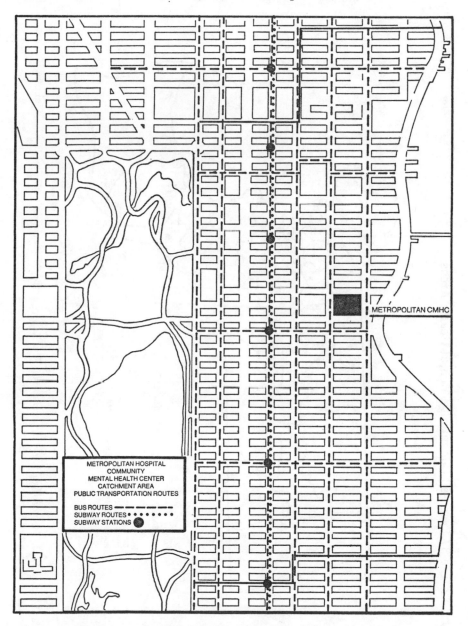

Source: National Institute of Mental Health, *Services to the Mentally Disabled of Metropolitan Community Mental Health Center Catchment Area,* Series B, No. 10 (Washington, D.C.: U.S. Government Printing Office, 1976), pp. 11-12.

Exhibit 3-22 The 37 Proposed Community Mental Health Areas

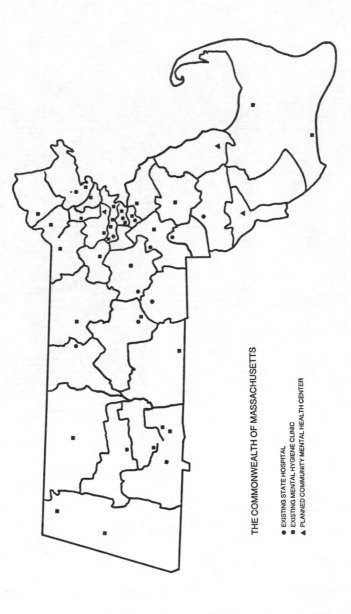

THE COMMONWEALTH OF MASSACHUSETTS

● EXISTING STATE HOSPITAL
■ EXISTING MENTAL HYGIENE CLINIC
▲ PLANNED COMMUNITY MENTAL HEALTH CENTER

Source: A. D. Spiegel, ed., *Mental Health for Massachusetts.* The Report of the Massachusetts Mental Health Planning Project (Boston: Massachusetts Department of Mental Health, 1965), p. 38.

Exhibit 3-23 Plotting on a Routine Geopolitical Map

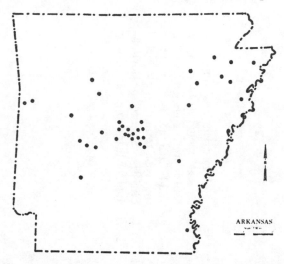

Source: Reprinted with permission from the *American Journal of Public Health,* vol. 6, 1976. Copyright 1976 by the American Public Health Association, 1015 Eighteenth Street, N.W., Washington, D.C. 20036.

Exhibit 3-24 Same Data Plotted on a Population Based Map

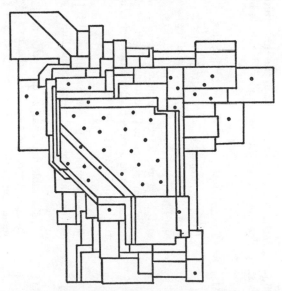

Source: Reprinted with permission from the *American Journal of Public Health,* vol. 6, 1976. Copyright 1976 by the American Public Health Association, 1015 Eighteenth Street, N.W., Washington, D.C. 20036.

Exhibit 3-25 Health Resources Inventory Legislative Review
PL 93-641 (National Health Planning and Resources Development Act of 1974)

Title XV: National Health Planning and Development

The following sections are those relevant to the undertaking of an inventory. Bracketed interpolations and underlining have been added.

Sec. 1513:   Functions of Health Systems Agencies

(a)   (4)   [For the purpose of] preventing unnecessary duplication of health resources, each health systems agency shall have as its primary responsibility . . . planning . . . and . . . promotion of the development . . . of health services, manpower and facilities which meet identified needs, reduce documented inefficiencies, and implement the health plans of the agency.

(b)   [To carry out this primary responsibility] . . . a health systems agency shall perform the following functions:

(1)   . . . assemble and analyze data concerning . . . (D) the number, type, and location of the area's <u>health resources</u>, including health services, manpower, and facilities . . . . .

In carrying out this paragraph, the agency shall to the maximum extent practicable use existing data (including data developed under Federal health programs) and coordinate its activities with the cooperative system provided for under section 306(e).

<u>Definitions</u> (Sec. 1531)

(4) the term "health resources" includes health services, health professions personnel, and health facilities, except that such term does not include Christian Science sanatoriums operated, or listed and certified, by the First Church of Christ, Scientist, Boston, Massachusetts.

(f) To assist State health planning and development agencies in carrying out their functions ..., each health systems agency shall review and make recommendations to the ... State ... agency respecting the need for new institutional health services proposed to be offered or developed in the health service area of such health systems agency.

(5) The term "institutional health services" means the health services provided through health care facilities and health maintenance organizations (as such facilities and organizations are defined in regulations prescribed under section 1122 of the Social Security Act) and includes the entities through which such services are provided.

(g) (1) ... each health systems agency shall review on a periodic basis (but at least every five years) all institutional health services offered in the health service area ... and make recommendations to the State ... agency ... respecting the appropriateness in the area of such services.

(2) A health systems agency shall complete its initial review of existing institutional health services within three years of [its] ... designation ...

(h) Each health systems agency shall annually recommend to the State health planning and development agency ... projects for the modernization, construction, and conversion of medical facilities ... [See definition of medical facilities].

Sec. 1523:   State Health Planning and Development Functions

(a) (4) [Each State Agency shall] serve as the designated planning agency of the State for the purposes of section 1122 ... and (B) administer a State certification

Exhibit 3-25 Continued

of need program which applies to new institutional health services proposed to be offered or developed . . . Such program shall provide . . . that only those services, facilities, and organizations found to be needed shall be offered or developed . . . . In performing its functions under this paragraph the State Agency shall consider recommendations made by health systems agencies . . . .

(5)   After consideration of recommendations submitted by health systems agencies . . . respecting new institutional health services proposed to be offered . . . , make findings as to the need for such services.

(6)   Review on a periodic basis (but not less often than every five years) all institutional health services being offered in the State and, after consideration of recommendations submitted by health systems agencies . . . respecting the appropriateness of such services, make public its findings.

Sec. 1532:   Reviews of Proposed Health System Changes

(c)   Criteria required . . . for health systems agency and State agency review shall include . . . :

(5)   The relationship of services reviewed to the existing health care system of the area in which such services are provided or proposed to be provided.

(6) In the case of health services proposed to be provided, the availability of resources (including health manpower, management personnel, and funds for capital and operating needs) for the provision of such services and the availability of alternative uses of such resources for the provision of other health services.

Title XVI: Health Resources Development

The following sections are those relevant to the undertaking of an inventory. Bracketed interpolations and underlining have been added.

Sec. 1603:

(a) [In order to receive assistance for modernization and construction projects under this Title] ... the State Agency ... must have submitted to the Secretary and had approved by him a State medical facilities plan ..... a State medical facilities plan for a State must--

(4) set forth ... on the basis of a statewide inventory of existing medical facilities, a survey of need, and the plans of health systems agencies within the State--

(A) the number and type of medical facility beds and medical facilities needed to provide adequate inpatient care to people residing in the State, and a plan for the distribution of such beds and facilities in health services areas throughout the State.
(B) the number and type of outpatient and other

Definitions (Sec. 1633)

(13) The term "medical facility" means a hospital, public health center, outpatient medical facility for long-term care, or other facility (as may be designated by the Secretary) for the provision of health care to ambulatory patients.

(3) The term "hospital" includes general, tuberculosis, and other types of hospitals, and related facilities, such as laboratories, outpatient departments, nurses' home facilities, extended

Exhibit 3-25 (Continued)

medical facilities needed to provide adequate public health services and outpatient care to people residing in the State, and a plan for the distribution of such facilities in health service areas throughout the State, and (C) the extent to which existing medical facilities in the State are in need of modernization or conversion to new uses . . . .

care facilities, facilities related to programs for home health services, self-care units, and central service facilities, operated in connection with hospitals, and also includes education or training facilities for health professional personnel operated as an integral part of a hospital, but does not include any hospital furnishing primarily domiciliary care.

(4) The term "public health center" means a publicly owned facility for the provision of public health services, including related publicly owned facilities such as laboratories, clinics, and administrative offices operated in connection with such a facility.

(6) The term "outpatient medical facility" means a medical facility (located in or apart from a hospital) for the diagnosis or diagnosis and treatment of ambulatory patients (including ambulatory inpatients)--

(A) which is operated in connection with a hospital,

(B) in which patient care is under the professional supervision of persons licensed to practice medicine or surgery in the State, or in the case of dental diagnosis or treatment, under the professional supervision of persons licensed to practice dentistry in the State; or

(C) which offers to patients not requiring hospitalization the services of licensed physicians in various medical specialties, and which provides to its patients a reasonably full-range of diagnostic and treatment services.

(7) The term "rehabilitation facility" means a facility which is operated for the primary purpose of assisting in the rehabilitation of disabled persons through an integrated program of--

(A) medical evaluation and services, and

(B) psychological, social, or vocational evaluation and services,

under competent professional supervision, and in the case of which the major portion of the required evaluation and services is furnished within the facility; and either the facility is operated in connection with a hospital, or all medical and related health services are prescribed by, or are under the general direction of, persons licensed to practice medicine or surgery in the State.

(8) The term "facility for long-term care" means a facility (including a skilled nursing or intermediate care facility) providing in-patient care for convalescent or chronic disease patients who required skilled nursing or intermediate care and related medical services--

(A) which is a hospital (other than a hospital

Exhibit 3-25 (Continued)

primarily for the care and treatment of mentally ill or tuberculous patients) or is operated in connection with a hospital,

or

(B) in which such care and medical services are prescribed by, or are performed under the general direction of, persons licensed to practice medicine or surgery in the State.

Source: Health Resources Administration, *Guide to the Development of Health Resources Inventories* (Washington, D.C.: U.S. Government Printing Office, 1976), pp. 161– 165.

Chapter 4

Generating and Considering Alternative Courses of Action

With knowledge about the input data and the resources available, health planners next must consider alternative courses of action to resolve their particular problem. In most instances, health planners will face limited resources and, therefore, the need to determine the most efficient utilization of the scarce resources. This dilemma necessitates creativity and innovation among those individuals involved in the planning process. In discussing this point about business management by creativity and innovation, F. D. Barrett[1] noted the following generalizations:

- Increasingly, more businesses practice a deliberate style of management that emphasizes creativity and innovation.
- Considerable research has investigated the mental processes that engender invention, creativity, and innovation; that knowledge is available and usable.
- There are a variety of methods and techniques that can be used to enable people to be successfully creative.
- Individuals can be trained to be creative and innovative, making use of new methods and techniques.
- Results as a product of creative thinking tend to be many times the value of time invested and costs.

Generating alternatives with a flair for the creative and innovative approach can aid health planners in visualizing the most efficient path to the objective. Psychological research clearly indicates that all aspects of creativity are within the normal abilities of the average human being. To upgrade and increase this creative output, the individual requires practice, confidence, and encouragement.

E. Raudsepp and G. P. Hough, Jr.[2] developed six guideposts to creative problem solving. These are listed along with suggestions expanding each guidepost:

1. Stretch your horizons.
   > Set time aside to read in other fields.
   > Collect and file clippings, notes, and ideas that seem original.
   > Attempt to work or write on a problem outside your own field.
   > Move about and exchange ideas with others.
   > Listen to comments and complaints.
   > Cultivate hobbies like puzzle solving, chess, and bridge.
2. Cultivate your field.
   > Seek out all available sources of information.
   > Read and examine the literature in your field.
   > Question every accepted assumption about your problem.
   > Don't be too quick to throw out unorthodox or unusual ideas.
   > Look for the key factors of your problem and try to isolate them.
3. Pinpoint the problem.
   > State your problem in a simple, basic, broad, general way.
   > Keep asking yourself: What are the problem's actual boundaries?
   > Break down the problem's variables through analysis.
4. Hunt for ideas.
   > List the ideas and various approaches that might solve the problem.
   > Beware the dangers of early commitment to an idea or strategy.
   > Refuse to be downed by initial failures.
   > Do not be discouraged if you experience stress when looking for a solution.
   > When you tackle your problem again, go over the approaches and ideas you had listed previously.
   > If you still do not make progress toward a solution, reexamine your problem definition(s).
5. Boost your lagging enthusiasm.
   > Suspend judicial thinking.
   > Set idea-quotas for yourself.
   > Always carry a notebook with you.
   > Proper mood is important for creative problem solving.
   > During the creative process, practice empathic involvement.
   > If you are not making any headway, even after your "second wind," drop your problem and do something different.
   > Organize your time with long periods when you can engage in hobbies or be completely alone and silent.
   > Sometimes it is inadvisable to discuss your problem solving

ideas with others—particularly before you have had a chance to develop and crystallize them to some degree.

Sometimes discussing your difficulties with people unfamiliar with your problems or line of work can give you a new slant.

Determine the physical conditions during which you regularly do your best thinking.

During problem solving, avoid distractions and intrusions as much as possible.

Develop a "retrospective awareness" of the periods when you solve your problems creatively.

Schedule your creative problem solving periods for those times when you have your most favorable mental set for producing ideas.

Be prepared and alert for the "moment of suprise."

6. Prepare for premiere.

With these principles in mind, examine the perception exercises in Exhibit 4-1 and solve the problems.

Exhibit 4-2 illustrates a process of generating alternatives. The story was one of Aesop's fables, so the concept is certainly not new. Those who specialize in creativity would have advised the mice to generate a greater quantity of alternatives and to withhold discussion until after the ideas were all noted. Perhaps, some mouse would have come forward with the way to bell the cat.

In an article discussing whether creativity could be cultivated, J. W. Clark[3] detailed some of the more commonly used devices for cultivating mental attitudes, skills, and habits of the creative person. He listed the following:

- scientific problem solving,
- deferred or postponed judgment, and
- systematic self-questioning.

Scientific problem solving is the traditional mechanism that many health care providers learned in their respective professional schools. Usually a series of steps is involved, including a definition of the problem, data collection, appraisal of the information, formulation of a hypothesis, testing the hypothesis, and evaluation of the results. Training in scientific problem solving techniques should form the foundation for individuals to apply their creativity to the generation of planning alternatives.

A vital factor in the creative process, popularly known as "brainstorming," involves deferred or postponed judgment. One of the

Exhibit 4-1 Perception Exercises*

Imagine you are the chief health coordinator for your region and each of the nine dots below represents a health care agency.

Your job is to tie them together using four straight lines (of cooperation). Your lines may cross but they must be connected (the federal guidelines so mandate). In other words, do not take your pencil off the paper when starting a new line.

You are the administrator of health care units physically located as indicated below—a row of three units and a row of four units. If you can relocate your units into two rows of four units each, the federal government will pay 90 percent of the costs of all the units.

O

O O O O

O

*Solutions at the end of this chapter.

Source: Health Planning and Public Accountability Workbook (Germantown, Md.: Aspen Systems Corporation, 1976), p. 1.

drawbacks of the scientific method is that the individual constantly evaluates as he proceeds through the process. When one delays thinking about advantages or disadvantages, no negative barrier is raised to inhibit the outpouring of alternative ideas in a spontaneous and infectious fashion. Such a tool could require some practice before scientifically oriented individuals become accustomed to the technique.

Systematic self-questioning utilizes the crutch of a prepared list of questions to ask relative to a specific problem. These checklists serve to start the creative juices flowing and enable the individual to generate ideas within a structured framework. This tool could be employed by individuals wanting some practice before moving into the free association type of creative thinking.

Vertical and lateral thinking are identified by E. deBono[4] as he comments on the virtues of zigzag thinking. Barrett[5] calls these convergent and divergent thinking, respectively.

Exhibit 4-2 The Mice in Council, by Aesop

[From *Aesop's Fables,* Revised by J. B. Rundell, 1869]
(c. 620–560 B.C.)

A certain Cat that lived in a large country-house was so vigilant and active, that the Mice, finding their numbers grievously thinned, held a council, with closed doors, to consider what they had best do. Many plans had been started and dismissed, when a young Mouse, rising and catching the eye of the president, said that he had a proposal to make, that he was sure must meet with the approval of all. "If," said he, "the Cat wore around her neck a little bell, every step she took would make it tinkle; then, ever forewarned of her approach, we should have time to reach our holes. By this simple means we should live in safety, and defy her power." The speaker resumed his seat with a complacent air, and a murmur of applause arose from the audience. An old grey Mouse, with a merry twinkle in his eye, now got up, and said that the plan of the last speaker was an admirable one; but he feared it had one drawback. He had not told them who should put the bell around the Cat's neck.

Source: Fragments of Heracleitus, *Heracleitus, On the Universe,* English translation by W. H. S. Jones (London: William Heinemann Ltd., 1931).

Vertical thinking follows three basic steps:

1. It is a stepwise process. Each step follows on from the previous step in an unbroken sequence.
2. It must be correct at every step. Perhaps this is the essence of the process.
3. It selects and deals with only what is relevant.

Vertical thinking is neat, orderly and rational.

Lateral thinking, as the name implies, moves sideways (zigzag), bringing alternative patterning to a problem. The three basic characteristics of lateral thinking run contrary to vertical thinking, as follows:

1. It is not sequential. Individuals can take a single step or jump over steps to reach a point.
2. It does not have to be correct at each stage. A frame of reference that allows for wrong steps to be taken while still seeking the right step is required.

3. It is not limited to relevant information. Deliberate use is made of random or unrelated data in an effort to generate creative alternatives.

Using vertical thinking, planners built toll booths at each end of a bridge. Traffic increased, and crowds occurred at both ends of the bridge. A lateral-thinking planner realized that most cars use the bridge to go into the city as well as leave the city. His solution was to double the toll, but to collect the money only one way.

Reversal is a technique that lateral thinkers use to generate ideas. Obese patients are constantly told to eat less and to follow a strict diet. Reversing this approach, a lateral thinker might recommend eating more, particularly sweets or food calculated to lessen the appetite before meals. This solution has been merchandized by some private companies.

But whether the thinking is called vertical, lateral, divergent, or convergent, the health planner has to strive to develop an atmosphere that supports the generation of creative alternatives, even though most public organizations and business firms were established with bureaucratic patterns that discourage innovation and reward conformity. Barrett[6] cites several features of the organizational climate that inhibit creative thinking:

- undue respect or reverence for existing policies and practices;
- frequent reference to past precedents and experiences;
- lack of strong orientation toward the future;
- excessive caution, coupled with severe criticism for errors and mistakes; and
- dislike of the different or unusual and preference for the customary, the orthodox, and the established.

Conversely, the innovative organization accepts skepticism toward existing policies and practices, follows future-oriented decision-making directions, tolerates minor errors, and has an appetite for the unusual.

This condensed introduction discussed some aspects related to the need for health planners to stimulate creative thinking and to generate ideas. Included in the possible techniques are simple idea generation, brainstorming, forced association, self-interrogation checklist, think tanks, and the Delphi technique. Obviously, these are not all-inclusive methods. It is to be hoped that health planners will generate their own mechanisms and bend those mentioned to their own devices.

SIMPLE IDEA GENERATION

If all participants can be creative, everyone should participate in the generation of ideas relative to a specific activity. An atmosphere in which all can think up ideas without criticism is vital to the success of this technique, as it is in all other methods for generating ideas. Individuals will not participate with enthusiasm if they believe that their output will be summarily rejected.

Having created a conducive atmosphere, the following steps are involved in this simple idea-generating technique:

- Explain what kinds of ideas are needed and the process for achieving them. Stress the freedom to express any idea without criticism.
- Each person is given paper and pencil and told to list as many ideas as possible. Sometimes a time limit is established, but this is flexible and can be adjusted depending on how the flow of ideas seems to be going.
- When everyone has finished their list, go around the table and ask each person to state one idea. At this point, there should still be no criticism allowed. However, other participants can add ideas suggested by any other person to their own lists.
- As the ideas are given, list each one on large sheets of paper with felt pens or other marking devices; paste up the large sheets so everyone can see. Continue asking for ideas and listing them until all are recorded.
- After the list is complete the suggestions can be considered critically. At times, it is best to allow for some mulling time before getting down to critical appraisal.

This technique can quickly generate ideas for alternative activities to be considered in the planning process. Although the steps are similar to other techniques for generating alternatives, this method still allows the individual to maintain some control over what his input will be to the listing of ideas. Perhaps, the pace of idea generation is a bit more controlled because each person is writing an individual list rather than shouting out an idea and being caught up in enthusiastic interplay among the participants. Health planners will have to judge which method is best suited for their agencies and the people who are going to think up the alternatives.

Another adjustment to this method could be to have the individuals prepare their list of alternatives prior to the meeting. However, such a method would still require that each individual be given the information in step one and the enthusiastic lift required to work by themselves.

BRAINSTORMING

Generally, the concept of brainstorming in action throws caution to the wind; any stimulus is used to generate a large quantity of unquestioned alternatives to solve problems. This method involves mentally "storming" a task from all possible facets with the combined brainpower of all participants—hence the term "brainstorming." The method usually involves the following steps or rules:

- Anything goes. Participants must be completely free to propose any suggestion. Think freely; the wilder the better. It is always easier to tone down ideas.
- Postpone judgment and/or criticism. Participants should not make any negative comments or adverse points about any ideas during the spontaneous idea generation session.
- Hitchhike on other ideas. Seek combinations and improvements. Participants do this by calling out "hitchhike" during the brainstorming session and adding their own adaptation.
- Seek quantity. Ideas should be generated as quickly as possible in great number. This stimulates all the participants, and there is a greater likelihood of creating useful alternatives.
- Record all suggestions. Every idea should be written, tape recorded, or noted in some other manner to be utilized in the process of screening, evaluating, and developing the ideas.
- Set a time limit. Use a timing device with an audible buzzer, bell, or chime that rings when the time is up.
- Analyze later. The ideas can be evaluated at your leisure, to determine what suggestions to consider.

Suppose about 100 ideas are generated at a group session of five minutes duration. If only one usable alternative emerges, the amount of staff time utilized is still within reason. (In all probability, more than one useful idea will emerge from 100 suggestions.) The time-saving aspects of the method are numerous. Since no idea is discussed relative to its merits until the total list has been produced and examined, a great deal of time is saved. During the analysis stage, discussion will only be directed toward the most promising alternatives. This division of labor in itself also stimulates greater productivity, since the participants are free to concentrate on the separate tasks one at a time. First they concentrate on the creative problem of the task, and second on the judicial aspect.

Health planners who use brainstorming might find the concept of free-wheeling, unconstrained idea generation alien to their scientific training. But individuals who can be freed from the fear of ridicule and/or the prospect of being evaluated against some standard can be more unrestrained in their creative efforts. Ridicule and evaluation foster the need for the individual to be defensive. Therefore, for brainstorming to work the health planner must ensure psychological safety and psychosocial freedom of expression as the basic conditions for stimulating creativity among the participants.

FORCED ASSOCIATION

This technique for generating alternatives tends to force individuals out of their ruts of habitual thinking: that things are bound together in the real world. Examples of usual associations are hospital and patient; doctor and nurse; ambulance and accident; dentist and drill. Since these things are associated in pairs, people conclude that it must be so in the future. Obviously, if the health planner wishes to stimulate creative approaches to thinking about alternatives, these habits must be broken down and new associations formulated.

Forced association deliberately seeks to break down the habitual associations to establish new relationships. This technique forces the participants to move from conventional and orthodox modes into new thinking. One method for using forced association to generate alternatives goes through the following steps:

1. Take the activity or thing that needs improvement. For this exercise, let us use continuing education.
2. Use free association to generate a list of ten words or phrases usually associated with continuing education training. These might be professional credit, instructors, lecture halls, films, case studies, students, paper, blackboard, notes, question and answers.
3. Choose an entirely different activity such as skiing. Use free association to generate another list of ten words, as above in step 2. Words could include: winter, cold, snow, boots, ski-tow, instructor, speed, chalet, north, parties.
4. List the words in two parallel columns as below:

Continuing Education	Skiing
professional credit	winter
instructors	cold
lecture halls	snow
films	boots
case studies	ski-tow
students	instructor
paper	speed
blackboard	chalet
notes	North
questions and answers	parties

5. Force your mind to work back and forth between the two columns and between the items in each individual column.
6. List the alternatives and ideas generated. Examples might include:
   a. Have parties for those who achieve professional credits for taking continuation courses.
   b. Questions could be sent up to the instructor on cards attached to a ski-tow that moved up to the lecturer for him to answer.
   c. Warm up the cold students with a party before the continuing education course.
   d. Schedule the education session in the north at a chalet with sessions in the morning and skiing in the afternoon.
7. Critically analyze the ideas to choose those that might be useful.
8. Repeat the forced association by:
   a. Using free word association to generate another list of things usually connected with continuing education.
   b. Choose another unrelated activity such as football, movies, or eating to generate an association list.
   c. Force relations again across these two new columns.

Identification of the problem to be considered should pose no problem for health planners since this is familiar territory. Listing the components involved in the activity should also flow easily. Choosing the other activity for the forced association might emerge from thinking about successful commercial businesses or popular attractions in the theatrical world such as hit movies, sports attractions, or travel lures. In any event, the participants have to expand their scope and allow their ideas to run wild as they go back and forth between the two listings of key words. At no time during the generation of alternatives should evaluation or negative comments be given. This will impede the flow of the ideas and put a damper on those who might otherwise propose worthwhile suggestions.

A variation on forced association is a device designed to trigger new and original ideas. This device is a large eight inch sphere with a clear window, a base, a shuffling device, and two knobs (see Exhibit 4-3). Inside the sphere there are 13,000 different words printed on small plastic chips. By turning the two knobs the words are throughly mixed to give a random selection of printed words that appear visible in the window. When you work on a particular problem, the words are mixed, and the planner writes down the visible words. Then, the health planner can utilize free and/or forced association between the problem and the random words to generate new ideas and alternatives. This Think Tank sold for $45.00 and in itself is probably a product of random association.

Random stimulus using a dictionary was illustrated by E. de Bono[7] as applied to city traffic. From a table of random numbers, 295 and 26 were chosen. The 26th word on page 295 in the dictionary turned out to be "freezer." In a timed three-minute period the following thoughts were generated:

> freezer; frozen; traffic jam; change of temperature to get things moving; different colored signal lights along streets to indicate traffic density, perhaps different permissible speeds according to the prevailing color at different times of day, perhaps different license plates for using different density areas; route indicators at junctions to indicate which routes frozen by traffic; signal system to freeze all traffic movement within a street, i.e., not just at traffic lights.

> recirculate and expand; some sort of movement reservoir which can be switched into use to even out traffic flow, or to break up jams.

> preserve; take out of time dimension?

> accumulate; cut down shopping journeys by accumulating foodstuffs in a freezer; could one accumulate work in this way by a block system, plus efficient home communications?

One of these ideas as applied to hospitals and other health care facilities results in the use of different color lines painted on floors so patients and others can follow a color to a particular destination in the institution.

Exhibit 4-3 The Think Tank

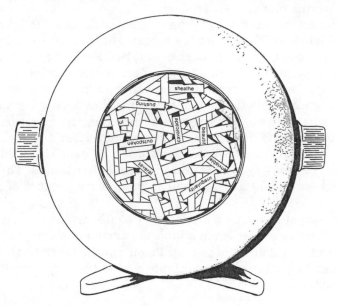

Source: As advertised by Think Tank Corporation, Scarborough, Ontario, Canada.

Forced association, random association, random stimulus, or free association all use a contrived technique to stimulate the mind to seek new alternatives and ideas. These techniques allow any individual to hold his own creative thinking session as well as the ability to hold group creativity sessions. These techniques have been impressively used in industry for problem solving, imagination, innovation, inventions, brainstorming, and seeking out new products and processes. There is no reason to doubt that health planners could make effective use of these same methods to generate planning alternatives related to specific activities.

SELF-INTERROGATION CHECKLIST

A self-interrogation checklist uses questions to prod the mind to develop new perspectives related to a problem. Four different types of questions have been identified as cited below:

Problem	*Type of Question*
Define and uncover problems	Can we do more things with this service?

	Can we identify and eliminate excess task components?
Secure extra facts	Can we use material elsewhere?
	Can we make a profit on the service?
	Can we handle the task ourselves?
Decision making	Does it reduce costs?
	Is it practical?
	Does it improve safety?
Generating ideas	(example given below)

In his famous book *Applied Imagination,* A.F. Osborn[8] presents lists of self-interrogation questions that can be adapted by the health planner who wishes to use this method. In utilizing the self-interrogation checklist, the health planner must continue to withhold judgment until after the ideas are listed. In addition, the principles of association are helpful in stimulating the mind to search for alternatives. As the questions are applied to the problem, the individual should be alert to similarities, contrasts, and a continuation or extension of the idea. Keeping these points in mind as the checklist is used allows for a systematic exploration while still maintaining the necessary spontaneity.

As an exercise, let us apply a question checklist to the problem of improving medical records.

Modify?	New twist? Changing meaning, color, motion, sound, odor, form, shape? Other changes?
	Use different colored paper in records for the parts of the problem-oriented record.
	Use audio cassettes with a background on the disease for attending health care providers.
Magnify?	What to add? More time? Greater frequency? Stronger? Higher? Longer? Thicker? Extra value? Duplicate? Multiply? Exaggerate? Plus ingredient?
	Add larger size lettering for major problems.
	Provide stronger bindings so pages do not get mixed up.
Substitute?	What else instead? Who else instead? Other place? Other ingredients? Other material? Other process? Other powers? Other approach? Other tone of voice?

Have medical record prepared by aides from phoned in
notes to central recording.

Have records prepared on microfiche.

Combine?   How about a blending, an assortment, an ensemble?
Combine units? Combine purposes? Combine ideas?
Combine appeals?

Combine medical records with quality review and
third party insurance needs.

Combine medical records with case illustrations for
teaching purposes.

Additional questions relate to adapt? minify? reverse? rearrange? in
the same fashion as illustrated above.

A checklist of questions serves as a spur to the imagination and not
as a substitute for creative thinking. As health planners experiment
with the use of systematic self-questioning, the checklists will emerge
and serve for future situations.

THINK TANKS

Think tanks, used here as opposed to the commercial variety already
discussed, are simply a number of people getting together to apply
their energy to a problem. Methods for conducting think tanks as well
as for organizing them vary greatly, but all usually feature the creative processes of the participants and cross-fertilization among the
participants. Several requirements are vital to effective think tanks:

- Selection of the participants is vital. Think tank members could be
  from the same hospital or organization, or it could be a mixed
  group representing varied viewpoints. It has been suggested that
  no less than five people and no more than eight people should be in
  a think tank. Fewer than five does not provide enough variety of
  views. More than eight impedes participation and may cause the
  group to divide into subgroups.
- A proper meeting place is needed. While a conference room is
  adequate, it is often true that an exotic meeting place lends impetus to the creativity of the participants. A sound argument can
  be supported as to the beneficial effect of a meeting in a relaxed,
  unique, strange, or different physical environment for the
  generating of divergent and unusual ideas. Think tanks have met
  in the bottom of an abandoned mine shaft, on a boat in a harbor,
  and at a swimming pool.

- A specific problem or goal must be stated as clearly as possible for the participants to try to solve.
- Members of the think tank must come together often enough to give the idea's pollinating, germinating, and flowering processes the opportunity to take root.
- Administrative tolerance is required. Think tank members might do things quite differently from other employees in terms of dress, working hours, and adherence to the rules and regulations of the organization.

Starting a think tank is the first and perhaps largest hurdle. Only people who believe in the power of the imagination and the rewards of innovation will be tempted to try to establish a think tank. Furthermore, people who establish think tanks have to know that the status quo is not the desired end. Future-oriented people who realize that constant change is the norm will be motivated to start think tanks.

Health planners may question the value of a think tank to produce alternatives or ideas relative to problems in the planning process. However, the technique has been effectively used by private contractors to government agencies to deal with health situations, and there should be no reason to doubt that the method would not be useful in the planning process. A think tank is an extension of the other creative methods mentioned for generating ideas. A major difference is the intensity of the effort. Think tank members should devote more time and energy to the problem.

Faith in the ability of the participants and the anticipated outcomes form the cornerstone for the acceptance of the think tank as a sound method.

Synectics,[9] a method of creative thinking that uses deliberate metaphors, has been used by think tank participants in their sessions. Participants could imagine that they were a pill being swallowed by a patient and trace their way through the body, as if they were a ship sailing in the bloodstream. Their problem might be related to drug absorption, retention in the body, and excretion. This method follows an open stream of consciousness as thoughts are vividly expressed somewhat like the following:

I'm moving swiftly down into the toe. I don't want to go there. What can I do? Start paddling backwards. How can I stay here? What can I adhere to? If only I had hooks. I could hook on to the artery wall. How can I get hooks?

From this could come the need to develop a pill that does not move through the body so rapidly or, as is in existence now, the slowly dissolving pill to last longer periods of time.

This technique might appear far-fetched. Faith in the creative ability of think tank members to produce is most needed in this situation, which often contains elements of humor and disbelief.

DELPHI TECHNIQUE

Although the Delphi technique has already been mentioned in another chapter, this technique can also be used to generate creative alternatives. C. R. McLaughlin and his associates[10] note that the Delphi method can be used for at least five applications in health organizations: prediction, survey of views and attitudes, simplified problem solving, airing controversial views, and strategy formulation.

To review, the Delphi technique involves the following steps:

- Selection of a group of experts in the area under consideration. Three, four, or sometimes more experts can be chosen.
- The experts react to a questionnaire anonymously using whatever method they wish to respond with their opinions.
- Each expert receives the feedback analysis of all the responses anonymously.
- This process is repeated as often as necessary until a consensus is reached with regard to the problem.

Suppose that the panel of experts were given the task of coming up with alternatives to solving the following problem:

It is extremely difficult to transfer patients from one unit to another and still insure continuity of care as well as the simple task of having the patient's records accompany him. What alternatives can you suggest to resolve this?

During the first round of responses the experts come up with the following solutions:

1. Have the health care providers come to the patient rather than the patient go to the provider.
2. Give the patient his own records to carry with him when transferred.
3. Have the patient's doctor render care at the transferred unit.

4. Assign a paramedic to provide continuity of care for the patient regardless of which unit he goes to for care.
5. Use a Telex machine to transmit records from one unit to another and have the attending doctor call for the additional information.

During the next Delphi round of responses, items 3 and 5 were eliminated because of the low priority given those two by all the experts. All experts are informed of the deletion due to low priority ranking and asked to consider responses 1, 2, and 4 for a final choice.

In this last Delphi round, the experts came to the consensus that suggestion 4 was the most appropriate at this time and 5 might be considered for future implementation.

Although this is a simplistic example, the Delphi method has been used to elicit alternatives to health planning problems and can provide an added input for comprehensive planning of health care. In some cases, this technique has even been used where the experts respond by mail. In any event, the Delphi technique does offer a reasonably quick method for generating alternatives needing the critical element of evaluation.

CONSIDERING ALTERNATIVE COURSES OF ACTION

Although considering alternative courses of action could be covered in the chapter on priorities, the reason for its inclusion here is to relate the methods to the generation of alternatives. Often, thinking about the criteria for possible activities can lead to a new approach and new alternatives.

One of the more familiar mechanisms for the consideration of alternative courses of action relates to an examination of the costs and benefits of each alternative. This is nothing new; some claim that it began in the Garden of Eden and that the problem from the onset has been to avoid an underestimation of the costs and an overestimation of the benefits. Costs usually include a dollar value for all the manpower, materials, and resources required for the activity. Benefits commonly relate to mortality, morbidity, changes in health services, and improvement in the quality of life. J. E. Veney[11] observes that health is affected by a number of factors expressed in the equation $H = f(I,E,N,M,X)$, where health H is some function f of income I, environment E, nutrition N, medical services M, and several unspecified factors X. The problem is to determine the alternative mixtures of I,E,N,M, and X that yield the greatest benefits at least cost.

Benefits sometimes are placed into direct, indirect, and intangible categories, as by H. E. Klarman.[12] Calculations are made to put dollar values on the lives saved and the amount that people will spend to avoid illness. A difficulty arises with using dollars that relates to the value of the money and the need to adjust for the future worth. Furthermore, the calculation of the value of life is frequently linked to the loss of productivity (Rice[13]), and there are disagreements about this technique. Evaluating the dollar equivalent of the unmeasureables such as discomfort, grief, rehabilitation, and emotional suffering also complicates the benefits picture. What data to use and how accurate the information is are also bones of contention. In addition, A. Wildavsky[14] raises the issue of who is making the determinations, who benefits, and for whose welfare the activities are undertaken.

Cost measurements that the health planner are likely to encounter include the following:

Average costs	These are most often the total dollars spent on the activity divided by the total end product. Cost per patient day would be the result of dividing the number of patient days into the total expenditures of the institution. Cost per active case of tuberculosis would result from dividing the number of new active cases of tuberculosis into the total case finding expenditures.
Sunk costs	These costs are usually not altered by a decision since they refer to expenditures already made for existing equipment or facilities. The cost would not be relevant to the consideration of alternative uses of the equipment or facility.
Incremental costs	These costs occur when an activity is changed. If the pediatric clinic added two more days to its schedule, the incremental costs would include salaries and supplies, but not depreciation since this is already figured in the facility costs.
Opportunity costs	When available resources are being used for one activity that prohibits their use when an opportunity arises to initiate a different activity of potential value, this is an opportunity cost. If the value of the existing activity is less

than the opportunity cost of a desired alternative, the health planner should consider drop-
ping the old and substituting the new.

Obviously, this is a simplistic approach to the benefits and costs
situation, and the method does not cover all considerations. This material is merely serving as an introduction to the examination of a cost–
benefit and a cost–effectiveness methodology that relates more closely
to the consideration of alternatives. However, a good deal of work has
considered the costs of specific diseases and conditions such as alcoholism,[15] cancer, [16] digestive diseases,[17] heart disease,[18] heart disease, cancer, and stroke,[19] heart and circulatory diseases,[20] influenza,[21] mental illness,[22] peptic ulcers,[23] and syphilis.[24] Other investigators have developed methods for attaching dollar values to illness
and the loss of life (Fein,[25] Mushkin,[26] Weisbrod,[27]). In continuing to
focus on the burden of illness in the United States, D. P. Rice and her
associates[28] updated their thinking about the costs of health care and
related that factor to decision making.

COST-BENEFIT ANALYSIS

In general terms, cost-benefit analysis has been variously defined as
providing more explicit and logically organized information on the
effects, or outcomes, of specific programs or projects,[29] or as an attempt
"to secure an efficient allocation of resources produced by the governmental system in its interaction with the private economy,"[30] or "as a
process whereby a public agency in pursuit of economic efficiency allo-
cates its resources in such a way that the most 'profitable' projects are
executed and developed to the point where marginal benefits equal
marginal costs."[31]

These definitions have in common the attempt at discovering ways
to better use limited resources, linking the use of these resources to
some goals, coordinating a wider range of information or data in a
systematic way on the goals being sought, and, finally, identifying
when a decision point for use of the resources has been reached. Motivation for the use of cost-benefit analysis is derived from the imperfec-
tion of the market place and the limited resources necessitating
choices. Concepts of efficiency become important when there are too
few resources to meet all needs. In that situation, cost-benefit analysis
serves to provide alternatives. Choices can be analyzed when the costs
and benefits of each possibility can be stated in monetary terms, pref-

erably dollar figures. Merits of widely differing objectives can be compared at that time.

Cost-benefit analysis is used for the following three major reasons:

1. Planners are forced to prepare alternative choices and background analysis in the use of scarce resources for the decision making process. Cost-benefit analysis acts as an aid to the decision making and does not replace that process.
2. Cost-benefit analysis is an excellent tool for conflict management. With many competing interests, proponents of different objectives and programs would be faced with a method that enabled decision makers to assess their demands, gain perspective, and support their decision. Although the political or value factors are not eliminated, the decision maker acquires additional technical knowledge on which to base a decision.
3. Cost-benefit analysis helps to integrate the planning–budgeting process by proposing alternatives based on technical analysis and greatly improves the analytical capacity required in systems such as the PPBS (Program Planning Budgeting System) which was in vogue in the mid- and late 1960s.

A number of limitations to the use of cost-benefit analysis should also be considered by health planners wishing to utilize this method for examining alternatives. These limitations will be noted before the method itself is explained and illustrations are given. Limitations include the following:

- Difficulty in finding agreement on objectives because of the values applied to them.
- Difficulty in dealing with important intangible values because they cannot be quantified or measured in comparable terms.
- Difficulty in identifying a common measure.
- Variances between the statistical accuracy of predicted behavior of important variables and the ability to predict what will really happen to a variable in the real world.
- Difficulty in knowing when actions taken will produce results because of constraints that occur during the implementation process. Constraints may be related to facilities, legal barriers, or administrative, political, financial, social, or religious problems. All can delay the implementation of a program.
- Cost-benefit analysis cannot be taken to mean that a "cause-effect" analysis has been undertaken. A thorough examination of all the major and minor contributions to a problem is not usually

attempted because of the time required. A best choice among those
alternatives analyzed may result, but not the best of all possible
alternatives that could have been considered.

Yet, while these limitations to cost-benefit analysis must be considered, the method remains a valuable tool for the health planner. Cost-
benefit analysis serves to enhance the health planner's already well-
developed intuition, experience, and knowledge with which decisions
are rendered.

Four steps are usually involved in the process of cost-benefit
analysis:

1. Program objectives should be specified in terms that are clear and
   not open to misinterpretation. Does the planning group want to
   improve the ambulatory care and/or the referral system for low
   income residents and/or the reduction of hospital costs?
2. Once the objectives are specified, the output for the program becomes necessary. Is the concern with how many persons a clinic
   handles per year, or how many are kept well enough to perform
   normal functions at work, home, or school? Or is the concern with
   how many low income persons receive various types of health care
   or the manner in which the health care is offered?
3. After the various objectives and the outputs of the program have
   been identified, the total costs of the program for both the first
   year and several years thereafter should be undertaken. First
   year expenditures for an ambulatory health system will be costly
   since it includes both capital expenses and maintenance costs.
   After the facilities have been constructed, renovated, and
   equipped, the operating costs may be lower. For this reason, the
   costs should be considered over the life of the project or a suitable
   time period.
4. It is necessary to analyze the alternatives to determine which
   have the greatest impact in accomplishing the various objectives
   or which achieve a given objective at the least cost. Thus, an
   analysis could be made of how best to spend a billion dollars of
   new public funds: should it all go to ambulatory care, a referral
   system or a reduction of hospital costs? Or should it be some
   combination of these? Cost-benefit analysis should help to determine on which single objective or combination of objectives to
   spend the billion dollars. On the other hand, if the objective is to
   improve health services for the ambulatory patient, then the
   question becomes one of economics or how such a program can be
   offered at the least expense. Such considerations as issuing credit

cards so each individual may seek his own health care provider, or building clinics to offer direct service in convenient locations, or purchasing hospital-based mobile health units would require evaluation.

Through feedback evaluation techniques, it becomes possible to measure the effectiveness of objectives and programs chosen. In this way, cost-benefit analysis becomes a cyclical process and modifications and adjustments can take place. Also, indirect side effects must be taken into account, whether positive or negative. For example, a side effect of building ambulatory health clinics in low income communities could result in pressure by the community leaders to assume the policy role of operating the clinic; it could also result in more jobs for local residents, and it could raise the wage levels of local businesses making them unable to compete with the higher wage structure of the tax-sponsored health facility. There may thus be benefits to local residents and harm (costs) to local businessmen.

Another aspect of cost-benefit analysis that should be considered is the effect of time on the program, referred to as discounting. Discounting is the assignment of a value or discount rate to the present value of the programs so it is possible to compare different programs by their costs and benefits at any future time period. For example, the current value of someone agreeing to pay $100 in one year is around $95 because if one were to deposit that money at a five percent interest rate tomorrow, one would have earned $5 in one year to return a total of $105. All future costs and benefits should be discounted to their present values.

Furthermore, the benefit-cost ratio should be based on the increments to the existing projects that are being considered rather than on the total project. Thus, a $10,000 increment to an existing $100,000 clinic program is based on the benefits that are attributable to the additional $10,000 and not from the total $110,000. If it is a new program, the total costs are computed and compared with the total benefits. A second way of comparing programs is to subtract costs from benefits to attain the net benefits. This method is preferable when different programs or objectives with different values that cannot all be put into a dollar figure are compared. A third method of comparing costs and benefits is the use of a ratio. A ratio would be used, for example, in determining whether a higher rate of satisfaction with services rendered and a subsequent higher rate of kept appointments were achieved by the use of indigenous outreach workers or by the physician making the appointments.

D. F. Bergwall and his associates[32] note that cost-benefit analysis is related to the scope of the comparison. They divide the comparisons into intrasystem, intersystem, intraprogram, and interprogram as follows:

- Intrasystem analysis compares alternative methods for a given system. Should the patient transport system move patients by helicopters or by conventional ambulances?
- Intersystem analysis compares alternative systems within a program. Should medical care be delivered with a curative medicine system or a preventive medicine system?
- Intraprogram analysis compares alternative combinations of systems that are aimed at the same general objective such as to maximize health during an entire life span.
- Interprogram analysis deals with competing goals. Should the health program or the welfare program be given additional funds?

As the cost-benefit comparisons move from the consideration of systems to programs, the alternatives change from very precise quantitative choices to choices of a much more qualitative nature. This may be due, in part, to the more complex details of the programs and to the difficulty in developing output measures. Patient transport can be measured in time differences and the condition of the patient. However, the relative values of a high school education and the eradication of venereal disease can not be compared that easily.

Cost-benefit analysis of the treatment and prevention of myocardial infarction through different alternatives was undertaken by Cretin.[33] Coronary care units, mobile coronary care units, and screening and intervention units were compared as related to an existing ten-year-old population. In projecting the alternatives into the future, cost-benefit analysis indicated that none of the alternatives was clearly preferable to the others.

In August 1965, President Lyndon Johnson directed that a PPBS be installed throughout the Executive Branch, to be supervised by the Bureau of the Budget. Cost-benefit analysis was an integral part of the PPBS. Built into the PPBS are procedures designed to improve rationality in decision making. These procedures can be summarized as follows:

- establishing goals and objectives after observations,
- designing alternative means to arrive at established objectives,
- predicting the consequences of each alternative, and

- selecting preferable alternatives in terms of the most valued ends and the least costs.

Utilizing PPBS, the Department of Health, Education, and Welfare examined eight alternative methods for reducing motor vehicle injuries:[34]

1. Seat belt use—to encourage people to use seat belts.
2. Restraint devices—to educate people to obtain and use additional safety restraining devices.
3. Pedestrian injury—to educate "accident-prone" pedestrians how to cross the street.
4. Motorcycle injury—to encourage motorcyclists to use helmets and eye shields to avoid fatal injury.
5. Reduce driver drinking—to educate people not to drink before driving.
6. Driver licensing—establishing a medical screening program for licensing.
7. Emergency medical services—providing grants to communities to aid in upgrading the quality of training and facilities available to accident victims from the general public, ambulance attendants, and in the hospital emergency rooms.
8. Driver skill improvement—establishing a nationwide driver training program.

Exhibit 4-4 shows the comparisons for eight alternatives with the benefit-cost ratio and cost per death averted as major indicators of the most appropriate alternative. Cost per death averted was determined by multiplying the cost of each alternative by the five years and dividing by the deaths averted. Benefit-cost ratio is achieved by estimating the expenditures that would have been required in medical care.

Obviously, the seat belt use alternative has the best pay-off, followed closely by restraint devices. However, a limitation arises because little is known about the true effectiveness of a program trying to motivate people to use seat belts or restraints. In fact, the current trend is to move toward passive belts and restraints requiring only that the driver purchase the automobile with the equipment. These alternatives could be supported on the basis of the low cost and the high potential benefits. On the bottom of the alternatives, emergency medical services and driver skills have the poorest pay-off in costs and benefits. The cost per death averted is astronomical when compared with seat belts. Yet, health planners may rationally support emergency medical services

Exhibit 4-4 Motor Vehicle Injury Control Alternatives 1968–1972

Program	PHS Cost[3] ($ millions)	Savings[2] ($ millions)	Benefit Cost Ratio[4]	Deaths Averted	Cost per Death Averted
Seat belt use	$ 2.0	$2728	1351.4	22,930	$ 87
Restraint devices	.6	681	1117.1	5,811	100
Pedestrian injury	1.1	153	144.3	1,650	600
Motorcyclist helmets	7.4	413	55.6	2,398	3,000
Reduce driver drinking	28.5	613	21.5	5,340	5,300
Improve driver license	6.1	23	3.8	442	13,800
Emergency medical services	721.5[1]	1726	2.4	16,000	45,000
Driver skills	750.5	1287	1.7	8,515	88,000

[1]Includes $300 million state matching funds.
[2]Discounted.
[3]Public Health Service.
[4]Numbers have been rounded to a single decimal point from three decimal points; therefore ratio may not be exact result of dividing column 1 into column 2 as they appear here.

Source: Selected Disease Control Programs, US DHEW, Office of Program Coordination, September 1966, p. 14, Table 1.

because the services would reach more than just victims of auto accidents.

As a method of generating and considering alternatives, cost-benefit analysis can be utilized by health planners as long as the system's limitations are kept in mind.

COST-EFFECTIVENESS ANALYSIS

Although some planners do not distinguish between cost–benefit analysis and cost effectiveness, there does appear to be a difference that is particulary relevant when considering alternatives. In most cases, cost effectiveness is used to choose the best alternative to reach a fixed level of output, such as to reduce the incidence of lung cancer by ten percent. Either the input or output is held constant in cost effectiveness. N. Doherty and B. Hicks[35] define cost effectiveness analysis as a technique for assessing and comparing the costs and effectiveness of alternative systems or programs; it is designed to assist decision makers in identifying a preferred choice or choices. Its contribution to the decision process is that it provides information and an analytical framework by which conclusions can be reached in a systematic and traceable way. M. C. Weinstein and W. B. Statson[36] add the specifics when they note that cost effectiveness is the ratio of the net increase of health care costs to the net effectiveness in terms of enhanced life expectancy and the quality of life. Net health care costs include all direct medical and health care costs plus costs associated with adverse side effects of treatment minus costs saved due to the prevention of disease plus costs of treating disease that would not have occurred if patient had not lived. Net health care effectiveness is the savings in life years plus life years from prevention minus life years lost from side effects. In general, cost effectiveness is used to select the alternative approach to the achievement of a benefit that has already been determined to be worthwhile. Planners review both monetary and non-monetary information in arriving at the optimum alternative based on cost and effectiveness.

Limitations related to cost effectiveness include the fact that the method simply shows which of the alternatives is better, not which is the best. In addition, this method limits quantitative comparisons to programs within the same health care system.

Cost effectiveness of cardiopulmonary resuscitation training programs were studied by G. A. Gorry and D. W. Scott.[37] Alternatives considered involved the critical distance covered by trainees, the retraining interval, the type of person trained, and the distribution of emergencies as related to the distribution of the population. The researchers attempted to discover the most effective answer in terms of cost to each of the alternatives.

Doherty and Hicks[38] studied the cost effectiveness of alternative health care programs for the elderly. Nursing homes, day care centers, and home care programs were compared on costs and effectiveness. Day care centers were preferred on the effectiveness criteria of physical, mental, and social functioning. Home care programs were preferred on overall cost criteria (Exhibit 4-5).

Analysis of the cost effectiveness of pharyngitis management and acute rheumatic fever prevention was undertaken by Tompkins and his associates.[39] This analysis was conducted for epidemic and endemic streptococcal pharyngitis. Three penicillin alternatives were compared:

Strategy A—throat culture and treat only patient with group A strep.
Strategy B—treat all patients.
Strategy C—no culture and no treatment for any of the patients.

Cost figures used in the analysis are shown in Exhibit 4-6. Note that

Exhibit 4-5 Tabular Display for Cost-Effectiveness Analysis of Day Care, Home Care, and Institutional Care

Program	No. patients in 1st assessment	Effectiveness criterion*						Per diem cost ($)			
		IADL		ADL		MSQ					
		No.	Ratio	No.	Ratio	No.	Ratio	Total	Primary	Secondary	Tertiary
Day care....	45	37	0.82	40	0.88	38	0.84	27.38	18.60	3.20	5.58
Home care ..	78	55	0.70	61	0.78	54	0.69	22.43	14.26	2.05	6.12
Institutional care	60	45	0.75	42	0.70	31	0.52	26.69	25.12	1.57	0

*Number and proportion of patients in first assessment whose function on each scale was maintained or improved in second assessment.
IADL—Instrumental Activities of Daily Living (social functioning).
ADL—Activities of Daily Living (physical functioning).
MSQ—Mental Status Quotient (mental functioning).

Source: Reprinted with permission from *Health Services Research,* Vol. 12, No. 2, Summer 1977, p. 198. Copyright 1977 by the Hospital Research and Educational Trust, 840 N. Lake Shore Drive, Chicago, Illinois 60611.

the costs are divided up into unit costs, medical care strategy costs, and adverse medical outcome costs.

Decision trees for each strategy are illustrated in Exhibits 4-7 and 4-8. Each decision tree shows the cost of the various alternative actions.

In the epidemic situation, it is medically most effective and least costly to follow strategy B—treat all patients. In the endemic situation, strategy B is also most cost effective when oral penicillin is used in the patient population where the positive throat culture is at least 20 percent. Strategy A is optimal when the positive throat culture yield is between 5 and 20 percent. Below a 5 percent positive yield, strategy C is appropriate.

ALTERNATIVES INFLUENCED BY IDENTIFIABILITY, ATTRIBUTABILITY, AND ACCOUNTABILITY

In considering alternatives, decision makers are probably influenced by whether the people affected are identified, whether the decision will be attributed to the decision maker, and whether the decision makers

Exhibit 4-6 Cost Figures Used in Analyses

Unit costs
Throat culture	$ 2.00
Oral or benzathine penicillin	3.00
Patient time per office visit	4.50
Diagnostic office visit	10.00
Therapy-only office visit	4.00
Daily cost hospitalization	94.00

Medical care strategy costs
Strategy A (culture, treat positives)
No treatment (culture-negative patients)	$ 16.50
Intramuscular benzathine penicillin	28.00
Oral penicillin	19.50

Strategy B (treat all patients, oral or intramuscular penicillin)	17.50
Strategy C (no culture or treatment)	14.50

Adverse medical outcome costs
Premature death	$72,000.00
Acute rheumatic fever	10,560.00
Serious allergic reaction	826.00
Mild allergic reaction	15.00

Source: Reprinted with permission from R.K. Tompkins, D.C. Barnes, and W.E. Cable, "An Analysis of the Cost-Effectiveness of Pharyngitis Management and Acute Rheumatic Fever Prevention," *Annals of Internal Medicine* 86, no. 4 (April 1977): 481. Copyright 1977 by the American College of Physicians, 4200 Pine Street, Philadelphia, Pennsylvania 19104.

will be held accountable for their actions. A single identified patient with kidney disease who needs a transplant appears to attract more resources than an other statistical death from air pollution, who joins hundreds who would already die of chronic lung disease. Decision makers who can attribute their choice of the alternative directly to the saving of a life appear to garner greater satisfaction from making the choice to provide the transplant for the identified patient. In addition, the decision maker appears to enjoy the fact that the mass media and the public might laud him for the decision to provide the transplant for the patient. Whether they should or not, personal emotions do color considerations about alternatives. In evaluating the health effects of societal decisions on programs, H. Raiffa and his associates[40] raise a sensitive question: Should identifiability and accountability enter into societal decisions involving human life and health?

Exhibit 4-7 Decision Tree for Strategy A (culture and treatments)

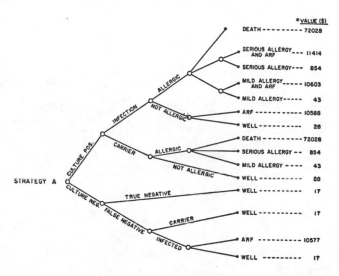

*The outcome values assume benzathine penicillin treatment; if oral penicillin were used, the values for the culture positive patients would decrease by $8.50. ARF = acute rheumatic fever.

Source: Reprinted with permission from R.K. Tompkins, D.C. Barnes, and W.E. Cable, "An Analysis of the Cost-Effectiveness of Pharyngitis Management and Acute Rheumatic Fever Prevention," *Annals of Internal Medicine* 86, no. 4 (April 1977): 481. Copyright 1977 by the American College of Physicians, 4200 Pine Street, Philadelphia, Pennsylvania 19104.

From observations of the behavior of society, it appears that the very fact that a potential victim is identified makes a difference in the alternative chosen. Possibly even more important is the degree to which the decision maker will be able to attribute his decision to the saving of a life or to a death. Consider the kidney transplant patient and the air pollution victims. Suppose that the pollution is expected to cause 1,000 deaths per year. In that same period, 100 patients might require transplants. Although statistically it is less costly to save those 1,000 statistical lives than to save 100 kidney patients, the identifiability factor could influence the choice of the alternative in the opposite direction.

A dying patient explicitly raises the identifiability issue in decision making. Without intervention, the identified person will surely die. Intervention might only reduce the risk slightly, perhaps from 1.000 to 0.999—from almost sure death to a slight chance of saving the pa-

Exhibit 4-8 Decision Tree for Strategy B (treat all patients) and Strategy C (no culture or treatment)

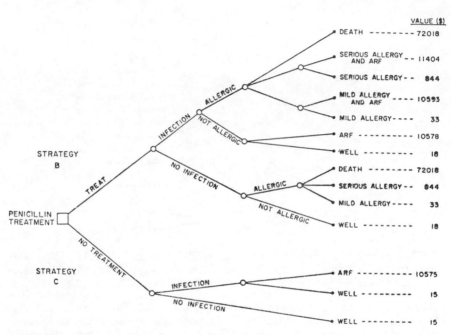

*ARF = acute rheumatic fever

Source: Reprinted with permission from R.K. Tompkins, D.C. Barnes, and W.E. Cable, "An Analysis of the Cost-Effectiveness of Pharyngitis Management and Acute Rheumatic Fever Prevention," *Annals of Internal Medicine* 86, no. 4 (April 1977): 481. Copyright 1977 by the American College of Physicians, 4200 Pine Street, Philadelphia, Pennsylvania 19104.

tient's life. Yet, quite often substantial resources are mobilized to try to save the life of a single identified person who is dying. To reduce the risk of another group of patients from .023 to .022—the same .001 reduction as with the dying patient—would hardly motivate the expenditure of a similar amount of resources. In part, this is related to the attributability factor. If the dying patient recovers, it will be attributed to the choice of the alternative to intervene. In the other case, the patients will probably live anyway and there may never be any attribution to the choice to reduce the risk.

Choices of alternatives appear to be affected by whether the risks faced by a few people are affected a great deal by the decision or whether the risks faced by many people are affected a little by the decision.

Should the physician use a risky procedure to reduce the probability of death, even if the procedure introduces the limited risk of death from a new cause? It is quite possible that the physician will be blamed for the death related to the risky procedure, but the saving of the life might not be attributed to the intervention of the physician. This has resulted in the practice of defensive medicine by physicians who choose not to take the risky alternative.

Accountability relates to the public's association of decisions with the persons making the choices. Pressure groups try to influence health planners and decision-making bodies to choose alternatives that favor their cause. Potential victims of a rare hereditary disease can exert proportionately more pressure for increased research and services than can the potential victims of heart disease, who represent such a large percentage of the entire population. In addition, the decision makers must establish a public record. If they can point to the fact that their decisions saved lives, they will be praised and kept on the job. Therefore, the health planners and decision makers who are accountable to the public will tend to choose alternatives that maximize the visible saving of life and minimize the visible loss of life.

Some would contend that ethical, physical, and emotional concerns rightly play a superior part in the decision making process. On the other extreme, some would say that those concerns are not a rational part of the health planning procedures. Yet others claim that identifiability, attributability, and accountability ought to be considered along with the scientific data and the rational planning information. Health planners will have to arrive at some conclusion about the relative weight to give to the various concerns.

Solution to the Perception Exercises

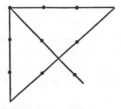

Some have connected all nine dots with three straight lines. Someone has even been able to connect all nine dots with *one* straight line.

```
      0
   ⊙ 0 0
      0
```

Move one unit on top of another in the row.

REFERENCES

1. F.D. Barrett, "Think Tanks: The Egnahc Makers," *The Business Quarterly* 36 (Summer 1971): 54.

2. E. Raudsepp and G.P. Hough, Jr., *Creative Growth Games* (New York: Harvest Publishing Company, 1977), pp. 183-195.

3. J.W. Clark, "Creativeness—Can It be Cultivated?" *The Business Quarterly* 30 (Spring 1965): 29.

4. E. de Bono, "The Virtues of Zigzag Thinking," *Think* 35, no. 3 (May-June 1969): 7.

5. Barrett, *op. cit.*

6. *Ibid.*

7. *Ibid.*

8. A.F. Osborn, *Applied Imagination* (New York: Charles Scribner & Sons, 1963), Chapters 16-19.

9. W.J.J. Gordon, *Synetics* (London: Collier-MacMillan Co., Ltd., 1961).

10. C.R. McLaughlin, A. Sheldon, R.C. Hansen and B.A. McIver, "Management Uses of the Delphi," *Health Care Management Review* 1 (Spring 1976): 51.

11. J.E. Veney, "Observations on Alternative Health Strategies," *Health Services Research* 8 (Winter 1973): 265.

12. H.E. Klarman, "Application of Cost Benefit Analysis to the Health Services and the Special Case of Technologic Innovation," *International Journal of Health Services* 4 (February 1974): 325.

13. D.P. Rice and B.S. Cooper, "The Economic Value of Human Life," *American Journal of Public Health* 57 (November 1967): 1954.

14. A. Wildavsky, "The Political Economy of Efficiency," *The Public Interest* 7 (Summer 1967): 30.

15. A.G. Goltman, Jr., "Estimating the Demand for Public Health Service. The Alcholism Case," *Public Finance* 9 (April 1964): 4.

16. T.A. Hodgson, "The Economic Costs of Cancer," *Cancer Epidemiology and Prevention*, D. Schottenfeld (Springfield, Ill.: Charles C. Thomas, 1973).

17. "Second Conference on Digestive Diseases as a National Problem," *Gastroenterology* 68 (1975): 1345.

18. H.E. Klarman, "Socioeconomic Impact of Heart Disease," in *The Heart and Circulation*. Second National Conference on Cardiovascular Diseases (Washington, D.C.: Federation of American Societies for Experimental Biology, 1965), p. 693.

19. D.P. Rice, "Economic Costs of Cardiovascular Diseases and Cancer, 1962," Health Economics Series No. 5 (Washington, D.C.: U.S. Government Printing Office, 1965).

20. J.P. Acton, "Measuring the Social Impact of Heart and Circulatory Disease Programs: Preliminary Framework and Estimates" (Santa Monica, Calif.: Rand Corporation, 1975).

21. J. Kavet, "Influenza and Policy," unpublished dissertation (Harvard University, School of Public Health, 1972).

22. D.S. Levine and S.G. Willnes, "The Cost of Mental Illness, 1974," Mental Health Statistical Note No. 125 (Washington, D.C.: U.S. Government Printing Office, 1976).

23. I.S. Blumenthal, "Social Cost of Peptic Ulcer" (Santa Monica, Calif.: Rand Corporation, 1967).

24. H.E. Klarman, "Syphilis Control Program," *Measuring Benefits of Government Investments* edited by R. Dorfman (Washington, D.C.: The Brookings Institution, 1965).

25. R. Fein, *Economics of Mental Illness* (New York: Basic Books, 1958).

26. S.J. Mushkin, "Health as an Investment," *Journal of Political Economy* 70 (October 1962): 129.

27. B.A. Weisbrod, *Economics of Public Health* (Philadelphia, Pa.: University of Pennsylvania Press, 1961).

28. D.P. Rice, J.J. Feldman and K.L. White, *The Current Burden of Illness in the United States* (Washington, D.C.: National Academy of Sciences, 1976).

29. B.M. Gross, "The New Systems Budgeting," *Public Administration Review* 29, no. 2 (March-April 1969): 113.

30. A. Wildavsky, "Rescuing Policy Analysis from PPBS," in *Public Expenditures and Policy Analysis*, edited by J. Margolis and R.H. Haveman (Chicago: Markham Publishing Co., 1970), p. 293.

31. M. Hill, "A Goal Achievement Matrix for Evaluating Alternative Plans," *Decision Making in Urban Planning*, edited by I.M. Robinson (Beverly Hills, Calif.: Sage Publications, 1972), p. 186.

32. D.F. Bergwall, P.N. Reeves and N.B. Woodside, *Introduction to Health Planning* (Washington, D.C.: Information Resources Press, 1974), p. 180.

33. S. Cretin, "Cost/Benefit Analysis of Treatment and Prevention of Myocardial Infarction," *Health Services Research* 12 (Summer 1977): 174.

34. E.B. Drew, "HEW Grapples With PPBS," *The Public Interest* 7 (Summer 1967): 10.

35. N. Doherty and B. Hicks, "Cost-Effectiveness and Alternative Health Care Programs for the Elderly," *Health Services Research* 12 (Summer 1977): 174.

36. M.C. Weinstein and W.B. Statson, "Foundations of Cost-Effectiveness Analysis for Health and Medical Practices," *New England Journal of Medicine* 296 (March 1977): 717.

37. G.A. Gorry and D.W. Scott, "Cost Effectiveness of Cardiopulmonary Resuscitation Training Programs," *Health Services Research* 12 (Spring 1977): 30.

38. Doherty and Hicks, *op. cit.*

39. R.K. Tompkins, D.C. Barnes and W.E. Cable, "An Analysis of the Cost-Effectiveness of Pharyngitis Management and Acute Rheumatic Fever Prevention," *Annals of Internal Medicine* 86 (April 1977): 481.

40. H. Raiffa, W.B. Schwartz and M.C. Weinstein, "Evaluating Health Effects of Societal Decisions and Programs," *Decision Making in the Environmental Protection Agency. Volume 11b. Selected Working Papers.* (Washington, D.C.: National Research Council, 1977), pp. 66-76.

Chapter 5

Priority Determination

INTRODUCTION

The National Health Planning and Resources Development Act of 1974 (PL 93-641) requires that priorities be determined among goals and objectives of health systems plans. Likewise, the Special Health Revenue Sharing Act of 1975 (PL 94-63) calls for a needs assessment of programs and providing services on a priority basis for those with mental disorders. Although Congress has been concerned with setting priorities for all of its programs, the health and mental health fields are a primary focus because of the great disparity between demonstrated needs and scarce resources. With regard to health priorities, PL 93-641 spelled out ten such priority concerns in Section 1502.

NATIONAL HEALTH PRIORITIES

Sec. 1502. The Congress finds that the following deserve priority consideration in the formulation of national health planning goals and in the development and operation of Federal, State, and area health planning and resources development programs:

(1) The provision of primary care services for medically underserved populations, especially those which are located in rural or economically depressed areas.

(2) The development of multi-institutional systems for coordination or consolidation of institutional health services (including obstetric, pediatric, emergency medical, intensive and coronary care, and radiation therapy services).

(3) The development of medical group practices (especially those whose services are appropriately coordinated or integrated with institutional health services), health maintenance organizations, and other organized systems for the provision of health care.

(4) The training and increased utilization of physician assistants, especially nurse clinicians.

(5) The development of multi-institutional arrangements for the sharing of support services necessary to all health service institutions.

(6) The promotion of activities to achieve needed improvements in the quality of health services, including needs identified by the review activities of Professional Standards Review Organizations under part B of title XI of the Social Security Act.

(7) The development by health service institutions of the capacity to provide various levels of care (including intensive care, acute general care, and extended care) on a geographically integrated basis.

(8) The promotion of activities for the prevention of disease, including studies of nutritional and environmental factors affecting health and the provision of preventive health care services.

(9) The adoption of uniform cost accounting, simplified reimbursement, and utilization reporting systems and improved management procedures for health service institutions.

(10) The development of effective methods of educating the general public concerning proper personal (including preventive) health care and methods for effective use of available health services.

The act did not spell out the methodology by which Congress set these priorities, but the findings in the preface to the act make it clear that the criteria used in choosing priorities were based on cost containment, maldistribution of services, and quality of care. The ten goals relate to one or more of these criteria. Furthermore, the act requires the secretary of HEW to provide a statement of goals: "A statement of national health planning goals developed after consideration of the priorities, set forth in section 1502, which goals, to the maximum extent practicable, shall be expressed in quantitative terms" (Section 1501). Goals thus are strongly related to priorities.

Determining priorities, of course, forces decision makers to decide which goals should be pursued first and which need greater financial and community support. Choices must be made. Within this framework, four components can be considered: priority determination, criteria for priority determination, use of priority determination, and components of the priority-setting process.

Priority Determination

While it is said that statistics do not lie, provided they are valid, neither do they tell the whole story. Statistics may show that area A receives twice as much money as area B for outpatient health services. However, they may not reveal that the needs of area A are four times as great as area B. Neither will such statistics illuminate the fact that the cultural composition of the population is such that residents will only go to physicians who come from their ethnic or racial background. Statistics are important in priority determination and helpful in mapping out directions and pitfalls, but they often do not take into account the quality and environmental factors, the sociocultural interests, or the psychological readiness of a people to want or to use health or mental health services.

However, taking the needs of people into account can lead to problems. There are probably as many differences within area A as there are between areas A and B. How people feel about different health and mental health problems is important. Should the elderly be given preference over youth? Mental health over health problems? Inpatient over outpatient services? Treatment over health education or prevention services? The list could go on. Statistics can set the parameters of the problem, but the values and attitudes of people are what really matter in the end. Without decision makers coming to agreement on which of the array of statistics represents the community's priorities, little will be done to translate the need identified in the data into real programs.

Priority determination is thus a method of imposing a people's values and judgments of what is important onto the raw data. The easiest way of achieving this is for those in the position of authority to take the responsibility themselves. In essence, this would be an elite imposing its wishes on the people by stating that they know what is in their best interests. To be sure, a great deal of priority setting is done in exactly this way. However, a number of new faces have joined the inner circle of decision making in health and mental health planning. Consumers from all walks of life, public officials, and a wider array of providers not previously involved in decision making have been required by law to deliberate about the health and mental health needs of their region and its subcommunities. Thus, there is a great emphasis on egalitarianism in setting priorities. Representation from this wider population spectrum makes it more difficult to come to agreement on health priorities. The values and interests of these groups that must be taken into account must include, according to A. F. North,[1] at least the following four sets of priorities: (1) patients, (2) physicians, (3) institutions, and (4) the community. He goes on:

> Failure to recognize each set of priorities as a separate issue, often competing with the others, has been responsible for at least part of the "crisis" in health care delivery.

While North believes the community priorities should be given the highest preference in decision making, he is realistic enough to know that "it is the institutional priorities of agencies, hospitals, medical schools, health departments etc., that override all three other sets of priorities."

Criteria for Priority Determination

There are at least three important criteria that should be used in setting priorities, the first being fairness. Fairness begins with the selection of representatives from all interest groups in the decision-making process. It guarantees that both those in the decision-making body and the general public have an opportunity to participate openly. Fairness also assures that choices are made in an impartial manner through the adoption of methods and procedures to guarantee that all will have an equal opportunity to make their choices without undue influence or pressure.

A second criterion is that the process should foster community participation. Not only the leaders and board members, but the users of health and mental health services should have some opportunity to be involved. In any large health service area or mental health catchment area, regionwide priorities might not always be consistent with the needs of subarea priorities, and these differences must be brought to light. A third criterion of the priority-setting process is that it be capable of linking quantifiable data with community values. Both should be used and taken into account.

Use of Priority Determination

Priority determination can be used for several different purposes. It can be used for setting priorities among problems elicited through needs assessment. It can be used for ranking solutions to problems identified by alternative ways of dealing with them. This is another way of setting goals and objectives. Finally, it can be used to select specific programs for achieving goals and objectives. However, the emphasis in this chapter is on determining priorities among goals and objectives.

Components of the Priority-Setting Process

There are three essential components involved in the priority-setting process: the inputs, the process itself, and the outputs. The components of the input are the information or data that are given to the decision-making group, the identification of decision elements, a complete list of decision criteria, and a format for setting down decisions that are made. The information or data refer to the knowledge that is needed for making value judgments. It could be mortality data, number of people living in an area, or the rate of admissions to hospitals. In this step of the planning process, data are related primarily to the goals and objectives the group or agency is interested in prioritizing.

The decision element refers to all the goals and objectives to be prioritized. They should be specifically identified so everyone accepts the list and has no additions to make to it. It is essential to bring closure on what should be included in the list before any decisions are made. Adding new items after the process is fairly well along will result in confusion and raise questions about the fairness of the process.

The decision criteria are those measures that are used to judge the importance or value of the decision elements, or goals, by each individual. Examples of such criteria are "percentage of people affected by goal," "costs of achieving the goal," or "availability of service to special target populations, such as the elderly." These decision criteria should have some relevance to the goals under consideration.

The format refers to the manner of capturing the decisions made by the decision-making body. It may be a chart or table or a simple tabulation of "yes" or "no" votes and should be appropriate to the priority setting methods and process involved.

The priority-setting process consists primarily of the rules for involving the group in an orderly decision-making process and adoption of mathematical procedures for scoring the decisions. With regard to the rules, one should take into account such factors as the size of the group, who should be involved in making decisions, how the voting will proceed, and naming a leader or chairman for the meeting. Procedural rules generally follow what the body has used to render decisions in the past. However, it may be necessary to make some changes to adapt to different priority-setting methods. With respect to the computational rules, the group should decide how it will arrive at a group consensus. Simple addition, multiplication, or averaging might be used. Because of the importance of individual preferences for ranking goals and objectives, complicated statistical measures are not appropriate for arriving at a measure of the group's thinking.

The output aspect of the process has already been mentioned. Its major element is a ranking of a list of goals and objectives that captures the thinking of the decision-making body. Second, but potentially almost as important, outputs relate to the group's making decisions about the relevance of the list of decision elements or the criteria used to judge these. It may be the list is too long or that the elements are written in too general a manner to discriminate the importance of one from another. The priority-setting process should identify information that will be beneficial in making decisions in the next iteration of the planning process. These secondary outputs should lead to more sophisticated and valid decision making in future cycles of the planning process.

These three elements of the priority-setting process (inputs, the process itself, and the outputs) are generic to all the methods for setting priorities to be discussed in the pages that follow. This rational, systematic approach is consistent with the planning process that has been adopted as the general framework for linking methods to the components of the planning process. In the pages that follow, a number of important methods for determining priorities are presented.

PRIORITY SETTING METHODOLOGIES

The Simplex Method

In the Simplex method,[2] board perceptions are gathered using questionnaires. This method can help a decision-making group work more effectively by providing them with structured questions to analyze each problem or proposal before them. The answers they arrive at for these questions are scored and the results totaled. Top priority is given to the problem or proposal with the highest number. The others follow in order.

A variety of data can be employed in conjunction with this method.

Sample Questions for Considering Problems

Questions that bear on the problem being considered might, for example, fall into three main categories: (1) nine questions concerning impact on the community's health; (2) six questions concerning issues of more general social concern; and (3) five questions of a health planning nature. Exhibits 5-1 through 5-3 present these questions. Each set of questions is presented as an illustration. Both the questions and categories may be expanded or otherwise modified as circumstances require.

Sample Questions for Considering Solutions

Sample questions that bear on the solutions being considered might fall into four categories: (1) six questions concerning impact on the community's health; (2) seven questions concerning issues of more general social concern; (3) nine questions of a health planning nature; and (4) six questions concerned with political factors. Exhibits 5-4 through 5-7 present these questions. Again, each set of questions is presented as an illustration. It, too, may be expanded or otherwise modified.

A Step-By-Step Example of the Method

The Simplex method can be used to rank order either problems or solutions. If the board is faced with a decision on which one of several proposals should be chosen to deal with an identified problem, the board would answer the 28 questions bearing on selection of proposed solutions. If, however, the group has not yet clearly identified the problems it wants to address, the group of 20 questions bearing on problem prioritizing would be used to select the most important problems from a list of all recognized health problems.

The process by which the three proposed solutions are rank ordered is as follows:

Step 1: Develop a Simplex Questionnaire   The questions listed in Exhibits 5-1 to 5-7 are generally useful in a proposed selection process. Yet it is likely that conditions unique to one area might dictate that certain questions be added and others deleted. The basis for such actions is the knowledge that some members of the decision-making group have about the immediate area, which the developers of these questions do not have.

Exhibit 5-1 Problems Being Considered: Community Health Questions

---

1. This problem affects:
    1. very few people
    2. a minority of them
    3. half the people
    4. a majority
    5. everyone

2. This problem's effect on the community health environment is:
    1. negligible
    2. very slight
    3. moderate
    4. significant
    5. very detrimental

3. In the next ten years, this problem is going to:
    1. get much better
    2. get better
    3. stay the same
    4. get worse
    5. get much worse

4. Left unattended, this problem:
    1. will go away
    2. is likely to go away
    3. will stay the same
    4. is unlikely to go away
    5. will not go away

5. The number of premature deaths (those deaths caused before the end of the normal life span) caused by this problem is:
    1. none
    2. few
    3. some
    4. many
    5. very many

6. The pain, discomfort, and/or inconvenience caused by this problem is:
    1. none
    2. little
    3. appreciable
    4. serious
    5. very serious

7. The amount of distress or danger to others caused by this problem is:
    1. none
    2. little
    3. appreciable
    4. serious
    5. very serious

8. The extent of disability caused by this problem is:
    1. negligible
    2. mild
    3. appreciable
    4. serious
    5. total

Source: Exhibits 5-1 through 5-7 are from J. Drake, P. McCann, S. Adams, and J. Isaacs, *Methods for Priority Setting in Area Wide Health Planning* (Washington, D.C.: Arthur Young & Co., 1977), pp. IV 1-40.

Exhibit 5-2 Problems Being Considered: General Social Concerns

1. If unattended, this problem lasts for:	1. days 2. weeks 3. months 4. years 5. life
2. Public interest in this problem is:	1. very low 2. low 3. average 4. high 5. very high
3. Public dissatisfaction with this problem is:	1. very low 2. low 3. average 4. high 5. very high
4. Public attitude toward groups affected by this problem is:	1. antagonistic 2. disapproving 3. indifferent 4. sympathetic 5. deeply concerned
5. The estimated amount of lost work time caused by this problem is:	1. none 2. little 3. appreciable 4. serious 5. very serious
6. The extent to which racial or other segregation is involved in this problem is:	1. none 2. slight 3. noticeable 4. significant 5. great

By whatever means chosen, a list of questions should be developed and categorized in the appropriate fashion and approved by the whole decision-making group. It is suggested that the approval vote require a two-thirds or greater majority. Any disagreements concerning the list should be fully negotiated before the process starts.

The questionnaire can be as long or specific as desired, given constraints on time, available data, and the like. It should be noted that the larger the number of questions, the greater the possibility that the

Exhibit 5-3 Problems Being Considered: Health Planning Concerns

1. The attitude of local political bodies toward efforts to solve this problem is:	1. antagonistic 2. indifferent 3. complacent 4. interested 5. very interested
2. Trained health care manpower available to cope with this problem is:	1. extremely short 2. less than adequate 3. sufficient 4. abundant 5. overabundant
3. Of the health care manpower, facilities and money currently available, this problem consumes:	1. much less than its share 2. less than its share 3. its share 4. more than its share 5. much more than its share
4. In attempting to deal with this problem, the HSA has for its consideration:	1. No proposals or programs which might help solve 2. One or more rough ideas concerning possible solutions 3. One or more preliminary draft proposals or program ideas concerning possible solutions 4. One or more final proposals or recently initiated programs that seek to solve the problem 5. One or more existing programs aimed at solving the problem.
5. For this problem, present technology can:	1. do nothing 2. do little 3. control it 4. improve it 5. eliminate it

responses to them will overlap or that other distortions might occur. Further, should the group decide to use more complex methods of evaluating the answers, greater difficulty could arise with larger numbers.

Step 2: Familiarization with Proposal Background Information Prior to completing the evaluation questionnaire, group members should review all proposed solutions and all other information avail-

Exhibit 5-4 Solutions Being Considered: Questions On Community Health

1.	This solution will benefit:	1.	few people
		2.	some people
		3.	half the people
		4.	a majority
		5.	everyone
2.	This solution would make manpower, facilities, and money available to:	1.	very few
		2.	minority
		3.	half the people
		4.	majority
		5.	everyone
3.	The effect of this solution on premature deaths (those deaths before the end of the normal life span) will be:	1.	none
		2.	slight reduction
		3.	reduction
		4.	great reduction
		5.	elimination
4.	This solution's effect on the community health environment will be:	1.	very harmful
		2.	harmful
		3.	without effect
		4.	improvement
		5.	great improvement
5.	This solution will probably solve the problem:	1.	never
		2.	eventually
		3.	in good time
		4.	soon
		5.	immediately
6.	The effect of this solution on pain, discomfort, and/or inconvenience will be:	1.	an increase
		2.	no change
		3.	moderate reduction
		4.	substantial reduction
		5.	great reduction

able to them concerning the intent, scope, probable effectiveness, and overall value of each proposal.

Step 3: Complete the Simplex Questionnaire The Simplex questionnaire on the solution(s) being considered is distributed to group members and is completed for each proposal being considered. The group members complete the questionnaires independently, answering each of the questions by choosing one of the possible responses. When complete, all questionnaires are returned to the staff for tabulation.

Step 4: Tabulation of "Solution(s) Questionnaire" Results The tabulation process consists of averaging the numbers that correspond

Exhibit 5-5 Solutions Being Considered: Questions On General Social Concerns

1. The effect on lost work time by this solution will be:	1. an increase 2. no effect 3. a reduction 4. a great reduction 5. elimination
2. The distress or danger to others caused by this solution will be:	1. increased 2. not affected 3. moderate 4. reduced 5. eliminated
3. This solution will:	1. create many other problems 2. create few other problems 3. create no other problems 4. solve a few other problems 5. solve many other problems
4. This solution's impact on a patient's employability will be:	1. a substantial reduction 2. a moderate reduction 3. no change 4. a moderate increase 5. a substantial increase
5. The aesthetic effect of this solution will be:	1. bad 2. poor 3. fair 4. good 5. excellent
6. Public attitudes toward this solution are:	1. antagonistic 2. disapproving 3. tolerant 4. sympathetic 5. whole-hearted support
7. Public opinion toward financing this solution will be:	1. antagonistic 2. negative 3. indifferent 4. favorable 5. highly favorable

with each selected answer from each member of the group. Multiple choice questions are arranged in an order that guarantees that the higher the number (1-5) the better the solution for that criterion. Therefore, when all the members' answers for one question are totaled and then averaged, the resulting figure represents the group's assessment of how good the proposal is with regard to that question. Then this assessment can be numerically compared with the group's assessment of the other proposals.

Exhibit 5-6 Solutions Being Considered: Questions On Health
Planning Concerns

1. In practice this solution would be:	1. difficult to change 2. inflexible 3. somewhat rigid 4. fairly easy to change 5. highly flexible
2. This solution will benefit:	1. few at high costs 2. few at moderate costs 3. many at moderate costs 4. majority at low costs 5. everyone at low costs
3. The return for the dollar spent on this solution will be:	1. a losing proposition 2. break-even 3. moderate 4. substantial 5. very high
4. This solution's effect on manpower requirements will be:	1. a great increase 2. an increase 3. no effect 4. a reduction 5. a substantial reduction
5. The phases of the problem attacked by this solution will be:	1. one 2. few 3. many 4. a majority 5. all
6. The amount of beneficial side effects produced by this solution will be:	1. none 2. few 3. some 4. many 5. very many
7. The amount of health care manpower, facilities, and money used by this solution will be:	1. unacceptable 2. excessive 3. acceptable 4. minimal 5. negligible
8. Necessary technology for this solution is:	1. unavailable 2. difficult to find 3. accessible 4. largely available 5. completely available

9. There are many other solutions to this problem---------------1
    There are several other solutions to this problem-------------2
    There are a few other solutions to this problem---------------3
    There is another solution to this problem--------------------4
    This is the only solution to this problem-------------------5

Exhibit 5-7 Solutions Being Considered: Questions On Political
Factors

1.	The political attitude toward this solution is:	1. 2. 3. 4. 5.	antagonistic indifferent complacent concerned very interested
2.	This solution will affect public opinion toward health planning:	1. 2. 3. 4. 5.	very adversely adversely not at all favorably very favorably
3.	Because of this solution, coordination among official agencies will be:	1. 2. 3. 4. 5.	greatly discouraged slightly discouraged unaffected slightly encouraged greatly encouraged
4.	Because of this solution, coordination among public and private agencies will be:	1. 2. 3. 4. 5.	greatly discouraged slightly discouraged unaffected slightly encouraged greatly encouraged
5.	Community participation and support in this solution will be:	1. 2. 3. 4. 5.	negligible slight moderate high very high

The second step of the tabulation process is to total all the averages for all the questions. The resulting total figure for each proposal, which in this case ranged on a scale from 28-140, can then be compared with the other proposals. The proposal with the highest number would then be considered the most desirable.

Step 5: Evaluation of "Problem Questionnaire" Results The questionnaire results can be evaluated in several ways. The simplest way is to compare the score for this problem with the scores for other problems identified by the group to arrive at a rank ordering of problems in terms of severity. Or, the group might establish an arbitrary cutoff score (for example, 60) below which problems can be postponed. Or, it might establish "ranges" that indicate the problem's severity. For example, 80-100 might mean the problem requires immediate attention, 70-79 the problem should be dealt with in one year's time, and so forth. The method chosen, however, is somewhat arbitrary. It should be adapted to the needs and abilities of the members of the group.

Weighting Techniques (Optional)

Each of the questions in both questionnaires is implicitly accorded equal weight. However, in many areas the importance of each question may vary. "Return for dollars spent" can, for example, be viewed as much more important than "aesthetic value." If the group believes the various questions should be weighted to express relative importance, weighting can be accomplished in several ways. One of the easiest is to assign each question a value expressing its comparative importance. This expression of "relative importance" can be determined through a polling process. Each member assigns a value to each question, (within a specified numerical range, e.g., 1 to 3), and the results are averaged. The average score for a given question is employed as that question's weight.

To illustrate, suppose that the group rates the relative importance of each question on the "Questions On The Problem Being Considered" on a scale of 1 (low importance) to 10 (high importance). Suppose for the first question, numbers of people affected, the average rating turns out to be 7, indicating relatively great importance. When tabulating the questionnaire results, this weight would be multiplied by the response given by each group member. If a given group member judged the problem at hand to affect "half the people" for example, this response (#3) would be multiplied by the weight (7) to result in a weighted response (21) for the question. The sum of each of these member weighted scores would be divided by the number of members, thereby resulting in an average weighted score for that question as related to a particular proposal.

All other question responses are weighted in the same fashion. The sums of all questions for each proposal are still comparative, and the highest weighted score is still the most desirable.

Application of the Method for Prioritizing Problems

The same steps are used to rank order the identified health problems in the area. The only change is that a set of problem-oriented questions is used instead of solution-rating questions.

THE NOMINAL GROUP PLANNING MODEL

The Nominal Group Planning Method,[3] as described by its principal developers, is applicable in a variety of ways for exploring problems and problem dimensions. The developers, A. L. Delbecq and A. H. Van de Ven, list the following applications:

- problem exploration,
- knowledge exploration,
- priority development,
- program development, and
- program evaluation.

The mechanics of the process are essentially the same in each application. A variety of data can be employed in conjunction with the method. It is, however, essentially a process for employing collective opinions and values more systematically in decision making.

Although each of the above activities relates to a decision process, this description will deal only with the slight variation of the nominal process as applied to prioritizing problems and alternative solutions.

The major premise of the nominal process is based on the fact that the decision-making body is made up of people with diverse backgrounds, expertise, and perceptions. Hence, the successful completion of a planning process involves assimilating the diverse inputs of the participants into a decision consensus.

Of the several priority setting methods available today, this one involves a lesser amount of mathematical procedures and a greater amount of group discussion and information exchange. The key phase is information exchange.

The process itself is one of having the participants identify elements of the subject under discussion. For example, the subject could be problem identification, in which case the elements would comprise a list of all the health care problems in the area perceived by the participants. If the subject matter were development of decision-making criteria, the elements would form a list of individual criteria on which an evaluation of the success of the health care system would be based. Once the elements are listed, information regarding them is exchanged, and consensus is reached on the question by a simple voting process.

Step-by-Step Example

The board or decision-making group in this example must choose those problems, out of all possible problems, which within a budget constraint should receive priority with regard to the allocation of efforts and resources. The method is presented in detail in the following step-by-step example.

Step 1: Set Up the Structure of the Decision-Making Group   The questions to be resolved at this point are:

• How large should the group be?
• Should the group be broken down into subgroups?

The answers to these two questions relate to both the size and complexity of the subject under consideration and the existence of subtopics within the subject area around which different decision-making groups can be formed.

In some cases, a subject might be of such complexity that it is necessary to break the decision down into components and assign each component to a subgroup of participants. Then after a consensus has been achieved by each subgroup, the full group will begin its nominal group process based on the collected consensus of the subgroups. As a general rule, however, nominal process results can be improved by first achieving subtopic consensus.

The actual selection of the subgroup members can be achieved in several ways. For example, the board may already have certain committees which correspond to the component subject areas of the question and thereby could form the subgroup. There are, however, some advantages in exposing the subgroup as a whole to a wide range of perspectives through the inclusion of noncommittee members in the subgroup. If the board does not have a topic-oriented committee structure, members of subgroups may be randomly selected or assigned according to background or expertise. Again the best results occur when the members of the group or subgroup contribute the broadest possible perspectives and knowledge to a given question.

A minimum group size for a nominal process is six to ten. The size of the decision group can be larger. The larger the number of participants the better the results will be, but the time requirements and complexity of the process also increase. Should a group of 15 to 20 members wish to come to a consensus on the question at hand with a single attempt, as is the case in this example, the process remains very workable.

Step 2: Define the Main Dimensions of the Decision Question   Each group will be run by a coordinator whose responsibility is to explain how the process works and outline the question being considered. Having identified the working group structure and membership, each participant is given a preprinted "Nominal Group Task Statement Form" which specifies an exploratory question about which the group is seeking a consensus. More than one form and question may be used in the course of reaching an overall consensus.

On each statement form, in addition to the overall decision question, there will be a statement indicating the type of input sought from each of the participants. In this example case, statements which might be used to elicit input are:

- List all the problems which you perceive to be affecting the delivery of health care
- List the criteria by which you would judge the seriousness of a problem.

These two statements are included in the example Task Statement Forms I and II shown in Exhibit 5-8.

Each participant will independently complete the Task Statement Form(s) within a predetermined time limit. On Task Statement Form I, each participant lists as many criteria that he/she believes ought to be considered while reviewing health care delivery problems. The criteria might be drawn from any of the following sources:

- participant's personal knowledge and experience,
- staff suggestions,
- federal regulations (as well as state and local regulations), or
- public opinion.

Other sources should be used as are appropriate to the area and its health needs.

For the second form, the participants would list all the problems they perceive to be affecting the delivery of health care, subjective as well as objective ones. Objective problems may be defined as those problems relating to the organization, resources, or environmental barriers to meeting the areas needs. Subjective problems are those problems caused by emotions, feelings, and the like. An example of the latter would be a situation where a person presumed that he/she could not get treatment for lack of money when in fact he/she could.

At the end of the allotted time period, the coordinator brings forward a large flip chart for compiling a master list of problems and criteria. In a round-robin fashion, each participant contributes one problem (criterion) aloud from his list to be recorded on the flip chart. At this point there is no discussion. One participant after another reads an item from his list until all the items from all the lists have been recorded.

Step 3: Discussion of Decision Question   After all problems are recorded, the coordinator leads the group in a discussion of the ideas now before the group. The purpose of the discussion is to clarify, elaborate,

Exhibit 5-8 Example Task Statement Forms

NOMINAL GROUP TASK STATEMENT FORM I

TO IDENTIFY THOSE HEALTH CARE PROBLEMS THAT SHOULD RECEIVE PRIORITY WITH REGARD TO THE ALLOCATION OF EFFORT AND RESOURCES.

LIST THE CRITERIA BY WHICH YOU WOULD JUDGE THE SERIOUSNESS OF A PROBLEM AFFECTING THE AREA'S HEALTH CARE DELIVERY SYSTEM.

1.

2.

3.

4.

•

•

•

•

N

NOMINAL GROUP TASK STATEMENT FORM II

TO IDENTIFY THOSE HEALTH CARE PROBLEMS THAT SHOULD RECEIVE PRIORITY WITH REGARD TO THE ALLOCATION OF EFFORT AND RESOURCES.

LIST ALL THE PROBLEMS WHETHER SUBJECTIVE OR OBJECTIVE, WHICH YOU PERCEIVE AS EFFECTING THE DELIVERY OF HEALTH CARE IN YOUR AREA.

1.

2.

3.

4.

•

•

•

•

N

Source: J. Drake, P. McCann, S. Adams, and J. Isaacs, *Methods for Priority Setting in Area Wide Health Planning* (Washington, D.C.: Arthur Young & Co., 1977).

defend, or dispute existing items. New items may be added as well. No items may be eliminated at this point. The discussion proceeds one item at a time, until all items have been clarified to the satisfaction of the group. A specific time limit can be set.

Step 4: Problem Evaluation   Thus far the group has compiled a list of problems and a list of criteria. Each list has been discussed. At this point each participant will be asked to review and evaluate the list of problems in light of the list of criteria. The participants, based on their own preferences and the discussions, can choose any of the criteria listed for evaluating the problems. Another option would be for the group to first select a certain number of the criteria listed by some voting or ranking procedure. The selected criteria would then be used by the participants to review and evaluate the problems.

By whatever procedure the evaluation is conducted, the end result is that each member has come to a subjective decision as to the importance of each of the problems listed.

Step 5: Rank Ordering of Problems   During this step each partici- pant will list in rank order the ten most important problems as deter- mined by his evaluation. Each of the ten selected problems will be recorded on a separate index card by problem name and number. That problem which is considered the most important should then receive a rank vote of ten, which will be marked on the corresponding card. A nine will be marked for the second most important problem, and so on.

As the participants complete their rank ordering, they will individu- ally mark their votes on a voting tally sheet on the flip chart. Exhibit 5-9 provides an illustration of the tally sheet. The relative importance of each problem is shown by summing the participant votes for each problem.

Step 6: Discuss Ranking   After the participants' votes have been recorded and summed on the tally sheet, a discussion of the results is encouraged by the coordinator. At this point, participants can re- clarify, elaborate, defend, or dispute these preliminary results.

Step 7: Final Ranking   Following discussion of the initial vote, the coordinator asks the participants to review and change, if they wish, the ten priority items on their index cards. The participants are then asked to rate their priority items by assigning a value of 100 to the most important priority card and then assigning values between 0 and 99 on the other nine cards in their sets to reflect relative differences in importance between items. This final rating of priorities is collected by the staff coordinator.

These ratings are placed on a tally sheet similar to that in Exhibit 5-10. Again the individual ratings are summed. The problem with the

Exhibit 5-9 Vote Tally Sheet Example

| RANK ORDERING OF PROBLEMS ON MASTER LIST (RANKS ASSIGNED TO PROBLEMS BY EACH PARTICIPANT) | | | | | | | | |
MASTER LISTING OF PROBLEMS \ PARTICIPANTS	1	2	3	4	5	6	7	TOTAL
A	10	9	8	8	7	9	7	58
B	–	2	–	4	–	–	–	6
C	9	10	7	6	5	7	5	49
D	6	–	–	5	4	–	6	21
E	8	7	6	7	6	6	4	44
F	5	8	5	9	–	5	–	32
G	7	–	–	–	–	4	3	14
H	–	3	–	–	2	3	1	9
I	4	4	3	2	–	–	2	15
• • • • • •	(2,3)	(1,5,6)	(1,2,4, 9,10)	(1,10)	(3,8,9, 10)	(1,8, 10)	(8,9, 10)	
(N)	1	–	–	3	1	2	–	7

Source: J. Drake, P. McCann, S. Adams, and J. Isaacs, *Methods for Priority Setting in Area Wide Health Planning* (Washington, D.C.: Arthur Young & Co., 1977).

highest ratings represents the group's consensus as to the most important problem to be solved within the area's health care system.

Comments

This example has dealt with one group, but it is possible and often desirable to break the decision-making body into subgroups of eight to ten participants. These groups can include outside members with expertise in the subtopic area or consumers, thereby achieving a desirable size and breadth of input.

These subgroups can be directed to achieve a consensus on the matter before that group. Such matters might include:

Exhibit 5-10 Final Rank Tally Sheet Example

WEIGHTED RANK ORDERING OF PROBLEMS ON THE MASTER LIST.								
MASTER LIST OF PROBLEMS \ PARTIC-IPANTS	1	2	3	4	5	6	7	TOTAL
A	90	100	85	88	76	78	92	609
B	–	85	–	70	–	42	–	197
C	83	65	55	100	100	100	72	575
D	100	–	–	48	59	–	95	302
E	95	92	86	82	70	64	100	589
F	85	90	100	80	–	45	–	400
G	81	–	–	–	56	42	30	209
H	–	32	21	10	–	91	15	169
I	65	78	41	30	–	–	22	236
J	32	65	27	–	29	–	61	214
K	–	51	91	82	73	60	87	444
L	22	10	–	–	51	18	45	146
M	–	–	31	–	57	–	–	88
N	15	–	16	42	22	45	–	140

Source: J. Drake, P. McCann, S. Adams, and J. Isaacs, *Methods for Priority Setting in Area Wide Health Planning* (Washington, D.C.: Arthur Young & Co., 1977).

- subtopic-related criteria,
- subtopic pertinent information, and
- subtopic-related problems.

When each subgroup has completed its work, having followed the step-by-step procedure shown above, the product of their efforts can be combined into a whole group master list (problems, criteria, etc.) The whole group would begin by asking each participant to make any additions to the master list and then discuss and rank order the items on the list. The process described proceeds from here.

It should be noted that as this process relies heavily on the subjective analysis of the subject by each participant; the process itself is in fact flexible enough to be modified to meet the issue at hand, the preferences of the board, and the like. Yet the seven basic steps, though taking different forms, should be kept intact and in order.

CRITERIA WEIGHTING METHOD

The Criteria Weighting Method[4] is a simple mathematical process by which a set of decision-making criteria is applied to a set of decision elements to award a comparative value (significance level) to each alternative under consideration. The basic steps involved in this process are:

- assign weights to the criteria, which have been chosen as appropriate to the health care delivery system in the area;
- rate each problem or proposal under consideration according to each criterion;
- multiply the weighting value by the rating to obtain the comparative significance level; then
- review and compare each alternative in light of its priority ordering according to significance level values.

The final value ordering need not reflect the final decision. Yet higher rank ordered alternatives exhibit the belief in their definite merit and by the nature of the process have more of a consensus backing of the group.

A Step-by-Step Example of the Method

In this step-by-step example the board is required to choose one of three identified problems to which resources will be directed to improve health care in the area. Therefore, it has been assumed that the set of problems to be considered is known and that a set of criteria applicable to the determination of the priority problem(s) has been agreed upon.

If either the problems (proposals) or the criteria are undermined at this time, the first step in this method would be to identify them. A useful process for determining either list is a simplified nominal group process. This process is described in detail in the nominal group process presentation.

Step 1: Preparation of Criteria In this method, the criteria are grouped into topical categories. Although the number and topics of the categories are to be determined by the decision group, categories such as the following might be used:

- technological issues,
- community health issues,
- general social issues, or
- financial issues.

Under each of these categories the decision criteria agreed upon should be listed. Methods for development of these criteria (e.g., group process techniques) have been described in earlier sections.

Step 2: Establishing the Relative Importance of the Criteria   Once the criteria have been defined for each of the four categories, the group decides the relative importance of each criterion. This is done in two basic steps.

First, the criteria are discussed thoroughly ensuring that all participants understand them and that the appropriateness and validity of each can be ascertained.

Second, a single value expressing relative importance is assigned to each criterion by each participant. A scale of values (e.g., from one to five), can be used. The most important criteria receive the highest values. The values assigned by the group members to each criterion are then averaged. The result is a single value for each criterion that expresses its *relative* importance as viewed by the decision-making group. For example, the criteria weighting process might proceed as follows:

- Group members assign values of one through five to each of three criteria under a category (e.g., "technological issues").
- The members privately assign values in the following manner:

Criteria	Jones	Smith	Johnson
X	5	4	3
Y	4	3	2
Z	2	2	4

- The average of the members' scores for each criterion reflects the relative weights of each criterion to the others:

Criterion	Weight
X	4
Y	3
Z	2.6

The weighted criteria values show that criterion X should carry more weight in making the final decision than criteria Y and Z.

Step 3: Rating Problems (Solutions) by Criteria   Rating the problems or proposals under consideration is achieved by a subjective process similar to that which was used to assign weights for the criteria. In this case, each member will privately review each problem (proposal) successively in light of each criterion. The member's impression of the worth of a given problem based on one of the criteria is expressed by scoring the problem between −10 and +10. For example, suppose the board member believes that the problem requires very little technology and that the technology that *is* required is extremely well understood. That member believes there is no doubt as to the problem's "technological solubility," so he or she scores the problem as a +10 on this criterion. The use of negative numbers to indicate that a particular alternative is very unfavorably rated allows for more accurate distinctions between alternatives.

After all members have rated each problem, their rating scores for each criterion are averaged by problem. The results of this process are single numbers (+ or −) that reflect the consensus of the group on how important one problem is based on one criterion. Each combination of one problem and one criterion should have a number rating associated with it.

The results of steps two and three in this process are shown in columns 1 & 2 of Exhibit 5-11. Column 2 is broken down by the three problems (A, B, and C).

Step 4: Obtaining Criterion Significance Levels   For each criterion, the problem's rating is multiplied by the criterion's weight. The product of this step is a "significance level." Adding the positive and negative significance levels provides a total of significance points per problem. For example, suppose the group is considering a problem from the point of view of "community health issues." The criteria as weighted and the problem as rated are shown in the appropriately headed columns in Exhibit 5-11. The criterion, "accessibility to health services," has been assigned a weight of five. The average of the members' problem A rating for that criterion is +2. By multiplying weight by rate, the significance level for that criterion/problem combination is determined to be ten. The same process is followed for each criterion/problem combination (cell) in Exhibit 5-11 as shown.

Step 5: Summing and Standardizing Significance Levels   When a significance level has been compiled for each of the relevant criteria, they are summed. These totals are "standardized" by dividing them by the number of possible criteria listed for each problem on which ratings can be made. The total is divided by the number of criteria actually used, because not every problem is measured against all the possible criteria listed. The result is the average significance level for the prob-

Exhibit 5-11 Determining Significance Levels for Example
Community Health Issues Criteria

EXAMPLE CRITERIA	① Example Weights	② AVERAGE RATING			③ SIGNIFICANCE LEVEL		
		A	B	C	A	B	C
ACCESSIBILITY TO HEALTH SERVICES	5	2	3	1	10	15	5
HEALTH MANPOWER REQUIREMENTS	4	4	3	2	16	12	8
PUBLIC EDUCATION ABOUT TOPIC	2	-1	0	-2	-2	0	-4
PROBABLE DURATION IF LEFT UNATTENDED	2	3	3	1	6	6	2
MORTALITY IMPACT	2	2	1	3	4	2	6
MORBIDITY IMPACT	2	-1	-4	—	-2	-8	—
PREVALENCE OR ATTACK RATE	3	-3	-3	-2	-9	-9	-6
TOTAL HEALTH PLANNING SIGNIFICANCE LEVELS					23	18	11
DIVIDED BY THE NUMBER OF CRITERIA APPLIED TO EACH PROBLEM					7	7	6
AVERAGE STANDARDIZED SIGNIFICANCE LEVEL					3.29	2.57	1.83

NOTE: The criteria and weights used are merely examples and are not intended in any way to
represent any particular real-life situation. They are solely for the purpose of presenting
how the criteria weighting methodology operates.

Source: J. Drake, P. McCann, S. Adams, and J. Isaacs, *Methods for Priority Setting in
Area Wide Health Planning* (Washington, D.C.: Arthur Young & Co., 1977).

lem. The significance level is intentionally skewed by dividing by the
number of criteria applied rather than by the sum of the weights involved. The problems in each category can then be arranged in a priority sequence according to these significance levels. The higher the
significance level, the higher the priority.

Again referring to Column 3 of Exhibit 5-11, one can see this step being taken. The columns under each of the three problems are added and divided by the number of criteria used in the evaluation process. You will note that the criterion for "morbidity impact" was not used to evaluate problem C. Therefore the total of Column 3C is divided by six rather than by seven.

Step 6: Compare and Set Priorities   The results of the whole process for all three problems being reviewed are shown in Exhibit 5-12. Each of the cells corresponding to one problem and one group of criteria should contain a numbered value reflecting the consensus of the decision-making group as to the importance of that problem (or the effectiveness of the proposed solution) based on that group of criteria. For each problem the criteria group values are summed to produce the final problem valuation. The figure is comparable to any of the other problem values determined by this process.

The end result is a rank ordering of priority problems as follows:

Rank	Problem	Significance Level
1st	A	17.69
2nd	B	9.47
3rd	C	8.33

The consensus of the group is that problem A exhibits greater need and should be addressed first. Consequently, the other problems would probably then be dealt with by rank order given the limited resources available in the area. This process does not conclude that the highest ranked problem can be solved or should be solved in the final analysis. The process does indicate that given the criteria chosen and the other problems reviewed, the priority problem chosen as number "one" is considered the most serious and the most in need of resolution.

The rationale for this process is built on the assumption that with such an analytical tool decision group members will be more readily able to agree on complex decision issues. It is believed that by considering problems in light of relevant weighted criteria and then rating them to provide significance levels for each problem, groups can come up with reasonably acceptable decisions.

THE HANLON METHOD

The Hanlon Method[5] has three major objectives:

- to permit a decision-making group of health planners to identify explicit major factors to be included in the priority-setting process,

Exhibit 5-12 Significance Level Rating of Importance of Three Problems: Governing Board of Sample HSA Rating Results

CATEGORY OF EXAMPLE CRITERIA:	PROBLEM A	PROBLEM B	PROBLEM C
GROUP OF CRITERIA ON TECHNOLOGICAL ISSUES	+4	+2.1	+2
GROUP OF CRITERIA ON FINANCIAL ISSUES	+3	+2.5	+2.1
GROUP OF CRITERIA ON GENERAL SOCIAL ISSUES	+3.4	+2.3	+2.4
GROUP OF CRITERIA ON COMMUNITY HEALTH ISSUES	3.29	+2.57	+1.83
TOTAL SIGNIFICANCE LEVEL	17.69	9.47	8.33

Source: J. Drake, P. McCann, S. Adams, and J. Isaacs, *Methods for Priority Setting in Area Wide Health Planning* (Washington, D.C.: Arthur Young & Co., 1977).

- to organize the factors into groups that are to be weighted relative to each other, and
- to allow the factors to be modified as needed and scored individually.

The Hanlon Method groups the selected decision-making factors (criteria) into four components. Each of these components is assigned values by scoring each of the factors within it on a predetermined scale. Components are then inserted into two formulas that reflect the relative weight of each component in the decision-making process. Values derived from these formulas for each of the problems (solutions) being considered can be compared and a rank order determined: the higher the score, the more important the problem.

A particular relative weight of a component has a direct effect on a decision-making process. Without relative weights, choices in actions or priorities can remain unclear or undecided. For example, a problem that affects many people should take precedence over one that affects relatively few, but not if the former is the common cold and the latter is endemic hepatitis.

The relative weight of each component is a reflection of the types of factors grouped within it. That is, factors also have relative weights and ought to be grouped according to these relative weights. For example, consider the following factors which are grouped together: existence of scientific knowledge and techniques; economics; cultural acceptability; availability of personnel; and propriety and legality of the contemplated action. Other factors can be subjectively grouped in a like manner.

Based on repeated trials conducted in various health planning contexts whereby problems were prioritized or solutions selected based on numerous criteria, a consistent pattern became apparent. This pattern is reflected in the four components used in the Hanlon Method:

- component A = the size of the problem,
- component B = the seriousness of the problem,
- component C = estimated effectiveness of solution (solubility of the problem),
- component D = PEARL factors (to be explained).

These components, which will be discussed shortly, are a collection of one or more criteria that the decision-making group collectively believes is appropriate to the question at hand.

The scores expressing these four components are then inserted into the following two formulas:

- Basic Priority Rating (BPR) = $(A+B)C$,
- Overall Priority Rating (OPR) = $(A+B)C \times D$.

The difference between the two formulas is the presence of component D in the OPR formula. The reason for this distinction will become apparent as component D (PEARL) is defined.

As in the case of many evaluative procedures, a large amount of subjectivity enters into this process. The choice and definition of the factors in each component of the formulas and the relative weights assigned to them are based upon a group decision and are flexible. Application of the formula in the rating of programs and activities involves the judgments of individual raters. However, some scientific control may be achieved by the use of a representative sample of qualified raters, a precise definition of terms, the delineating of exact rating procedures, and the utilization of statistical data to guide ratings to the extent they are available.

Components

Component A—Size of the Problem

Generally, the factors of this component will be few in number, often only one. Yet the choice of factors remains open to the group. An example of the type of factor that could be used is the percentage of population directly affected by the problem. Each of the terms in the factor description must be defined carefully (e.g., for population, which individuals are to be counted).

Component B—Seriousness of the Problem

In this component, the group will establish a list of factors to be used to determine the seriousness of the problem. This list can best be developed by a group process in which each individual completes a list of factors that he/she believes to be pertinent to the problem. (Staff input in this process is valuable.)

A composite list is developed from the individual lists, and a vote is taken to determine those factors that most members believe are important in assessing the seriousness of the problem. The number of factors should be kept "reasonable," i.e., less than ten. A list of such factors might include the following:

1. *Urgency*
   - public concern
   - public health concern
2. *Severity*
   - mortality rates
   - morbidity—degree and duration
   - disability—degree and duration
   - accessibility—average distance to care
3. *Medical Costs*
   - to individuals directly affected
   - to third party payers

4. *Trends in Health Care Needs (forecasts)*
   • potential number of persons who may acquire problem or be affected by the problem, and relative degree of involvement.

The list can be structured in any fashion meeting the group's approval.

Having developed this list, each member individually indicates the seriousness of the problem by scoring each factor on a zero to ten scale, ten being most serious. For each criterion, an average of the members' score is determined. The average scores for all factors are summed, and an average value for component B is determined.

Having defined the factor to be scored, a table is developed that matches the factor (i.e., percent, or dollars) to a score. Using the percentage of population directly affected as an example, the board would first identify "break point categories." For example:

Percentage of Population Directly Affected
        75% or more
        50%–75%
        25%–50%
        10%–25%
        less than 10%

These breakpoints can be determined arbitrarily or by a collective group process. The number of breakpoints should not exceed ten and for ease should probably be kept to about five or six. They also should make up a large portion of the base figure. The top breakpoint would likely be considered the most serious possible category.

To each "breakpoint category" a score will be assigned, again either by an arbitrary or group deliberative process. The result would be a table as follows:

Percentage of Population Directly Affected	*Score*
75% or more	10
50%–75%	8
25%–50%	6
10%–25%	4
less than 10%	2

The participants should discuss the table and vote on its acceptability. If all members do not agree, revisions should be made until a predetermined acceptable number agree.

Having set up the table, each participant would estimate the size of the problem. (If sufficient data are available to determine the actual size of the problem, then by all means these data should be used). With the size estimated (or determined), the score corresponding to the size of the problem will be used as the value of that factor and placed in the formula. Where there are differences in board member estimates, an averaging process should be used to determine the value.

If more than one factor is designed for this component, the average score of the combined factors will become the component value and will be inserted in the formula.

Note, however, that each factor on the list may not be of equal importance in the decision process. For example, "mortality rates" may be considered a more important factor than "public concern." If the board requires a relative weighting of these factors, the weighting can be accomplished by having the members vote on the criteria factors before indicating the value of the factors applicable to the problem. The method described above would be used. A factor considered most important would receive a score of 10. The factor weight would be multiplied by the problem score (for that factor). These products would be averaged by problem and inserted in the formulas.

Component C—Effectiveness of the Solution (Solubility)

Effectiveness of the solution is defined as the improvement of the services offered (programs) in relation to current services as a result of the implementation of the suggested solution. In almost all cases the degree of improvement or the lack of it will be an estimate on the part of the group members, based on all information available to them. Effectiveness measurement, both prospective and retrospective, involves difficult evaluations for which valid measuring tools have yet to be developed. Estimates are necessary. When the group is considering problems rather than solutions, the question for component C should be changed to "How well can this problem be solved, if at all." Again this answer is an estimate.

This component will be scored within a range of .5 to 1.5. At the low end of the range, .5 signifies that the effect of the alternative implementation is not going to improve service levels to the currently desired level. On the other hand, 1.5 shows that service levels are expected to exceed desired levels upon implementation. A value of 1 indicates that services will be neither appreciably above nor below desired levels.

As in component B, each member will assign his estimated value for component C. The individual values will be tabulated to produce an average value. This value will be inserted in the formula. Note that in the formula, component C is multiplied by the sum of (A+B); a value of

.5 for C will reduce the product, and a value of 1.5 for C will increase the product. This concept is illustrated by the same scale shown below:

| will not achieve desired effectiveness | | | | will exceed desired effectiveness |

```
will not                                              will exceed
achieve                                               desired
desired                                               effectiveness
effectiveness    .5    .75    1.0    1.25    1.5
```

Component D—PEARL

PEARL consists of a group of factors that are not directly related to actual need or effectiveness but that determine whether a particular program or activity can actually be carried out:

P = propriety,
E = economic feasibility,
A = acceptability,
R = resource availability,
L = legality.

Each of these qualifying factors is appraised and the result expressed as a value equal to zero *or* one. Since together they represent a product rather than a sum, if any of them is rated zero (i.e., improper, infeasible, unacceptable, or illegal), it not only gives PEARL a total rating of zero but also makes the OPR score zero. Therefore, although the BPR might be high, the proposed activity or program is impossible or impractical at the moment. Certain intermediate steps are needed.

A Step-by-Step Example of the Hanlon Method

Let us consider a hypothetical situation. An HSA determined that that there are currently three major health issues facing the community. It was agreed that these three issues should be considered for incorporation into the HSA's Health Systems and Annual Implementation Plans.

Prior to the current meeting of the board, a number of staff studies were conducted which outlined the main dimensions of each of the three problems. Given a number of constraints, the board is aware that it cannot devote equal emphasis to all three. It is necessary to determine their relative priority.

Step 1: Determine Component A—Size of the Problem The board must decide which factors will be used to determine the size of the problem. In this hypothetical example, the board's deliberations result in the decision to use the following factors:

- percent of total population directly affected by problem;
- average economic loss for each person affected per month (medical costs, salary loss, other related costs); and
- estimated dollar loss to the community per month as a result of this problem (*not* including loss per person affected).

Tables are developed that break down each factor into an appropriate number of levels, which range from high to low. To each level, a representative score is assigned. This board's tables appear below:

Score	Percentage of Population	$ Loss/Person	$ Loss to Community/Month
10	25–35%	>$1000	>$100,000
8	15–25%	$ 500–1000	$ 50,000–100,000
6	10–15%	$ 300– 500	$ 25,000– 50,000
4	5–10%	$ 150– 300	$ 10,000– 25,000
2	2– 5%	$ 50– 150	$ 5,000– 10,000
1	< 2%	$ 10– 50	$ 1,000– 5,000

The board must determine factually or estimate the actual values of each factor for each problem under consideration. Based upon a review of the community situation, the factors are assessed by the Board in the following manner:

Problem	Percentage of Population	$ Expenses/Person	$ Loss to Community
A	11%	$350	$ 35,000
B	31%	55	22,000
C	4%	800	101,000

The board determines the factor score for each problem:

Problem	% Pop.	$ Loss/Person	$ Community	Total	Score Average
A	6	6	6	18	6
B	10	2	4	16	5.3
C	2	8	10	20	6.7

For each problem, the three factor scores are averaged to produce the value of component A.

Step 2: Determine Component B—Seriousness This second set of factors is extremely subjective and, therefore, not likely to be fully quantifiable in the same way as component A factors.

The board must choose a certain number of factors to be scored as to their "seriousness." The board's consideration of the situation leads it to choose the following factors:

• urgency,
• medical cost,
• trends in health care needs (forecasts), and
• severity.

Each member scores each factor on a scale from zero to ten, where ten is the most serious. The individual scores for each factor are averaged to produce a board assessment of seriousness by each factor. The results are:

	A	B	C
Severity	5	2	6
Urgency	10	8	5
Medical Costs	5	4	6
Trends	6	9	2
Sum	26	23	19

The problem scores, which are the average of the factor scores for each problem, are inserted in the formula as component B:

$$\text{problem A} = 26 \div 4 = 6.5,$$
$$\text{problem B} = 23 \div 4 = 5.75,$$
$$\text{problem C} = 19 \div 4 = 4.75.$$

Step 3: Determine Component C—Solubility The board must estimate the effectiveness with which these problems can be addressed. The question is: Can current resources and technology do anything about this problem? Each member ranks the problems between .5 and 1.5 according to his estimate of the problem's solubility in practical day-to-day local terms. The value of .5 suggests that the problem is not likely to be solved, whereas 1.5 indicates that the problem is well within current capabilities. The idea is illustrated by the sample scale shown below:

not likely to be solved currently					well within current capabilities for solution
	.5	.75	1.0	1.25 1.5	

The results of the individual board member scores are averaged:

problem A   1.1,
problem B   1.3,
problem C   .9.

Step 4: Appraise PEARL   PEARL, it will be recalled, consists of a group of factors that are not directly related to actual need or effectiveness, but that determine whether a particular program or activity can actually be carried out:

P = propriety,
E = economic feasibility,
A = acceptability,
R = resource availability,
L = legality.

Each of the problems must be appraised in terms of PEARL. The question to be asked by the board is: Do any of the factors in PEARL preclude pursuing solutions to the problem? Each member votes "yes" that it can be pursued or "no" that it cannot be for each element of PEARL by using the number one for a "yes" vote and a zero for a "no."

The votes for each element of PEARL are tabulated, and the results are discussed. Members may change their votes if they wish. The board as a unit must not come to a decision as to the value (one or zero) to be assigned to each element of PEARL. The example board chooses to assign the value that the majority of the board favored in the final vote count. The results are:

Problem	P	E	A	R	L
A	1	1	1	1	1
B	1	1	1	1	1
C	1	0	1	1	1

The scores in the rows corresponding to the problems are multiplied to produce a PEARL value (component D) to be inserted in the formula. Note that the presence of a zero eliminates that problem from further consideration. The sample problem results:

A	B	C
1	1	0

This shows C is dropped from further consideration because its viability is questionable.

Step 5: Compute BPR   Enter all the component values into the BPR formula for each problem, and solve it. The formula, it will be recalled, is

$$BPR = (A+B)C.$$

The results of these simple computations are shown below:

Problem A	BPR = (6 + 6.5)1.1	= 13.75
Problem B	BPR = (5.3 + 5.75)1.3	= 14.37
Problem C	BPR = (6.7 + 4.75) .9	= 10.31

A	B	C
13.75	14.37	10.31

Step 6: Compute OPR   Enter the value for the components into the OPR formula. This step has the effect of eliminating problem C, as it has a zero value for D, while the other two problems have a value for D of one. The formula is

$$OPR = (A+B)C \times D.$$

The resulting priority order is

$$B = 14.37,$$
$$A = 13.75,$$
$$C = 0 \quad (10.31).$$

Step 7: Evaluate Other Factors   A number of other factors, political or otherwise unquantifiable, exist that might be considered by the board. These could serve to change the rank order established and should be considered in this step. However, it would be better to incorporate such factors into one of the components of the method. Special care can be given to assigning weights to each factor.

The resulting prioritized list of problems or solutions provides the board with an organized framework for decision making. The board may choose to address the top ranked problem fully, and any combination of lower ranked problems as budget constraints allow.

THE DARE METHOD

The Decision Alternative Rational Evaluation (DARE) Method[6] for planning requires (1) the criteria to be used to evaluate the alternatives; (2) group members' views regarding the relative importance of each criterion; (3) the relative "worth" of each alternative solution with respect to each criterion; and (4) the "total worth" of each alternative having taken the relative weights of the criteria into account. DARE provides a means for making such evaluations and rank orderings.

The following is a description of how DARE is used for rank ordering alternative solutions. However, the method may also be employed for the rank ordering of problems and other decision elements. DARE may be employed as a means for evaluating diverse types of problems, matching them against the appropriate decision criteria that have been established. This rank ordering of problems will indicate the one perceived as the most "serious" of those identified (i.e., the problem deserving the highest priority attention).

The DARE process can be illustrated by the following algebraic equations:

$$\text{proposal A's total worth} = C_1 W_1 + C_2 W_2 + \ldots C_5 W_5,$$

$$\text{proposal B's total worth} = C_1 W_1 + C_2 W_2 + \ldots C_5 W_5.$$

In the first equation, five different criteria have been applied to proposal A. The scores for each criterion are shown as C_1, C_2, $\ldots C_5$. Each criterion has had a relative weight assigned to it (i.e., W_1 is the relative weight of criterion one, and so on). Thus, the total worth of proposal A is the sum of all the products of the criteria scores and their relative weights. The product of a criteria score and its relative weight is called a weighted score and is symbolized by $C_1 W_1$.

The other proposals under consideration are scored according to the same criteria. Their scores are multiplied by the same weights, and a total worth is determined by the same formula. The total worth of the proposals are then compared. The proposal with the highest score is seen as the most desirable for solving the identified problem.

A Step-by-Step Example of the Method

This step-by-step example assumes that the various proposals have been identified and that the decision makers have agreed on the criteria to be used to judge these proposals. For this example, three proposals are being considered. The criteria developed by the group and staff are:

- the initial cost of the proposal,
- the estimated number of persons to benefit from the proposal during the operating year,
- the time required to implement the proposal once it is approved,
- the desirability of the proposal from the community viewpoint, and
- its operating cost, once completed.

If the set of proposals (problems) to be considered is not clearly identified and if a set of criteria has not been developed and agreed upon, these would be the first steps the group would have to take. The method one can use for completion of these steps is described in the introduction. If these two activities have been completed, the following steps should then occur.

Step 1: Determine the Relative Weights of the Criteria Chosen to Evaluate the Proposals The first part of this step is to rank order the decision criteria. There are several ways to do this. Probably the simplest method is to have all the participants rank the criteria privately by scoring the criterion that they believe is most important with a higher number than they assigned to the next most important criterion, and so forth. To have the resulting rank order vary significantly from criterion to criterion there should be a larger scale of whole numbers than there are criteria. For example, with five criteria being used by the group, a range of scores might be one to seven. But, members must avoid ranking any two criteria equally. No two criteria should have the same value score on any one member's scoresheet.

The members' scores are then averaged. The criterion with the highest average score is considered the most important by the group, with the second highest score being considered second most important, and so on. Exhibit 5-13 shows this process and the results.

The second step in this method requires the group to agree on the *amount of importance* that should be attached to the various criteria. This is necessary since a particular criterion might be considered many more times important than the criterion ranked just below it, while another might be considered just slightly more important than the criterion just below it. To arrive at a consensus on these differences, the group proceeds as follows.

The criteria are considered in pairs starting with the two lowest ranked. By considering the relationship between the higher and lower ranked criteria in each pair, the group can determine its collective

Exhibit 5-13 DARE Sample Problem: Process for Rank Ordering of Criterion

DECISION CRITERION	MEMBERS						TOTAL	AVERAGE
	I	II	III	IV	V	VI		
INITIAL COST OF THE ALTERNATIVES	7	6	5	4	3	5	30	5.0
ADDITIONAL TREATMENT CAPACITY PROVIDED	4	5	6	5	5	4	29	4.83
TIME REQUIRED TO COMPLETE GIVEN GO-AHEAD	3	3	3	2	1	1	13	2.16
DESIRABILITY FROM LOCAL COMMUNITY VIEWPOINT	1	2	4	1	6	3	17	2.83
OPERATING COST ONCE COMPLETED	5	4	2	3	4	2	20	3.83

SCALE OF SCORES=X+2
X=# of CRITERIA

Source: J. Drake, P. McCann, S. Adams, and J. Isaacs, Methods for Priority Setting in Area Wide Health Planning (Washington, D.C.: Arthur Young & Co., 1977).

opinion as to how much more important the higher criterion is than the lower. This relative importance is expressed by a multiple of the latter (i.e., criterion X is higher than criterion Y, thus criterion X is 1.3 times more important than criterion Y). You will note that the relative importance for the lowest scored criterion must be 1.0 due to the fact that there are no criteria scored lower than it.

Having completed the first comparison and recorded the difference as shown in Exhibit 5-14, successive pairs must be compared. Note that in this process the relative importance of the higher criterion to the lower criterion is the multiple times the determined relative importance of the lower criterion. As in this example, the lowest scored criterion, "time requirements," is given by rule a relative importance of 1.0. The next highest scored criterion, "desirability," is determined to be 1.3 times more important than "time requirements." The multiple is 1.3. The relative importance of the "desirability" criterion is 1.3 × 1.0 = 1.3. The third highest scored criterion, "operating cost," is determined to be two times more important than the next lowest criterion, "desirability." Therefore, the relative importance is 2 × 1.3 = 2.6. This value, 2.6, in effect says that the "operating costs" criterion is 2.6 time more important than the "time requirements" criterion, the lowest scored criterion.

This process is continued for all successive pairs, and the results are recorded as in Exhibit 5-14. In this example, the board considered "desirability from the local viewpoint" to be 1.3 times as important as "time required to complete." It considers "operating costs" two times as important as "local desirability." It believes that the "additional number of persons benefiting" is only 1.1 times as important as "operating costs," and the "initial cost" of the alternatives as being twice as important as the "additional number of persons benefiting."

There are several methods by which the multiples can be determined. However, the commonly used method is to have each member determine a multiple for each pair, based on a scale of one to three, for example. These multiples are then averaged, and the group multiple is recorded on the table. Numbers can designate multiples in terms of fractions (e.g., 1.5, 2.3, etc.).

Although one could stop at the relative importance values, it is useful to standardize them by converting them to equivalent values that sum to one. To do this, the column values are added, obtaining 13.48. Each item of the column is then divided by this sum to obtain the figures for the "criterion weights" column in Exhibit 5-14.

Step 2: Evaluate Alternatives in Terms of the Criteria In this step, the alternatives are evaluated in terms of each of the five criteria. The

Exhibit 5-14 DARE Problem Derivation of Criteria Weights

DECISION CRITERIA	COLLECTIVE RANK ORDERING BY SCORE	MULTIPLE	TABULATION	RELATIVE IMPORTANCE	RELATIVE CRITERIA WEIGHTS
INITIAL COST OF THE ALTERNATIVE	5	2	2x2.86	5.72	.424
ADDITIONAL NUMBER OF PERSONS TO BENEFIT	4.83	1.1	1.1x2.6	2.86	.212
OPERATING COSTS ONCE COMPLETED	3.33	2	2x1.3	2.6	.192
DESIRABILITY FROM LOCAL COMMUNITY VIEW POINT	2.83	1.3	1.3x1.0	1.3	.096
TIME REQUIRED TO COMPLETE GIVEN GO-AHEAD	2.16	1.0	—	1.0	.074
TOTAL				13.48	1.00

Source: J. Drake, P. McCann, S. Adams, and J. Isaacs, *Methods for Priority Setting in Area Wide Health Planning* (Washington, D.C.: Arthur Young & Co., 1977).

procedure is analogous to obtaining the criterion weights. It is illustrated in Exhibit 5-15.

This table compares the three alternatives being considered in terms of each of the five criteria. Look first at the R column for criterion 1, initial cost. In this hypothetical example, data gathered by the HSA staff on alternative A show that it has an estimated initial cost two and a half times that of B, while B costs one-half as much as C. Data permitting evaluation of each alternative are obtained for each of the remaining criteria. For example, in comparing the alternatives on the second criterion, "additional number of persons to benefit," the HSA data indicate that A would result in one half the number of B, while B would result in the same amount as C. The results of these appraisals are entered in the R column of the table.

Step 3: Evaluate Cross Products of Criteria and Their Weights   The final step consists of summing the products of the criteria weights and criteria scores for each of the alternatives. It will be recalled that the formula for this operation looks like this:

$$A = C_1W_1 + C_2W_2 + \ldots C_5W_5,$$

$$B = C_1W_1 + C_2W_2 + \ldots C_5W_5,$$

$$C = C_1W_1 + C_2W_2 + \ldots C_5W_5.$$

In this formulation, C_1 is the project's "score" on criterion 1; W_1 is the relative weight of criterion 1 as compared with the other criteria. A project's "total worth" is simply the sum of its weighted scores from each of the decision criteria.

When defining the criteria for use in a priority-setting activity, the group should be aware of the values implied by the criteria phrasing. The scale of values must be applied in such a manner as to produce a consistently addable series of criteria scores for each factor. For example, the criterion "initial cost" has an inherent negative value (as with "operating cost" and "time required"), whereas with the other two criteria, the greater the criteria value (number to benefit, local desirability) the higher the score. For the three negative criteria (in this example), the greater the value is (more dollars of cost), the lower the attractiveness of that alternative and, therefore, the lower the score. There are two ways to treat this positive/negative criteria values problem. They are:

1. define and describe orally criteria for the voting members, to explain that
   - a high cost should be given a low score and, conversely, a low cost gets a high score; and

Exhibit 5-15 DARE Sample Program: Comparing the Alternatives Against Criteria

CRITERION	CRITERION SCORES R
1. Initial Cost	
A	1.25
B	0.50
C	1.00
2. Additional Number to Benefit	
A	0.50
B	1.00
C	1.00
3. Operating Cost Once Completed	
A	1.40
B	0.70
C	1.00
4. Local Desirability	
A	0.75
B	0.75
C	1.00
5. Time Required	
A	1.50
B	0.50
C	1.00

Source: J. Drake, P. McCann, S. Adams, and J. Isaacs, *Methods for Priority Setting in Area Wide Health Planning* (Washington, D.C.: Arthur Young & Co., 1977).

- a criterion should be expressed as one that "minimizes cost" or "affords savings," rather than simply "cost;" or
2. utilize negative numbers in the criteria scores to reflect the value of the "cost" criteria—the higher the cost, the less favorably the alternative should be viewed.

In this example, negative scores have been used. However, the other options open to the group should be recognized. When selecting criteria for this methodology, the group members and staff should be alert to identify such effects and compensate for them in the final total worth calculation.

The results of the entire process are shown in Exhibit 5-16. The relative criteria weights from Exhibit 5-14 are shown in column one. Corresponding criteria scores for each proposal from Exhibit 5-15 go under their appropriate headings. Multiplying the factors of the criteria score columns by the elements of the corresponding criteria weight columns and summing the products produces the final total score shown.

In this example, alternative B, which has the lowest negative score, is ranked as the first priority, alternative C is the second priority, and alternative A the last priority. The negative ratings are due to these facts:

- three of the five criteria are negative (i.e., costs and time necessary to initiate services), and
- the negative criterion "initial cost" also has the largest weight assigned to it.

ADDITIONAL METHODS FOR SETTING PRIORITIES

Size of Need Gap

Using this method, data are collected for the subject under discussion. Predetermined standards that are desired are agreed upon and set forth. Then the difference among the desired goal, the standard, and the current level of attainment are compared. Those goals with the greatest gap between the current level and the future level are given a higher priority than those with a lower level.

As an illustration, a health planning agency's plan development committee has identified four goals of concern to the region. These were selected on the basis of combined technical and value factors. The analysis of the data reveal the following:

1. There are 22 percent fewer general practitioners in the region than are needed based on a standard of one general physician per 4,000 persons.

Exhibit 5-16 DARE Sample Problem: Derivation of Overall Scores for Each Alternative

(criteria weights × criteria scores = weighted scores)

Criterion	Criterion Weights	ALTERNATIVE A		ALTERNATIVE B		ALTERNATIVE C	
		Criterion Scores	Weighted Scores (Product)	Criterion Scores	Weighted Scores (Product)	Criterion Scores	Weighted Scores (Product)
Initial Cost	.424	-1.25	-.530	-.50	-.212	-1.00	-.424
Additional Number to Benefit	.212	.50	.106	1.00	.212	1.00	.212
Operating COST	.074	-1.40	-.104	-.70	-.052	-1.00	-.074
Local Desirability	.096	.75	.072	.75	.072	1.00	.096
Time Required	.192	-1.50	-.288	-.50	-.096	-1.00	-.192
TOTAL SCORES	-	-	-.744	-	-.076	-	-.382

Source: J. Drake, P. McCann, S. Adams, and J. Isaacs, *Methods for Priority Setting in Area Wide Health Planning* (Washington, D.C.: Arthur Young & Co., 1977).

2. The venereal disease (VD) rate in the urban areas of the region is 50 percent higher than the state rate, which was used as the standard.
3. There is a deficit of 15 percent of physician extenders required to serve the rural area and inner cities of the region based on national averages.
4. There is seven percent more cancer in the region than in the state as a whole.

Based on the needs gap between what exists and the standards, the priorities among these four health issues would be:

First priority: reduction of the venereal disease rate.
Second priority: increase in the number of general practitioners in the region.
Third priority: increase in the number of physician extenders in the region.
Fourth priority: reduction of the cancer rate.

The basic strength of this method is that its simplicity permits easy use by almost any planning audience. Also, the use of a single, accepted criterion, size of gap, permits the group to avoid the difficult value differences that usually exist among participants. This is particularly true of a planning body where members are representative of their own professional organizations such as medicine, nurses, hospitals, mental health, rehabilitation, and so forth, as well as from special interest groups in the general public.

The main weakness of using the size of need gap relates to the oversimplification of what are complex issues. Although it may be true that in this illustration the greatest gap exists for venereal disease, other factors should be taken into account before a health planning body puts a great deal of its energy into this health issue as the highest priority. The group must answer such questions as: Is the problem amenable to complete or partial solution? Is this the most urgent problem in the region? Is the manpower available to make an impact on the problem? Does the problem depend on achieving other goals, such as increasing the number of physician extenders who would be expected to play a major role in reducing the incidence of venereal disease? When one takes these factors into account, the complexity of the problem may reveal that it should still be the number one priority, yet it appears little can be done about it in the five-year time frame of the plan because other factors must be settled first, such as the manpower ques-

Exhibit 5-17 Mental Health Status Indicators by Catchment Area, Town or Poverty Area

Status Indicator Description	Raw Score	Rank
1. Providence, age 0–18, inpatient	65	12
2. Providence, age 0–18, outpatient (ratio)	87	33
3. Statewide, age 0–18, outpatient	64	11
4. Northern Rhode Island (except Woonsocket), outpatient	75	21
5. Statewide, age 65+, outpatient	51	1
6. Woonsocket (poverty), female, outpatient	86	30
7. Washington County, age 0–18, inpatient	55	2
8. Washington County, age 0–18, outpatient	66	13
9. Pawtucket, outpatient	91	37
10. Statewide, age 19–64, outpatient (ratio)	86	29
11. Woodsocket, age 65+, outpatient	61	9
12. Westerly, age 65+, outpatient	58	4
13. Pawtucket (poverty), outpatient	85	28
14. Pawtucket, age 0–18, outpatient	67	17
15. Woonsocket (poverty), age 65+, outpatient	59	5
16. East Bay, age 19–64, outpatient	83	25
17. East Providence, female, outpatient	86	31
18. Washington County, married/remarried	94	44
19. East Bay, divorced/separated	90	36
20. Newport, females, outpatient	93	41
21. Providence (poverty), never married, inpatient	83	26
22. Woonsocket, female, outpatient, poverty	86	32
23. Cranston, age 65+, outpatient	65	13
24. Providence, never married, outpatient	102	48
25. Newport, never married, outpatient	93	40
26. Cranston, age 19–64, inpatient	79	24
27. Cranston, age 0–18, inpatient	62	10
28. Providence (poverty), never married, outpatient	93	37
29. Kent County, age 0–18, inpatient	61	7
30. Warwick, age 0–18, inpatient	61	8
31. Kent County, age 0–64, poverty, outpatient	84	27
32. Pawtucket (poverty), age 0–18, outpatient	70	20
33. East Bay, age 65+, outpatient	66	16
34. Pawtucket (poverty), age 19–64, outpatient	94	43
35. Statewide (poverty), age 65+, outpatient	55	3
36. Northern Rhode Island, female, outpatient	89	34
37. Woonsocket, outpatient	103	50
38. Providence, divorced/separated, outpatient	98	45
39. East Bay, divorced/separated, outpatient	93	38
40. Washington County, never married, outpatient	77	23

Exhibit 5-17 Continued

Status Indicator Description	Raw Score	Rank
41. Providence, married/remarried, outpatient	103	49
42. Cranston, married/remarried, outpatient	99	47
43. Westerly, married/remarried, inpatient	69	18
44. Western Rhode Island, inpatient	69	19

Source: Rhode Island Department of Mental Health, Retardation and Hospitals. Final Report on Rhode Island Mental Health Systems Plan. Cranston, R.I. June 1978, pp. 6–7, Section III. Unpublished

tion and the feasibility of changing the life style of those who are carriers of the disease.

The validity of the method also is questionable if the issues being compared are not essentially similar. Physicians and venereal disease are two entirely different types of problems. One affects the performance of the health system and the other the health status of people. The method has more validity for comparing different population groups within the region, such as teenagers and young adults, males and females. The difference in the gap based on a common standard and basis for comparison then permits a more realistic manner of setting priorities.

Cluster Method of Prioritizing

The cluster method of prioritizing starts with the size of need gap but adds a further dimension. The group involved in planning becomes involved in determining the importance of the array of issues before them. The members know the facts and have identified the size of the need gap. They now must determine the importance of the issues compared with each other. Using a simple three-step continuum, they are asked to assign to each issue a high, medium, or low value regarding its importance in meeting the health needs of the region. If a region has identified a large number of high priority issues, these high priority rankings themselves must be clustered.

Exhibit 5-17 identifies 44 items from a larger list regarding mental health needs in the state of Rhode Island. Based on an initial ranking by a planning group, they were ranked based on the sum of the scores of each person voting. However, because the committee could not deal with all the issues within the five-year period, it became necessary to cluster them. One method was simply to divide the initial priority rankings into thirds. The first 15 priorities would be given first priority, issues ranked 16 to 30 second priority, and the rest third priority. This, in fact, is what happened.

After initially ranking them on the basis of the size of the need gap, the planning members then ranked them on the basis of the importance of the issues. This process produced a different set of priorities. For example, while the need gap was highest for item 5, "the needs of the elderly in the state as a whole for mental health services," it was ranked lower in terms of importance than the needs of youth in the view of those voting. Either method results in the capacity of the planning body to cluster the mental health needs of the various populations in the state into first, second, or third priority clusters. Within the clusters, the initial rankings can be used to determine priorities among the issues with the highest priority ranking, or all the issues within the cluster can be treated as equally important.

This method of prioritizing gives members an opportunity to express their value differences so the final clustering of issues by high, medium, or low priority results from a blend of technical and human value considerations. It also places final decision making on the community decision makers rather than the planners. In many situations where the data base is weak, planners tend to use quantitative analysis techniques to produce rankings, imposing on those rankings an aura of authority. There is little validity to attach such importance to them; as much if not more validity accrues from arriving at a consensus among the members of the committee even if that decision is based on the subjective opinions and personal experiences of the members.

Another advantage of the clustering method is that it produces a double ranking process, which tends to narrow the highest priorities by weeding out the less desirable alternatives. Thus, there is an opportunity to rethink or take into account new dimensions that were not originally considered in the first round of priority setting.

But the same weaknesses noted in the discussion of the size of gap method are relevant for the clustering method. Yet, because clustering takes into account a second criterion for setting priorities, it addresses a little more of the complexities of the issues than does the previous method. It should also be noted that those voting for priorities based on importance usually vote their bias. Consequently, the final choices are based on the self-interests of the members of the group. Those with the most influence or who make up the largest block of common values are more likely to have their priorities named the most important.

Preference Survey Method

In the preference survey method, each person in the group states his or her preference in considering the alternatives under consideration. As this method is based on the subjective attitudes and experiences of each participant, the preferences are not based on any explicit criteria. Typically 15 to 20 persons would consider the alternatives, voting a "one" or "zero" for each. For example, among the alternatives cited in the size of gap illustration, the preference ranking of a single participant would be shown as follows:

| | Alternatives | | Issues | | |
	Physician	Para-professionals	VD Control	Cancer	Total
Physicians	—	1	0	0	1
Para-professionals	0	—	0	0	0
VD Control	1	1	—	0	2
Cancer	1	1	1	—	3

Rank: physicians, third; paraprofessionals, fourth; VD control, second; cancer, first.

This illustration shows that the physician issue was preferred only over increasing the number of paraprofessionals. It was not preferred over VD or cancer control. Paraprofessionals were not preferred over any of the others; VD control was preferred over physician and paraprofessional needs, but not over the reduction of cancer. The cancer issue was preferred over all other alternatives. Consequently, this participant ranked cancer as the most important alternative to be dealt with first, followed by VD control, physicians, and paraprofessionals. The sum of the scores for each of the participants is added to determine the total group score and the final ranking.

The preference survey method is easy to administer, requiring only a list of the alternatives placed in a matrix as in the illustration. By relying on the subjective evaluations of each participant, it does not require weighting or measuring the alternatives against predetermined criteria. The final preferences will be clustered around a group consensus with the extremes tending to cancel each other out. Another advantage of this method is that since each person makes his own preferences privately, there is a minimum of influence that will be exerted by other members of the group. Finally, to the extent that the group is representative of the community at large, the end rankings will reflect community concerns. Yet, preference survey is best used when there are no more than ten alternatives to be considered because the matrix becomes unwieldy when a large number of alternatives are to be evaluated.

There are some disadvantages in this method. The final rankings as expressed by the sum of the preferences represent the consensus of the participants. In most instances this will be a limited reflection of the large number of differences that normally make up a community, particularly a 200,000-population catchment area or a 500,000 to 3 million-population of a health service area. Also, the method has poor reliability, even though it has some validity as an expression of community priorities of health and mental health issues or goals. This is because it is unlikely that the same persons would reappear at a second meeting in which preferences were determined. Consequently, the rankings of the first meeting would be changed by the different preferences of those who came to the second meeting. Finally, since many plan development committees typically must deal with many more than the ten health and mental health issues, preference survey is usually not the recommended method. It is best used in subcommittees or task forces dealing with six or seven alternatives related to a specific subset of the total range of health and mental health issues, such as ambulatory care, utilization of inpatient services, or environmental control.

Priority Determination Based on Timing of Implementation

Using this method, the staff typically identifies the constraints that will inhibit the implementation of each alternative as well as forces that are promoting such implementation. These positive and negative forces are assessed, and a determination is made of how long it may take to implement the alternative. The various time dimensions are then considered by the planning group to take into account other factors possibly overlooked or given too much emphasis by the planners. Through this collective thinking of plan development members and staff, adjustments are made for each of the alternatives in terms of the length of time required to achieve the objectives. Factors such as fiscal resource availability, legislative readiness to support the required change (such as certificate of need laws), scientific and technical knowledge and applicability to deal with the issue, and social acceptability by the target populations at large must be taken into account in determining the length of time required to achieve each alternative. On the basis of this discussion, a consensus is reached on the amount of time required to implement and achieve an objective.

Criteria then must be established for determining the priorities. Should a criterion such as importance of the topic be considered? Is dealing with cancer more important than adding more physicians in the community, regardless of how long it takes? A second criterion that must be agreed upon is whether those objectives that can be completed first are to be given an automatic higher priority than those requiring more time to achieve? For example, the education and training of a physician takes eight or more years, but a paraprofessional can be trained in less than one year. If both will eventually be needed, it would be more important using this method to give higher preference to the objective of educating physicians than paraprofessionals. Similarly, the causes of cancer are still unknown, so an indefinite time period must be attached to that objective. If one accepts that cigarette smoking and air pollution due to certain chemical emissions are the most prevalent causes, it might be possible to determine how long it would take to apply smoke emission controls and how long it may take to change personal life habits related to smoking. On the basis of this type of thinking, criteria are agreed upon by the group. If time alone were used as the criterion for determining priorities, and the group was more interested in alternatives with fast implementation potentials, an illustration using four alternatives might look like this:

Alternative	Time for Implementation	Rank
Physicians	8–10 years	4th
Paraprofessionals	1 year	1st
VD control	2–5 years	2nd
Cancer control	4–10 years	3rd

Based on quickness of implementation only, and taking into account the inhibiting and positive factors related to such implementation, the group concluded that training paraprofessionals was the most important alternative and reducing the deficit of physicians the lowest priority. However, it is most likely that the group would impose other criteria on this "time" criterion to take into account other factors. If cancer morbidity were unusually high in the region, the group might well want to consider giving added weight to this factor and give it a higher priority, while lowering the priority of paraprofessionals. If cost became a criterion, the group could well have considered it more costly to achieve cancer control, particularly if it involved expensive factory emission controls, than the education of physicians. This would result in a shift between these two alternatives. However, paraprofessionals as the least costly and quickest goal that was achievable would still be ranked first.

Seldom is length of time alone a criterion to be used for determining priorities. It is best used as a first criterion for setting priorities, but other criteria must be added to adjust for factors the group considers important. If a group is concerned with achieving credibility by showing quick results (for example, so legislators can build a record within their limited 2 to 4-year time span in office), this may be an important criterion to use. However, it is a very limited one, and that fact must be borne in mind.

Social Area Analysis Method

The Biometry Division of the National Institute for Mental Health has developed a method for using 1970 U.S. Census data to develop needs assessment and set priorities for identifying needed mental health services. Basically, the method calls for identifying those census characteristics that most closely correlate with mental disorders and adding to them utilization or pathology rates, which are directly or indirectly linked to treating those disorders. The rates for different census groups, utilization, and pathology factors can logically be grouped into clusters. Each of the clusters is given both a weight and a rank. The sum of the ranks of the clusters produces the final ranking of need. Finally, the resources available to meet the needs of those with mental disorders are also ranked, and the cross correlation between needs and resources produces the final priorities.

Many variations of this method have been developed over the last seven years. The aim is to discover the irreducible minimum number of census and utilization factors for determining which mental health catchment areas should receive what share of the scarce mental health dollar. An example that illustrates one method for determining priority determination was used in the development of an early Massachusetts State Mental Health Plan.[7]

The planners in Massachusetts identified four clusters that are linked in varying degree with mental disorders. Each cluster has its own subset of indicators. The clusters are socioeconomic, social pathology, welfare, and mental and physical illness indices. The indicators that make up each cluster are as follows:

Socioeconomic indicators

median income per family
number families having income less than $3,000

unemployment in civilian labor force

median value one-unit housing

percentage total housing units considered deteriorating or dilapi-
dated

median education completed by people over 25

percentage of people over 25 with less than five years education

Social pathology

total number of arrests by local and state police

number of commitments to youth service facilities

number of arrests for drunkenness

number of arrests for violation of narcotics laws

Welfare indices

old age assistance recipients

medical aid to the aged

disability assistance

aid to dependent children

general relief

Mental and physical illness indices

number of admissions to mental hospitals

number of mentally retarded children in special classes

number of physically handicapped children in special classes

The data related to each of these clusters were identified by the
subsets. Thus, the "median income per family" for each mental health
catchment area was ranked on this indicator. Likewise, that value was
ranked for the other subset indicators of the socioeconomic cluster. The
ranks for each indicator were summed to produce the total, which in
turn determined the rank of the catchment area.

A committee of staff and advisory board members came together and
assigned weights to the clusters since it was agreed that the clusters
were not equally important. As a consequence, the weights assigned
were as follows:

Category	Weight
Socioeconomic indicators	3
Mental and physical illness indices	4
Social pathology	4
Welfare indices	3

The committee believed that actual pathology should be given a higher weight than the factors that might contribute to such pathology as low income, poor housing, or unemployment. The weights were applied to the mental health catchment area rankings for the respective clusters. The new rankings were summed to produce the final ranking of need for the areas. Exhibit 5-18, taken from the Massachusetts plan, shows the rankings of need by catchment area and their individual rankings for each cluster.

The 37 areas were then divided into thirds, with the 13 catchment areas with the highest needs grouped together, the next 12 given a medium rank, and the last 12 the lowest priority. On the basis of these criteria, the Boston University catchment area was ranked first in terms of need and the Reading area ranked last.

Next, the staff made an analysis of the resources currently available to treat children and adults with mental disorders for all catchment areas. These were then divided into three groups: limited resources, average resources, and major resources. The resources were cross tabulated with the need to produce a new priority determination of those mental health catchment areas requiring most urgent attention. Exhibit 5-19 of the Massachusetts Plan produces a table that identifies the new priorities. Barnstable, which was ranked tenth in terms of "need," became part of the group with the highest priority for assistance because of their limited resources. On the other hand, Boston University's catchment area fell to a lower rank because it has major resources to serve the needs of its highest priority population. This cross tabulation clearly demonstrates how priorities change when important new criteria are taken into account.

There are several strengths to this method. The number of indicators involved in the method give surface credibility to important decision makers who only cursorily examine the methodology. Consequently, the results produced are believable and have the ring of authenticity and validity. Also, the method uses data that are readily available and, for the most part, are highly reliable. Another advantage is that this method is based more on technical, quantitative methods that committee members can readily understand and accept than it is on the subjective attitudes and values of the committee members. Finally, the two-stage process of priority determination produces rankings that are more reflective of real needs and resouces than if it were based on one criterion or the other.

But it must be remembered that there is no consensus in the mental health field that correlates one set of indicators or clusters better than another set with mental disorders. Several investigators have dis-

Exhibit 5-18 Rank On Each Category of Need and Total Need

Area	Socio-economic (Wt. 3)	Illness (Wt. 4)	Social Pathology (Wt. 4)	Welfare (Wt. 3)	Total Need
Barnstable	19.5	10	6	21	10
Berkshire	16	36	20	15	27
Boston State	25	31	10.5	17	22
Boston University	4	1	1	1	1
Brockton	22	8	16	20	14
Cambridge	26	9	5	10	8
Concord	34	34	30.5	34	35
Danvers	28	23	26	27	29
Fall River	1	26	25	4	13
Fitchburg	13	13	17	25	16.5
Foxborough	23	25	32	28	32
Franklin	12	22	23.5	16	20
Gardner	5	2	18.5	22	7
Government Center	8	27	2	6	6
Grafton	15	24	36	26	30
Haverhill	7	11	15	9	4
Holyoke	17	35	9	24	25
Lawrence	10	20	23.5	13	18
Lowell	18	33	18.5	11	23
Lynn	27	7	10.5	7	9
Malden	24	28	21.5	8	24
Mass. Mental Health Center	29	30	3	5	16.5
Medfield	31	19	37	36	34
Metropolitan	32	5	13	30	19
Mystic Valley	36	32	35	35	36
New Bedford	2	12	21.5	3	3
Newton	37	14	34	37	33
Northampton	11	29	28	31	28
Plymouth	14	18	12	12	11
Reading	35	37	33	32.5	37
Southbridge	9	21	14	18.5	15
South Shore	30	4	27	29	26
Springfield	21	17	7	18.5	12
Taunton	6	15	30.5	23	21
Tufts	3	3	4	2	2
Westborough	33	16	29	32.5	31
Worcester	19.5	6	8	14	5

Source: A.D. Spiegel, ed., *Mental Health for Massachusetts: The Report of the Massachusetts Mental Health Planning Project* (Boston: Massachusetts Department of Mental Health, 1965), p. 18.

Exhibit 5-19 Area Priorities in Program Development

Resources

		Limited (11)	Average (14)	Major (12)
O V E R A L L	High (13)	Barnstable Haverhill Lynn New Bedford Plymouth Springfield	Fall River Gardner	Boston University Cambridge Government Center Tufts Worcester

	Medium (12)	Franklin
		Lowell
		Malden
		Southbridge
			Brockton
			Fitchburg
			Holyoke
			Lawrence
				Boston State
				Massachusetts
				  Mental Health
				  Center
				Metropolitan
				Taunton

N E E D	Low (12)	Reading	Berkshire Concord Danvers Grafton Mystic Valley Newton Northampton South Shore	Foxborough Medfield Westborough

Source: A.D. Spiegel, ed., *Mental Health for Massachusetts: The Report of the Massachusetts Mental Health Planning Project* (Boston: Massachusetts Department of Mental Health, 1965), p. 30.

covered that poverty or unemployment rates correlate as well with those who have had mental illness as the rest of the indicators combined. Yet, there is no agreement among those who use such indicators. Consequently, the set of indicators used, whether one or many, remains open to questions of validity. Also, the data might not be completely reliable (though the use of computers and the training of persons to enter the basic information accurately and precisely continues to raise the level of reliability). The issue is more with validity than reliability at this time.

Impressive as the priority determination may seem, it does not take into account important implementation factors such as cost, readiness of the community to accept responsibility for establishing community mental health centers, or the availability of the numerous services required to develop such centers.

The final disadvantage to this method is that the set of indicators used for each cluster was generally determined by the staff in conjunction with key members of the advisory body. The advisory body was essentially composed of providers or consumer elites who would not normally use the services being provided. The real consumers were, for the most part, excluded from consideration in assisting the staff and board to determine which indicators to use in setting priorities. Studies in health planning have shown that consumers and providers tend to have different emphases when considering their priorities, and using this method it is usually only the providers whose voice is heard in the final determination.

SUMMARY

Although there are many more methods that can be identified in determining priorities for goal selection, the ones discussed in this chapter are the most relevant and easily used. As with many other facets of the health and mental health planning process, the field is still in its early stage of development. Priority determination is ultimately a balance of the technical and subjective.

The methods studied in this chapter embrace both elements. Some, such as DARE, are complex combinates; other, such as Simplex, are relatively easy to comprehend and use. There is no one perfect priority method, but these represent the range that exists and can be used appropriately by administrators, planning staffs, and boards to select priorities from a range of alternatives.

REFERENCES

1. A.F. North, Jr., "Competing Priorities in Health Care," *Medical Care* 14 (January 1976): 91.

2. J. Drake, P. McCann, S. Adams and J. Isaacs, *Methods for Priority Setting in Area Wide Health Planning* (Washington, D.C.: Arthur Young & Co., 1977), pp. IV 1-40.

3. A.L. Delbecq and A.H. Van de Ven, "The Nominal Group as a Research Instrument for Exploratory Health Studies," *American Journal of Public Health* 62 (March 1972): 337.

4. H.L. Blum, *Planning for Health: Development and Application of Social Change Theory* (New York: Human Sciences Press, 1974), Ch. 6.

5. J.J. Hanlon, *Administration of Public Health* (St. Louis, Mo.: C.V. Mosby Company, 1974), pp. 284-287.

6. A.J. Klee, "Let DARE Make Your Solid Waste Decisions," *The American City* 85 (February 1970): 85.

7. A.D. Spiegel ed., Mental Health for Massachusetts, *The Report of the Massachusetts Mental Health Planning Project* (Boston: Massachusetts Department of Mental Health, 1965), pp. 14-18.

Chapter 6

Promoting
Implementation

After all the discussion and the detailed energy involved in identifying the problem, finding the resources, considering the alternatives and determining priorities, the time comes to implement a program. Simply stated, implementation means that you are now going to utilize your materials, methods, and resources to do what you said you were going to do about a particular problem.

FIRST CONSIDERATIONS

In almost all implementation strategies, consideration will have to be given to the desired changes that the planner hopes to achieve. This consideration requires the ability to step back and see the whole forest, as well as the individual trees. An ecologic approach to comprehensive health planning as represented in Exhibit 6-1 suggests the broad spectrum of individuals and organizations that could be involved in the implementation process.[1] The author uses the term "ecologic" to indicate the teamwork that will be required between man and his environment to achieve comprehensive planning—note the elements in the wheel in Exhibit 6-1. Attention is directed in the diagram to the planning levels (national, regional, state, and community) as well as the evaluation of the process and the areas for analysis in the evaluation process. Of course, the overwhelming number of agencies and organizations could lead to the conclusion that a "philosopher-king," or a "Solomon" is needed as a planner. But social change manages to take place, though there may be a chance of reducing the "cottage industry" image through sustained planning efforts.

In planning for change, the health planner must consider the following dilemmas:[2]

Exhibit 6-1 An Ecologic Approach to Comprehensive Health
Planning

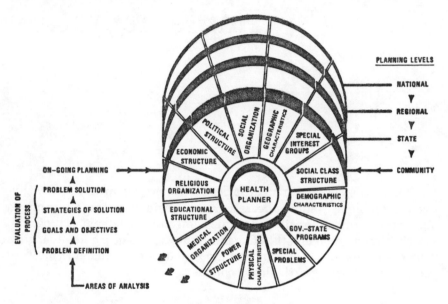

Source: Reprinted with permission from J. G. Bruhn, "Planning for Social Changes:
Dilemmas for Health Planning," *American Journal of Public Health* 63 (July 1973): 604.

- He must be an advocate for the beneficial effects of planning in a
  society that has been uninterested in social planning.
- He must plan in the context of a changing system while he is
  trying to effect change, realizing that his insights and knowledge
  about the system are also changing.
- He cannot deny his professional role and cannot become too en-
  tangled in the politics of planning, yet he must be a participant
  with the community in the planning process.
- The perpetual cycle of planning, which creates new needs and thus
  more planning, places him in the difficult position of needing to
  know when to leave the community system.

From the viewpoint of R. H. Murray,[3] "muddling through" with irrational, hit-or-miss planning is not enough. Four *sine qua nons* were
cited to create conditions for change:

1. We must recognize that there will be a pervasive reformation of
   the health care system.

2. We must accept the federal government's major role in this change but work to restrict its power.
3. We must develop an open organization for the creation of a coherent national health policy and a strategy for implementation.
4. National health policy should be implemented through local agencies by managing the muddling-through process.

Although these *sine qua nons* could refer to a national health insurance plan, a PSRO, or an HSA, they could just as easily be related to any implementation effort. Certainly the system will undergo reformation to some degree; there will be an interplay among organizations involved in the change; a need will exist for an overall implementation strategy; and, based on past history, the local agencies will want to control their own destiny.

Taking a behavioral approach, another concept of implementing change lists the characteristics of change that need consideration in the day-to-day working situation:[4]

- Above all, the model of implementing change should be practical.
- Parts of the model should be manipulatable.
- Economy of use should be a primary consideration.
- Ease of communication is important.
- The model should be comprehensive.
- Synergism—the force of factors working together—is important to consider. A general weakness of most models is that they seem to view, or at least report, changes as linear, rational processes.
- The model should lend itself to intervening in phases.
- Differential investment in working with the components of the model should be possible.
- The model should call attention to how the change process influences the rest of the system.
- The model should be flexible and versatile enough to apply to different organizational systems.
- The model should provide a basis for a subsequent evaluation of the effectiveness of change.
- The model should recognize the human qualities of the participants involved.

Incorporating these characteristics of change into a working model, a checklist for change was developed and is reproduced in Exhibit 6-2. The acronym "A Victory" is taken from the first letters of the eight factors considered to be required for organizational change.

Exhibit 6-2 A Checklist for Change Through Research Utilization

This checklist is intended to serve as a guide rather than as an outline for a systematic plan to bring about change. All factors interact, so that a given manipulation to increase the probability of desired results could influence more than one factor.

Ability

_____Are staff skills and knowledge appropriate to accommodate the desired change?

_____Are fiscal and physical resources adequate for the change?

Values

_____Is the change consonant with the social, religious, political, ethnic values of the beneficiaries?

_____Is the change consonant with the philosophies and policies of the program supporters?

_____Is the change consonant with the personal and professional values of staff?

_____Is the top man in the organization in support of the desired change?

_____Are the characteristics of the organization such as to render change likely?

Information

_____Is information on the desired change clear?

_____Does information about the idea bear close relevance to the improvement needed?

_____Is the idea behind the desired change one that is "tryable," observable, of demonstrated advantage, etc.?

Circumstances

_____Are conditions at this setting similar to those where the idea was demonstrated to be effective?

_____Does the present situation seem to be conducive to successful adoption of this particular plan?

Timing

_____Is this a propitious time to implement this plan?

_____Are other events going on or about to occur which could bear on the response to this change?

Obligation

_____Has the need for this change been ascertained through sound evaluation?

_____Has the need for this change been compared with other needs in this program?

Resistances

_____Have all reasons for *not* adopting this change been considered?

_____Has consideration been given to what may have to be abandoned if this plan is launched?

Exhibit 6-2 Continued

_____Has consideration been given to all who would lose in this change?

Yield

_____Has the soundness of evi-

dence about the benefits of this proposal been carefully assessed?

_____Have possible indirect rewards for this change been examined?

Source: Reprinted with permission from S. E. Salasin and H. R. Davis, "A Practical Model for Planned Change." Paper presented at AHPA meeting, November 13, 1972.

An illustration of the "A Victory" approach can be seen in the following example for a mental health project:[5]

> A "weekend hospital" was proposed for patients who needed intensive help but who couldn't come regularly for a variety of reasons. Services would be provided from Friday evening through Sunday afternoon and continued for a period of 16 weeks. Techniques would include saturational group therapy, a marathon approach.

What factors caused the hospital to adopt and implement the project or to not adopt and implement the project?

Now, the checklist for change can be applied to this situation and the results of the examination noted.

Ability	Two kinds of resources needed; staff competence in conducting marathon therapy and up to $9,000 for staff time and incidental costs. These modest resource needs constituted the greatest barrier to implementation.
Values	Therapists had to commit themselves to be away from their families for 16 straight weeks, and this clashed with the personal values of most potential participants. Therapy methodology also provided some conflict in values as well as some agencies who were rigidly orthodox in their values and their consideration of implementing innovative change.
Information	Initially only 5% of the potential users were familiar with the weekend hospital idea de-

spite good traditional information dissemination. Adding an attractive brochure with concrete examples raised the information level to 55%. Information was felt to be limited in terms of relevance, relative advantage, and credibility.

Circumstances
The weekend hospital concept proved to be more relevant to families in suburban neighborhoods and areas where transportation was difficult.

Timing
New budget cycles, reorganizations, changes in decision-makers and crises offer opportunities for timely implementation of change. At the time the weekend hospital was promoted, the timing did not appear particularly appropriate.

Obligation
Hospitals did not indicate they were aware of any pressure from patients for an alternative to the traditional hours of service. A few staff members felt there was a need and others reflected a need to start something new. There was virtually no felt need to implement a program such as the weekend hospital.

Resistances
Almost everybody resists upsetting the apple cart when they can rationalize the good of their services. A new program will require that resources be allocated from existing programs and administrators resist losing budget money and/or staff. Therefore, resistance is built in to most systems except where the new service is added on. Then different resistances enter.

Yield
Few rewards were implied for implementing a weekend hospital. Job security, creativity, writing papers and the like didn't interest staff members. Some noted that the weekend hospital might be more convenient for certain patients.

This analysis of the responses of community mental health centers to the weekend hospital idea clearly indicates that implementation at that time did not have a reasonable chance of success. Implementation could not be advanced despite the fact that the weekend hospital had been developed, demonstrated, and thoroughly evaluated in a controlled design over a period of years. Patients served in the weekend hospital improved significantly more—both statistically and practically—than did control patients who were provided traditional outpatient treatment over the same period.

From another vantage point, that of the health systems engineer (also referred to as industrial or management engineers), barriers to implementation were noted in a survey of 240 health systems experts[6] (see Exhibit 6-3). Furthermore, four major problem areas were identified, along with the frequency that these problems act as barriers to the implementation and attainment of the goals of the health system. Note that planning and policy problems emerged as the most prevalent problem with 70 percent of the frequency (see Exhibit 6-4). Although the listing of barriers in Exhibit 6-3 concerns itself with aspects of quality, cost, and accessibility of health care services, this listing directly applies to the implementation of a project since those aspects are usually part of any project. In Exhibit 6-4, the health systems engineer, though mainly concerned with operational problems, replied that he spent more time on areas outside of operational functioning. Of interest to planners should be the fact that the health systems engineers are being called upon to fulfill many of the tasks and functions of health planners, for better or worse. All other problem types cited constitute an overwhelming majority of topics that the health planner should rightly be concerned with: educational problems 50 percent, research and development problems 20 percent, and planning and policy problems 70 percent.

In a specific example relating to the implementation of a university hospital ambulatory care evaluation, the impediments to implementation were documented with an emphasis on judging quality assurance. Six barriers were cited:[7]

1. The condition of clinic records and individual charts.
2. The lack of established criteria for care.
3. Problems of provider intercommunication during the evaluation process.
4. Manpower availability.
5. Choice of evaluation method.
6. The method of implementing resulting plans for corrective action.

The sixth barrier, implementation, pervades all the others and indicates the necessity for reflecting on implementation during all phases

Exhibit 6-3 Composite List of Important Barriers To Improving the Quality, Cost, and Accessibility of Health Care Services

Barriers	Problem impact		
	Access	Cost	Quality
Consumers lack understanding of preventive measures.	*	*	*
Consumers lack understanding of when services are needed.		*	*
Third-party payment policies do not adequately discriminate between poor and good quality care.			*
Incentives for quality care provided by competitors, governing boards, third-party payers, and consumers are minimal.	*	*	*
Lack of quality care standards.			*
Consumers and providers view service as a reactive rather than a preventive function.	*		*
Organization and coordination of all health services is inadequate.		*	*
Inability to agree on health goals.	*		*
Consumers lack means of providing incentives to improve quality.		*	*
Services are not accessible when needed.			*
Consumers hesitate to take issue with the physician.		*	*
Information and measures causally relating treatment interventions to outcomes are largely absent.	*	*	*
Fee for service system encourages an increase in the volume of services provided but not in the quality of services.	*	*	*
Consumers lack understanding of availability of services.	*		*
Providers lack skills to evaluate proposed innovations.	*	*	
Needed cost benefit information does not exist.		*	
The increasing and changing nature of demand for health services.		*	
Inflation.		*	
Implementation skills for cost reduction projects are lacking.		*	
Cost reduction projects have had the wrong forms.	*	*	
Providers lack management skills.		*	
Consumer problems in financing their health care.	*		
Incentives do not exist for physicians to locate in rural or ghetto areas.	*		
Services not reimbursed by third-party payers are not sought.	*		
Legal and educational barriers to use of paramedical personnel.	*		
Design skills needed to improve accessibility are not present.	*		
Economic barriers prohibit wide distribution of high cost/low demand services.	*		

Source: D. H. Gustafson, G. L. Rowse, N. J. Howes and R. S. Shukla, "Opportunities for Improvement in Health Systems Engineering," *Inquiry* 14 (March 1977): 97. Reprinted, with permission of the Blue Cross Association, from INQUIRY. Vol. XII, No. 1, p. 44.

of the health planning process. Why spin wheels if a method cannot be prepared to achieve the desired result? It might be better to let things go on as is until something can be done.

Another revealing example deals with an analysis of factors influencing the implementation of family planning services in the United States. A survey of hospitals and health departments in New York state showed that a majority of the hospital administrators (43 percent) and the health officers (63 percent) did not implement family planning services because they believed that the services were provided by another agency.[8] Additional reasons for nonimplementation

Exhibit 6-4 Problem Types and Extent of Prevalence

Problem type	Percent prevalence
Operational problems	25
Those that require the refinement of existing procedures to improve productivity or satisfaction in health systems. Projects of this type occur primarily in delivery settings and focus on techniques for establishing standards, improving work methods and personnel utilization, accomplishing facilities layout, developing simple communication and monitoring procedures, and locating and providing needed information for decision-makers.	
Planning and policy problems	70
These involve the need for identifying appropriate policies and procedures that alter the health system at an organization-wide or interorganizational level. Projects dealing with these problems are currently being undertaken primarily in planning agencies, but should in the future also be undertaken at the upper management levels of delivery systems. Usually these projects are of a complexity that would benefit from considerable data collection, analysis, and the interaction and agreement of many diverse types of professionals. Outcomes of these projects include identification and redistribution of inequitable services across delivery areas, increased emphasis on the provision of preventive services to consumers, better definition of and agreement on health goals, new consumer financing mechanisms, innovative reward and incentive systems for health professionals, improved types of delivery units, provision of new computer and other management service mechanisms, and better coordinative links among various health organizations.	
Educational problems	50
These involve the need to improve the knowledge and skills of consumers or providers involved with the health system.	
Research and development problems	20
Those for which considerable data need to be collected under rigidly controlled conditions in order to develop effective and optimal solutions.	

Source: D. H. Gustafson, G. L. Rowse, N. J. Howes and R. S. Shukla, "Opportunities for Improvement in Health Systems Engineering," *Inquiry* 14 (March 1977): 97. Reprinted, with permission of the Blue Cross Association, from INQUIRY. Vol. XII, No. 1, p. 44. Copyright © 1975 by the Blue Cross Association. All rights reserved.

are listed in Exhibit 6-5. Among hospitals, the low community demand and the feeling that family planning was an inappropriate responsibility to assume indicate that health planners would need to mount a promotional information campaign prior to implementing a service-type of implementation project.

Implementation planning is being affected by the continuing dissatisfaction expressed by a variety of individuals and organizations with the health care system. As innovations or changes are considered, the health planner must be aware of three dominant themes consistently identified in the literature:[9]

1. People, both professional and lay, are more frequently questioning commonly used medical procedures. Tonsillectomy and hysterectomy are among the surgical procedures increasingly criticized as ineffective, overly expensive, and, occasionally, as dangerous.
2. Consumers are demanding more services from hospitals. Services

Exhibit 6-5 Reasons for Nonimplementation of Family Planning
Services Named by New York State Hospital
Administrators and Health Officers

Reasons	Hospitals No.	%	Reasons	Health Departments No.	%
1. Provided by another agency	21	42.9	1. Provided by another agency	12	63.2
2. Low community demand	11	22.5	2. Did not answer	2	10.5
3. Inappropriate responsibility to assume	6	12.2	3. Lack of appropriations	1	5.3
4. Community needs met	4	8.2	4. Lack of board approval of funds	1	5.3
5. Opposition by board	2	4.1	5. Community needs met	1	5.3
6. In process of instituting	2	4.1	6. Opposition by physicians	1	5.3
7. Not enough time to institute	1	2.0	7. Not enough time to institute	1	5.3
8. Personal opposition by administrator	1	2.0			
9. Did not answer	1	2.0			

Source: Reprinted with permission from J.T. Gentry, et al, "A Comparative Analysis of Factors Influencing the Implementation of Family Planning Services in the United States," *American Journal of Public Health* 64 (April 1974): 376.

such as geriatric maintenance, counseling, and humane basic primary care are merely examples.

3. The health needs of the community are receiving increased attention, as well as the concept of preventive health services. Malnutrition, housing, stress, and a wide variety of additional factors affecting the health of the community will have to be dealt with by health organizations.

Implementation projects have to be considered within the environment created by these three dominant themes. Obviously, the chances for success in implementing a project are much better if the contemplated change is in keeping with current feelings among the individuals and organizations involved in the project.

Three types of organizational change were identified that relate to implementation planning: technical, adjustment, and adaptational.[10] Technical changes are those that are primarily changes in the normal and usual activities of a hospital, but not in the basic goals. These changes may vary in their cost and their impact on a hospital. A decision to replace a four-test blood analyzer with a twelve-test one presents a cost increase with little impact on the overall function of the laboratory. However, a decision to install a cobalt machine represents a substantial cost increase as well as making an impact on the distribution of resources and utilization of the services of the cobalt machine. Nevertheless, both of these changes are essentially technical in nature dealing with the same services and the integration of new technology.

Adjustment changes are those that require the currently existing mechanisms for delivering health care to change to provide a service not offered in the past. Movements of the hospital to act as a primary care provider to the community or to establish a nontherapeutic abortion service mean that the hospital will shift existing resources and personnel to provide the services. The means remain the same; the ends change.

Adaptation changes are those that involve changing not only the means but also the ends. This is the most drastic type of change because it means a complete modification of the existing system. A community hospital that shifts its emphasis from acute and chronic treatment services to preventive health services is an example of adaptive change. The hospital would have to reorient its staff, reallocate its services, and engage in community outreach, case finding, social work, family medicine, and prevention.

Tools that the health planner can use to implement change were categorized by A. Etzioni[11] as utilitarian, normative, and coercive controls. Utilitarian control has as its base the control of resources such as knowledge, skills, and/or economic capabilities. Obviously, any change that has to be implemented requires that the planner have something to say about utilitarian control of resources.

Normative control is based on the fact that the goals, values, and/or ends are shared and agreed to in essense by those doing the planning. There can be no doubt that if a consensus exists among the parties involved in any implementation activity, the activity will proceed smoothly securing whatever resources are needed to initiate the project.

Coercive control rests on the actual control or access to control of force that influences any decision. Every health planner will probably come up against some use of pure, brute force in implementation situations. It might be of a political, economic, or zealous nature. But the planner will have to abandon the rational decision for the coercive one since alternatives may not be forthcoming.

All three types of control seriously affect health planning and the promotion of implementation methodology. Bickering among bureaucrats is a common occurrence when utilitarian control is exerted. Traditional values that refuse to budge battle with the "young turks" trying to reform the health care system by bringing in the grass roots consumers to run services. Or, a local politician throws all the planning priorities out of kilter by demanding that a building and services be established in his home territory before anything else happens. All these examples have actually occurred and will occur again in the future. These types of control may be used subtly or with raw élan; but, in any event, the implementation strategy has to be readjusted, redirected, or modified to accommodate the planning goals.

Yet, despite the need to concentrate on the variables involved in implementation and the resultant change, some planners suffer setbacks for reasons beyond their control or influence. In a discussion about delivering health care amid change, J. J. McGuire[12] noted the following about changes in the system:

> The greatest problem we face is how to control change in a complex environment so that some of the fundamentals we stand for are not destroyed or whittled away by political ambition playing upon consumer expectation like a fine instrument.

In relating the above to implementation of health programs, H. M. Sapolsky[13] considers the market and the regulatory strategies. Both are being pursued to control costs, to promote quality care, and to redirect activities into ambulatory, preventive, and long term care—away from the traditional emphasis on acute care. Market strategy aims to induce physicians to conserve resources. Regulatory strategy aims to compel physicians to reorder their professional priorities. Sapolsky contends that neither strategy can succeed and suggests an alternative—bureaucratic competition, the pitting of one professional interest against another. Implementation of this strategy in health would allow three or four governmental agencies to compete for the management control of specific federal health programs. Each agency would have a specific value bias, such as preventive care, chronic care, primary care, or inpatient acute hospital care. Thus, each agency would be implementing a program with its own value system, and the possibility of competitive choices to be decided by the public or its representatives seems more likely. In theory, these preferences could resolve the health crises that were engendered with the professionals making the decisions alone.

In view of the emphasis on change discussed here, do providers and health care professionals have to gird themselves for a topsy-turvy health world? M. F. Doody[14] reviewed the literature in 1975 and considered the question of whether providers change the system. He concluded:

> The 1975 literature on health care delivery is largely "more of the same" and indicates a high degree of acceptance of the status quo by providers. To some extent, this situation is not suprising, considering the general economic climate and the uncertainty about impending legislative and regulatory proposals.

Past history appears to support the status quo concept. Health care providers have been able to maintain considerable influence over what does and does not get implemented. Health planners until now have been able to anticipate and meet most objections. Will the new legislation and regulatory proposals change all prior history? It is too early to tell, but this certainly bears watching as developments take place.

IMPLEMENTATION WORKSHEET

An implementation worksheet can be used somewhat like the traditional approach utilized by newspaper reporters. Rudyard Kipling summed it up:

> I keep six honest serving-men
> (they taught me all I know);
> Their names are WHAT and WHY and WHEN
> And HOW and WHERE and WHO.
> I send them over land and sea,
> I send them east and west;
> But after they have worked for me,
> I give them all a rest.
> "The Elephant's Child," Rudyard Kipling

For each implementation activity, the following questions have to be answered:

- Who does what for whom?
- In what order and when?
- With what resources?

Utilizing the implementation worksheet approach, the planner can be quite clear about the specific tasks, the time period required for completion, and for what individual or agency is going to be responsible. Of course, it is vital that the planner know the end goals. Exhibit 6-6 lists the steps in the development of an implementation strategy. Note that the logical determination of the details also includes dates and the identification of responsible persons.[15]

Two examples of worksheets are illustrated in Exhibits 6-7 and 6-8. One deals with the development and distribution of a training manual for patient educators; the other shows plans to implement a countywide detection and treatment center. Both worksheets operate within a deadline and cover more than eight months in the implementation process.

The implementation worksheet method is probably the most traditional, although the use of a worksheet adds a bit more structure. Generally, the planner takes the decision to implement the activity and figures out the details in a logical manner, answering the appropriate questions about who, what, where, when, and how. Why has already been answered by the policy decision to go ahead with the activity.

Another related technique calls for the development of an action plan (see Exhibit 6-9), which sets down the short term objective, the specific activities, identifies who is responsible, defines the purpose of the activities, and lists the methods and the media to be used in the implementation.[16]

An action implementation plan assumes that for every action there will be a reaction—if something is provided then there will be some outcome. Implementation in an action plan, as is true in considering all implementation plans, must weigh the available resources, timing, and effort required for success. Again, the approach has a kinship with the newspaperman's guidelines for writing a headline story:

- why—the effect of the objective to be achieved;
- what—the activities required to achieve the objective;
- who—individuals responsible for each activity;
- when—chronological sequence of activities and timing in relation to other community events;
- how—materials, media, methods, techniques to be used;

Exhibit 6-6 Development of Implementation Strategy

1. Specify clearly (who does what for whom).

2. Be sure someone is responsible for the whole activity and coordinates individuals who may carry out the different tasks.

3. Identify all preparatory steps prior to doing that activity (e.g., prepare materials, write article, acquire equipment, train volunteers, prepare training manual, determine treatment protocol).

4. List steps in the order in which they must occur.

5. Check for missing steps that must be added.

6. Determine when (date) each steps should begin and end.

7. Check your dates to make sure that the correct amount of time has been allowed.

8. Consult with organizations affected by the activity; identify potential problems, opportunities, etc.

9. Specify what resources will be needed and their source.

10. Specify what constraints need to be addressed.

11. Make sure all people involved know what is expected of them and by when.

Source: National Heart, Lung and Blood Institute. *Handbook for Improving High Blood Pressure Control in the Community* (Washington, D.C.: U.S. Government Printing Office, 1977), p. 36.

- cost—an estimate of materials and time; and
- feedback—when and how to tell if the activities are working and if adjustments are needed.

Sometimes a linear timetable is used to place the activities along the line and give visual shape to the overall program. In any case, most planners have the available data on hand to implement a program. The worksheet method or action plan technique opens the door for an examination of other techniques that require structured planning for implementation such as flow charts, network diagrams, decision trees, PERT, and gaming simulations.

Flow Diagrams

At times, the planning for implementation will involve services to clients in a clinic, hospital, health center, or other type of facility. When this occurs, a diagram showing the flow of the clients through the system is helpful in the implementation process. As the flow chart

Exhibit 6-7 Worksheet for Implementation Strategy: 1

```
Worksheet for Implementation Strategy

Activity: Develop and distribute training manual for patient educators
Constraints: Deadline of 7/30. Must be accepted by Committee.

Implementation Strategy:
        (who does what)                                    (when)

    1.  Committee develops methodology                     11/10
    2.  Educator prepares draft manual                     12/10
    3.  Committee reviews draft manual                     12/20
    4.  Nine practicing educators review draft manual       1/10
    5.  Educator prepares final draft                       1/31
    6.  Artist prepares graphics                            2/15
    7.  Nine practicing educators test manual               4/15
    8.  Educator evaluates test and makes revisions         5/15
    9.  Committee approves manual                           6/1
   10.  Manual is printed                                   6/30
   11.  Manual distributed to nurses and educators          7/30
   12.  Educator evaluates training manual                  7/30
   13.
   14.
   15.
   16.
   17.
   18.
   19.
   20.
   21.
   22.
   23.
   24.
   25.
```

Source: National Heart, Lung, and Blood Institute, *Handbook for Improving High Blood Pressure Control in the Community* (Washington, D.C.: U.S. Government Printing Office, 1977), p. 33.

is being put together, the logic of the steps can be mentally tested to see if the steps reach the end result.

Consider Exhibit 6-10, a listing of five alternatives in a decision grid for an executive heart care program. Elements under consideration include the effect on mortality and disability, cost, feasibility, desirability and acceptance, and a priority decision. Alternative 3 received the first priority. Note that an exercise test, a serology exam, a psychological test, and a maintenance regimen along with referral to the client's private physician are all part of the proposed program.[17]

Now examine Exhibit 6-11, which illustrates a flow chart for new outpatients. Does this flow diagram meet the requirements of the new executive heart program? Questions could be raised as to where does

Exhibit 6-8 Worksheet for Implementation Strategy: 2

Worksheet for Implementation Strategy	
Activity: Develop a county detection and treatment center Constraints: Residents of the county have to be stimulated to come in and to undertake follow-up. Deadline 1/1 of next year.	
Implementation Strategy: (who does what)	(when)
1. Director of Ambulatory Services develops proposal for detection/treatment center	1/1
2. County Board funds proposal	3/1
3. County renovates facilities	6/1
4. Director hires staff, including administrator and medical director	6/15
5. Administrator and medical director develop protocols and procedures, including special effort to motivate residents to participate and to follow-up	8/15
6. Administrator acquires equipment and supplies	8/15
7. Data specialist develops patient record forms	9/15
8. Health educator develops education materials	9/15
9. Staff and volunteers are trained by medical director, health educator and head nurse	10/1
10. Administrator tests methods and materials with county residents	10/15
11. Staff begins detection and treatment services to county residents	11/15
12. Administrator evaluates detection and treatment services	11/15

Source: National Heart, Lung, and Blood Institute, *Handbook for Improving High Blood Pressure Control in the Community* (Washington, D.C.: U.S. Government Printing Office, 1977), p. 37.

the exercise testing, laboratory work, and the psychological testing take place. Perhaps in the box labeled clinic or service.

Another example is Exhibit 6-12, which depicts an automated multiphasic health testing sequence. Does this flow chart meet the requirements of the executive heart care proposal? Perhaps a combination of the two answers the need. The executive heart care proposal

Exhibit 6-9 Implementation with an Action Plan

An action plan detailing activities, responsibilities, and methods might be set up in the following fashion.

Short Term Objective	Activity	Responsibility	Purpose	Methods & Media
Gain support of community leaders	Interviews, conferences, written documents and articles	Health leaders, social scientists	Bring facts to attention; enlist support in solving problems	Kit of materials with statistical evidence, case histories, examples
Gain support of service groups	Talks, discussions, programs	Educators, health professionals, youth leaders, agency-based members	Bring facts to attention, involve service groups in the study and solution of problems, enlist support	Talks reinforced with written materials, audiovisuals, newsletters
Help health and welfare agencies to anticipate change & begin planning change	Seminars, workshops, study groups, conferences	Administrators, experts, policy-level board and staff	Discuss data, study present practices and needed change, enlist community for change	Wide variety of media: face-to-face and small group discussions, audiovisuals, printed materials.

Source: S.G. Deeds, *A Guidebook for Family Planning Education* (Columbia, Md.: Westinghouse Population Center, 1973), p. 56.

does have some elements of multiphasic testing and routine clinic operations.

For implementation purposes, the flow diagram logically leads to the consideration about what manpower, materials, and funding are needed at each step in the process.

Look again at Exhibit 6-11, the flow chart for new outpatients. Start with the direct travel arrows and respond to questions such as:

Exhibit 6-10 Decision Grid, Executive Heart Care Program—Target Population 5,000

Alternative	Effect on Mortality	Effect on Disability	Relative Cost	Feasibility	Desirability and Acceptance	Summary	Decision
1. Present system: treatment of acute cardiac episodes vs. prevention; inadequate early detection by private physicians	120 deaths per year, 60% considered preventable	800 disability days per year, 50% considered preventable	Dollar cost of preventable portion of morbidity and mortality as expressed in actual dollars expended for medical service: $640,000 per year		Unsatisfactory because known medical and social interventions not used, upping cost	All interested parties persuaded to modify present practices	Not recommended
2. Early detection through screening 80% of target, serology exercise tests, referral of high risk patient to own physician	10% reduction of preventable deaths	15% reduction of preventable disability	Cost: $75,000 Return: $69,000	Excellent technology and personnel available	Poses minor acceptance problems with patients, but none with attending physicians	Cost high compared with return	Not recommended
3. Above screening plus psychological testing plus recommendation of maintenance regimen to own physician	25% reduction of preventable deaths	30% reduction of preventable disability	Cost: $125,000 Return: $300,000	Requires recruitment and training of clinical psychologists to give screening test	Some resistance on part of patient to be overcome	Greatest return compared with cost. Least coercion of patient or disturbance of doctor-patient relationship	First priority

Exhibit 6-10 Continued

Alternative	Effect on Mortality	Effect on Disability	Relative Cost	Feasibility	Desirability and Acceptance	Summary	Decision
4. Above program plus group education of high risk patient in personal care program, including diet, exercise, stress prevention, plus continuing education of attending physician	30% reduction of preventable deaths	50% reduction of preventable deaths	Cost: $150,000 Return: $350,000	Requires development of education aids, such as films and videotapes. Some delay in implementation	May be difficult to obtain full participation because of lack of interest	Embraces patient responsibility, greatest potential return if screening program discontinued since patient will be motivated to continue	Second priority
5. Above program except quarterly examination, supervised group exercise, education of spouse on diet	35% reduction of preventable deaths	65% reduction of preventable disability	Cost: $300,000 Return: $415,000	Places heavy burden on available manpower	Excessive control and coercion of patient. Voluntary participation not likely to remain at level needed to obtain results	Greatest total return but burden on system and patient excessive	Not recommended

Note: This grid can be used to arrive at a decision on any problem once alternatives are defined and elements selected. At option of the user the elements may be weighted. For example, the relative cost element could be assessed a weighting factor of 2.5 times any other element, which would support alternative 3 as being of first priority.

Source: American Hospital Association, The Practice of Planning in Health Care Institutions (Chicago: AHA, 1973), pp. 56–57. Reprinted with permission. © 1973 American Hospital Association.

Is there enough parking space for the additional clients?
Do we need public conveyances to travel to the clinic?
If the clinic is to operate at night, do we have lights?
Is a parking attendant needed?
Do we need signs to direct the clients?
Is there an information person in the vestibule?
Does the control officer check for insurance coverage?
How does the control officer communicate with the clinics?
How many interview cubicles are needed?
Who does intake screening?
Can we use physician assistants in the clinic service?
Is medical social service available to all clients?
Is there a discharge officer at check out?

These are only a few of the questions triggered by the flow diagram that relate directly to the implementation of the program. One method of plotting the implementation needs is to list the steps and then fill in the chart under each heading:

Step	Manpower	Materials	Funding
Parking	Attendant	Minibus Lights	Hospital budget
Vestibule	Information clerk	Signs Mimeo directions Phone	Hospital budget Volunteers
Control	Control officer Messenger	Phone Files Forms	Hospital budget

As each step is charted, the planner can add or delete activities and requirements as ideas occur. When the planner finishes following the arrows in the flow chart, the implementation process should emerge fully documented as to what is needed for the total effort.

Mentally, the staff can go through the process using the flow chart and the accompanying data about manpower, materials, and money and give the implementation plans a dry run. This should help find any rough spots and point out needed adjustments. Of course, once the program starts, the planner should be on hand to evaluate the validity of the flow chart and the other aspects of the implementation plan.

A variation of the flow chart is shown in Exhibit 6-13. This chart shows the client flow through a rehabilitation system with the four

Exhibit 6-11 Flow for New Outpatients

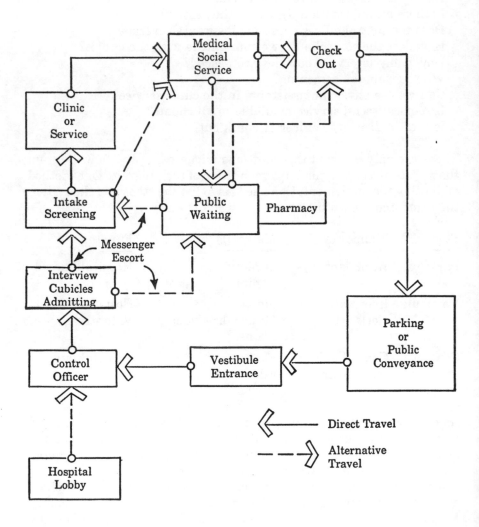

Source: Health Resources Administration, *Guidelines for Functional Programming, Equipping, and Designing Hospital Outpatient and Emergency Activities* (Washington, D.C.: U.S. Government Printing Office, 1977), p. 135.

Exhibit 6-12 Automated Multiphasic Health Testing Sequence

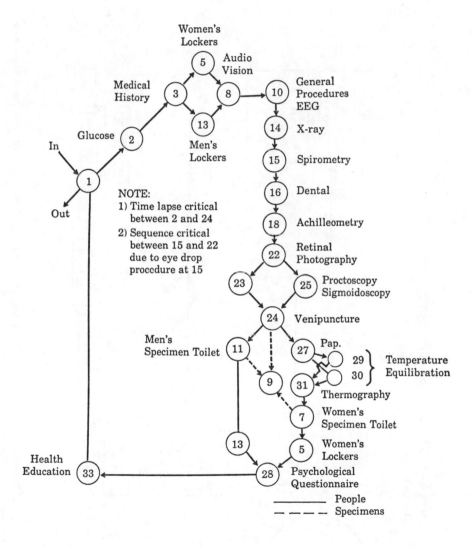

Source: Health Resources Administration, *Guidelines for Functional Programming, Equipping, and Designing Hospital Outpatient and Emergency Activities* (Washington, D.C.: U.S. Government Printing Office, 1977), p. 152.

Exhibit 6-13 Client Flow Through Rehabilitation System

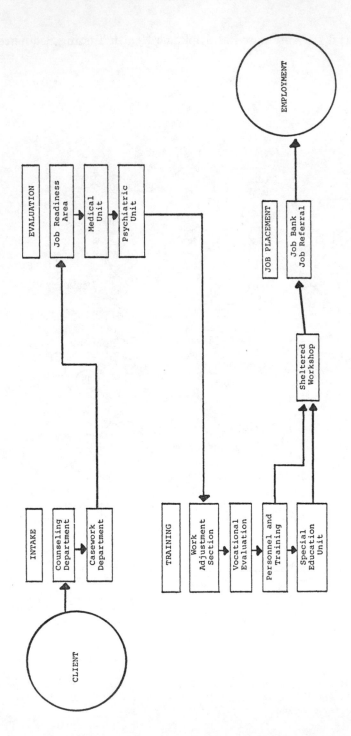

Source: G.T. Horton, V.M.E. Carr, and G.J. Corcoran, *Illustrating Services Integration from Categorical Bases*, Human Services Monograph Series of Project Share, No. 3, November 1976, p. 73.

components of intake, evaluation, training, and job placement. Each of the boxes under each of the four components could, and probably does, need a separate flow chart of its own. Each box has its own type of unit and is related to the others, yet each unit preforms a task that is different enough to require a separate method of thinking about implementation. Furthermore, each unit can have interactions with organizations outside the immediate facility, clinic, or hospital. Therefore, using a flow chart to depict an entire health care system including the public sector, the private sector, the volunteers, the social services, and all the actors in the system becomes much more complicated. In addition, many of the variables are no longer under the control or influence of the planner at the hospital or at any single agency. Nevertheless, it might be appropriate for a task force group of concerned planners to meet and work on the implementation process together. Then the same procedures utilized with the simpler flow charts could be used to everybody's advantage.

Another flow chart (Exhibit 6-14) shows the medical care appraisal model used in the state of Wisconsin and indicates the links to the PSRO and to the various committees.

A flow chart for optimum office efficiency has been developed by Hilton P. Terrell of Anderson, South Carolina.[18] Terrell, with tongue in cheek, diagrams the path of patients through a family practice center with attention to the efficiency pathway option, a few decision trees, and a time factor. Exhibit 6-15 shows this effort.

Going from a concrete example with a humorous twist to the generic abstract, Exhibit 6-16 illustrates a problem-solving technique flow chart. Five steps are covered in the flow chart: problem specification, fact finding, goals and criteria for solutions, evaluation of solutions, and implementation. Note the use of the yes/no decision and the resultant flow, as well as the use of the dead-end flow that occurs when parts of the process are rejected.

REFERRAL NETWORK DIAGRAM

A referral network diagram identifies all the organizations involved with a specific problem and diagrams the referral relations between them. In addition, the services provided by each of the agencies in what has now become a health care system are identified. For implementation purposes, this type of referral network diagram is important because all the actors and their services have to be integrated for a program to be sucessful. Furthermore, the points at which the client can enter this health care system are identified.

Exhibit 6-14 Health Service Data of Wisconsin Medical Care
Appraisal Model

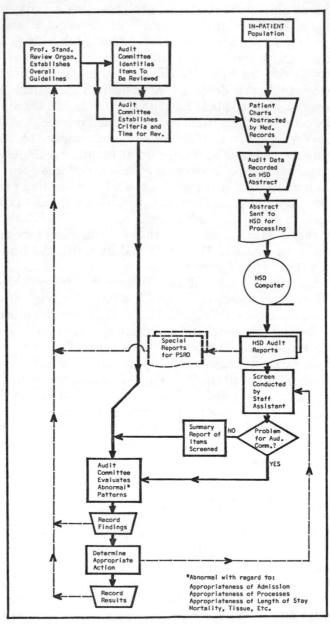

Source: S. Shindell, "The Elements of Professional Standard Review," *Journal of Legal Medicine* 1 (September-October 1973): 37.

Exhibit 6-15 Flow Chart for Optimum Office Efficiency

Tired of the same dull office routine? Then follow the protocol designed by HILTON P. TERRELL, MD, PHD, family physician, Anderson, S.C., to enliven the delivery of everyday care to ambulatory patients. FlowChart fans will find that placing the tongue firmly in the cheek before starting will further enliven the process.

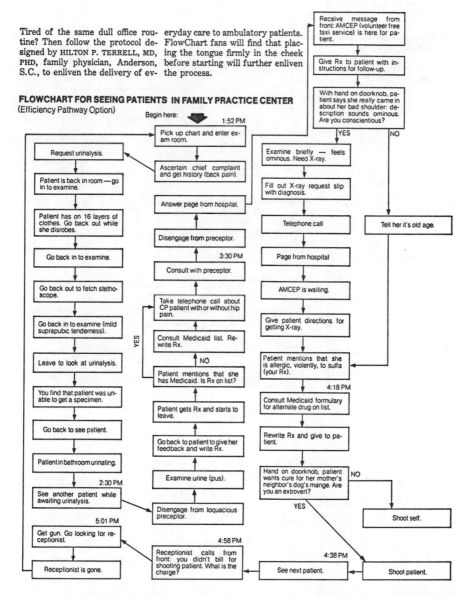

Exhibit 6-16 Problem-Solving Technique Flow Chart

I SPECIFICATION OF THE PROBLEM
II FACT-FINDING
   A. FACTUAL STATEMENT OF PROBLEM
   B. FACTUAL ANALYSIS OF CAUSES
III GOALS AND CRITERIA FOR SOLUTIONS
IV EVALUATION OF SOLUTIONS
V IMPLEMENTATION

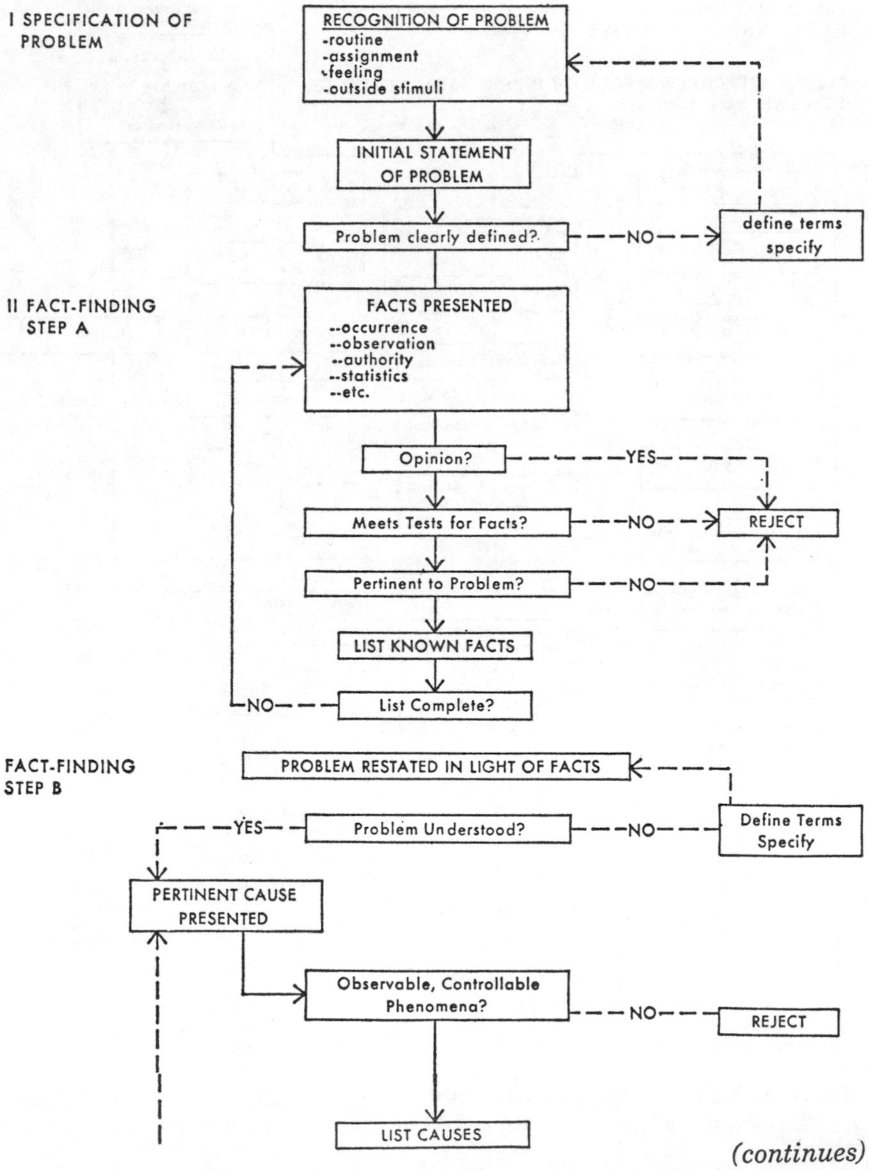

(continues)

Exhibit 6-16 Continued

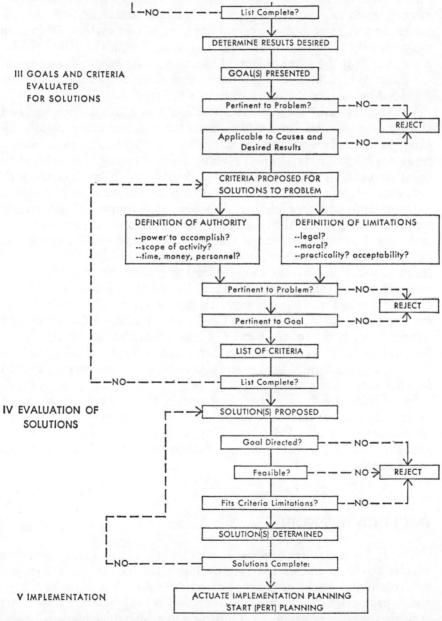

Source: M.F. Arnold, ed., *Health Program Implementation Through PERT* (San Francisco: American Public Health Association, 1966), pp. 28–29. Reprinted with permission. © 1966, American Public Health Association.

Consider Exhibit 6-17, a referral network dealing with illegitimate births. Note the two-way referrals in this system as well as the points of entry such as schools, welfare or health departments, and private physicians. Also note the criminal element in this system. (This does not mean that the health planner has to deal with the criminal element, but that the planner should be aware of its existence and possible effect on the implementation program being considered.) Services provided by each of the organizations are listed.

With the referral diagram, the points of entry into the system, and the services of each agency identified, the planner can consider the problem of implementing a program to improve health care for the newborn illegitimate child. Private physicians might be the focal point, except that the woman with an illegitimate child might not seek care early enough. Health and welfare departments also might be late entrants into the care picture. Schools could implement an educational campaign, but that would require postponed action since the girls might be too young or not ready to take action until they became pregnant. In this case, the focal point might be the hospital. True, the hospital would not see the women until they were ready to give birth, but this could still be the point at which all the other referral units cross and a logical program could be implemented. The implementation activity would have to deal with the newborn after birth and hopefully with the future health of mother and child. However, the hospital could interact with the other organizations and take the lead in initiating a program that would touch the entire health care system for this particular problem.

In utilizing a referral network approach, the planner secures more assistance toward determining the focus of an implementation effort rather than the actual details of implementation itself. Yet, this is valuable since a program that is launched from the wrong base might never succeed.

DECISION NETWORK

The decision network approach considers that implementation must involve the examination of all the decisions related to a specific project or program. A decision chart, logical flow diagram, branched logic chart, protocol, decision tree, or algorithm is diagramed in flow chart style with a beginning and an ending point within which is encompassed a complete action or sets of action where decisions are made. At each decision point, a "binary logic" form is used to answer questions with a

Exhibit 6-17 Referral Network — Illegitimate Births

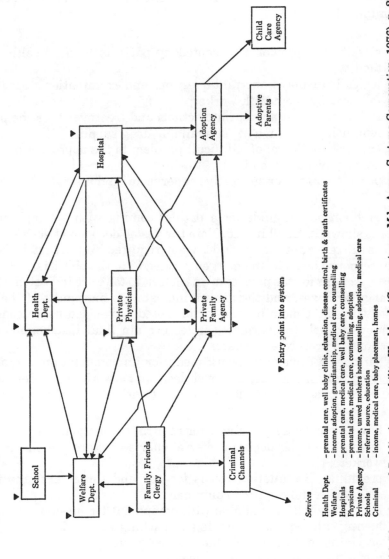

▶ Entry point into system

Services

Health Dept. – prenatal care, well baby clinic, education, disease control, birth & death certificates
Welfare – income, adoption, guardianship, medical care, counselling
Hospitals – prenatal care, medical care, well baby care, counselling
Physician – prenatal care, medical care, counselling, adoption
Private Agency – income, unwed mothers home, counselling, adoption, medical care
Schools – referral source, education
Criminal – income, medical care, baby placement, homes

Source: *Health Planning and Public Accountability Workbook* (Germantown, Md.: Aspen Systems Corporation, 1976), p. 270. Reprinted with permission.

yes or no, present-absent, more than-less than or another alternative to guide the patient's path through the clinic, service, or office.

Problem-action guidelines[19] for a physician's assistant illustrate a decision flow chart network. These decision networks help to accomplish the following:

- classify the problems presented by patients to the health care facility;
- logically display important questions and examination steps to be followed by the health worker;
- isolate the most appropriate actions and treatments for the problem, using a limited set of available drug supplies;
- encourage referral of a difficult problem to the appropriate workers or physicians; and
- provide a basis for supportive supervision and inservice training.

A problem action guide for a patient coming with a complaint of fever is shown in Exhibit 6-18. Note the yes/no decision at each step as well as the referral to other guides when required. At the first decision, a yes response leads to an emergency referral to the physician (shaded elipse). Actions for the physician's assistant to take are indicated in the rectangular boxes, and the arrows indicate the movement of the patient (with the time after the action noted). Six-sided boxes contain questions to ask the patient. Circles contain final instructions and directions to proceed elsewhere.

What does a decision network mean for implementation purposes? Referring to Exhibit 6-18, the fever decision network, implementation of this type of service means including attention to the following:

- having physicians available for referral of emergencies;
- having the other decision referral charts available for the health workers;
- providing examination rooms for ear and throat examinations along with the required equipment;
- having penicillin available with equipment for injections;
- having chloroquine available and packing materials;
- providing materials to do blood smears; and
- providing materials to treat fevers.

These aspects of the implementation relate only to the specific actions noted on the decision network. However, further consideration should raise other implementation activities, such as:

Exhibit 6-18   Fever Flow Chart

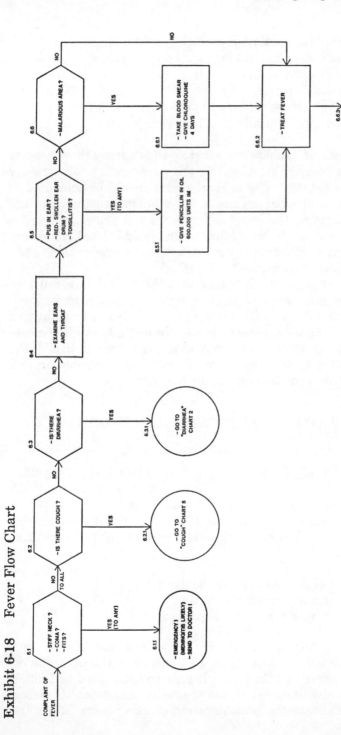

Source: Reprinted with permission of Management Sciences for Health, a nonprofit foundation, from N. Hirschhorn, J. Lamstein and R. O'Connor, *Problem-Action Guidelines for Basic Health Care,* 1974.

- charts required for medical records,
- additional personnel needed for laboratory analysis,
- how to store drugs and equipment,
- cleaning up the facilities,
- what to do about those allergic to penicillin, and
- how to assure inpatient admission for emergencies.

These implementation problems are merely illustrative; they indicate how a decision network chart allows for the consideration of a strategy for initiating the activity. The referral charts should be consulted to see if they raise additional elements to be integrated into any implementation program. The cough referral chart is shown in Exhibit 6-19. Immediately it can be noted that there are additional laboratory tests, medications, another emergency situation, and referrals to additional decision chart networks.

Utilizing a decision network means that the logical flow must be internally consistent, completely unambiguous, and the major decisions should be diagramed with all the yes/no decisions brought to a logical conclusion. All the alternatives must be plotted as well to create a comprehensive treatment diagram. Once this is accomplished, the planner can proceed to prepare the resources, money, manpower, and materials required to implement the diagramed project.

A PLANNING AND DEVELOPMENT FRAMEWORK (PADFRAME)

Although PADFRAME was designed for classifying organized medicine, the methodology can be applied to any existing group. PADFRAME[20] is designed to help organize, to clarify purpose, to set future directions, and to delineate specific activities, programs, and services. A framework and a process for implementation are provided by three main determinants:

- identification of segments of the health system,
- listing of program characteristics, and
- specification of implementation approaches.

Segments of the health care system have been cast in numerous classifications for a variety of reasons. In this case, the planning organization can choose one that suits it best, as illustrated in Exhibit 6-20. What this identification of the segments of the health system does is merely indicate the possible areas of interest for future im-

Exhibit 6-19   Cough Referral Flow Chart

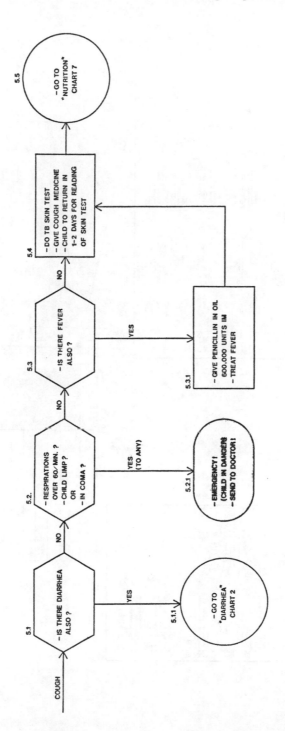

Source: Reprinted with permission of Management Sciences for Health, a nonprofit foundation, from N. Hirschhorn, J. Lamstein and R. O'Connor, *Problem-Action Guidelines for Basic Health Care,* 1974.

Exhibit 6-20 Program Development Worksheet and PADFRAME Dimensions. A, segments of health system; B, program characteristics; C, implementation approaches.

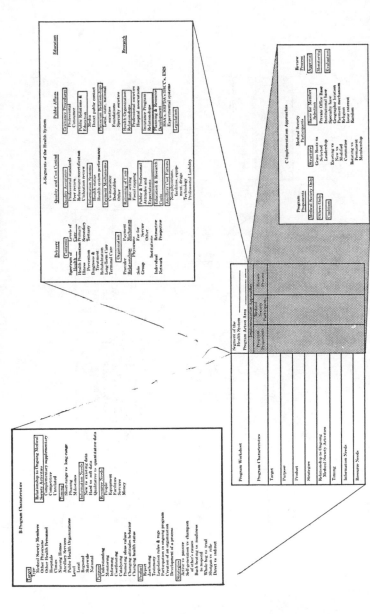

Source: G. Stuehler, Jr., "Organizing Organized Medicine Through a Planning and Development Framework (PADFRAME)," *Journal of the American Medical Association* 237 (1977):1591. Reprinted with permission. © 1977, American Medical Association.

plementation activities. Note that there are major categories with subsets and further divisions.

Program characteristics take a more direct approach to the implementation of activities. Exhibit 6-20 illustrates the type of information on a listing of program characteristics. Note that a target audience is listed along with the geographic level at which the program takes place. Under the heading of purpose, a generalized concept of the goal or objective can be noted. In addition, this listing calls attention to timing, resource needs, information needs, relationships, the product, and the strategies that might be used in program implementation.

Six strategies are noted, and each deserves some explanation. Each strategy is cited as the end point of a continuum, but there are, of course, shades in between that can take place.

- An *active* program means that the organization initiates and continues the program; a *passive* activity would generally respond to outside controls and influences.
- A *self-generated* activity would be conceptualized by the organization, led by it, and publicly identified with the agency. A *champion of other's causes* means that the organization supports the efforts of others, either publicly or privately.
- A *bush-beating* program tries to drum up interest and concern for the issue the agency wishes to address; a *readiness to respond* strategy requires that data and positions be developed in anticipation of questions or invitations to respond to the issue.
- Taking on the entire program at the begining is a *whole hog* strategy; a *trial* basis allows for taking on a part of a program on a small scale.
- A program directed at a large indiscriminate group or a number of different aspects indicates a *shotgun* approach. A *rifle* approach aims at a highly selective target or at a specific aspect of a program.
- Attacking an activity head-on seeking to affect it *directly* or attacking the problem *indirectly* through a secondary goal that eventually reaches the desired effect are two other strategies.

As noted, any of these strategies could be part of implementation planning; all should be weighed for possible use in a program.

Specification of implementation approaches takes into account the proponents of the program and the participants from both a structural basis and the basis for selection of participants (see Exhibit 6-20). Note the types of structures indicated. In addition, the implementation approaches include the review process, activities of monitoring, approval, and evaluation. In any implementation program, there must be a

Exhibit 6-21 Program Implementation Through PERT

1. DETERMINING SPECIFIC OUTCOME
2. DETERMINING PRECEDENT EVENTS
3. ORDER PRECEDENT EVENTS
   Include a Network
4. DETERMINATION OF ACTIVITY TIME
   Sub-PERT·if necessary
5. ALLOCATION OF PRIORITY EVENTS
   Include Major Computations
6. COMPLETION OF PROGRAM

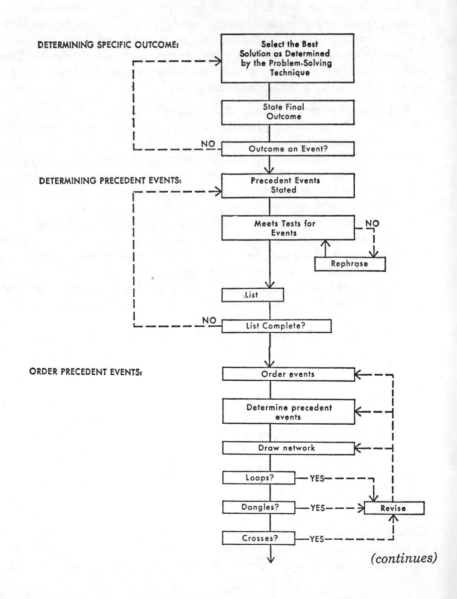

(continues)

Exhibit 6-21 Continued

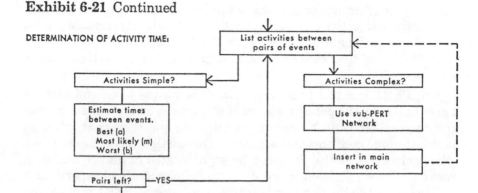

Source: M.F. Arnold, ed., *Health Program Implementation Through PERT* (San Francisco: American Public Health Association, 1966), pp. 44-45. Reprinted with permission. © 1966, American Public Health Association.

built-in ability to monitor the process and to make any required adjustments.

In totality, the PADFRAME technique acts as a stimulus to planning and as a creative effort toward the organization of the implementation activity.

PROGRAM EVALUATION AND REVIEW TECHNIQUE (PERT)

PERT is a tool to be used in planning. It is not a panacea or mechanized answer to how to do health planning. Generally, PERT is most useful in planning the implementation phase of a project. In essence, PERT allows the planner to develop a map plotting future activities that result in a network-type diagram so the flow of events can be seen in totality.

According to E.T. Alsaker,[21] PERT's graphic network analysis consists of:

1. the development of a model or activity network of a proposed program or part of a program;
2. the evaluation of the network and adjustment of it to provide a

degree of assurance that there will be a minimum of risk in reaching the objective on time and within the limits of acceptable cost if the implementation PERT plan is followed; and

3. the use of the network to monitor and control the activity represented.

Yet, PERT is a tool that emphasizes the means to an end already agreed upon by the policy makers. Management tools, no matter what they are called, cannot resolve the intricate questions that relate to political-value problems and decisions. There will always be executives who review the results produced by sophisticated hardware and then make their own decision based upon their judgment and experience.

However, once the decision is made, tools such as PERT provide the structured framework to produce a logical, ordered plan to carry out the decision. A flow chart showing program implementation through PERT is shown is Exhibit 6-21. This chart will be understood more clearly after checking the PERT terminology list (Exhibit 6-21A); explanation of the loops, dangles, and crosses (Exhibit 6-21B); and the step-by-step development of a PERT network (Exhibit 6-21C). Note that during the step-by-step development, there are additional references to other exhibits that illustrate how the steps are carried out.

In going over the steps in developing a PERT network, it is suggested that readers familiarize themselves with the exhibits and diagrams. This will certainly allow for an easier understanding of the methodology. In fact, as the steps are presented, it might be enlightening to refer back to the exhibit or diagram rather than to continue on through to the end of the procedure.

A PERT network for the development of an open heart surgery unit is illustrated in Exhibit 6-25. Starting with the decision to develop the capability, the PERT diagram follows through to the final event of having the equipment and team tested and ready. Note the critical path and the time estimates.

GAMING SIMULATIONS FOR IMPLEMENTATION

Games and simulations are common everyday situations. Monopoly is a familiar game and a part of the cultural scene, with jokes about owning Boardwalk or Park Place. Similarly, simulations became everyday occurrences as the space program progressed and the television stations broadcast simulations of rocket flights and moon landings.

Exhibit 6-21A PERT Terminology List

Final event or specific outcome—The event that signifies the completion of the program or the attainment of the goal.

Event—A factual statement of completion of an activity or series of activities. Events take no time or action and are not descriptions of an activity in progress. "Hospital clinic opened" is an event; "ordering supplies for clinic" is an activity in progress. Events are shown by numbers in network diagrams.

Activity—Actions between events that determine the time, effort, and personnel necessary to move from one event to the next. Represented on network diagram by the arrows between events.

Precedent event—An event that comes immediately before the event in question. All events but the first in a program have one or more precedent events.

Successor event—The event that comes immediately after the event in question. All events but the last in the program (final event) have one or more successor events.

Sequence number—The position of each event in the entire program and its relation to the other events.

Network—A system of diagramming the flow of events from the begining event to the final events. A network diagram consists of (1) sequence numbers indicating the sequence of events; (2) arrows designating activities required before proceeding to the next event; and (3) parallel paths representing a series of events taking place during a specific time sequence and an independent series of activities necessary in relation to the attached events.

Critical path—Series of activities and events that require the most time.

Source: Reprinted with permission from M.F. Arnold, ed., *Health Program Implementation Through PERT* (San Francisco: American Public Health Association), pp. 36-37. © 1966, American Public Health Association.

In combining games with simulations, the planner attempts to duplicate the real world and yet maintain the attraction of a game. Through the use of a gaming simulation technique, the health planner can test out a variety of implementation ideas and learn from a miniature dry run of the proposed activity. A number of alternative implementation strategies can be tested as well as a number of suggested implementation activities. With the knowledge acquired from the gaming simulation, the planner can then proceed to set the implementation process into the real situation. Gaming simulations can reveal the bugs and quirks of the proposed activity and allow the planner to

Exhibit 6-21B   Loops, Dangles, and Crosses

Three problems may occur in plotting the network diagram: loops, dangles, and crosses.

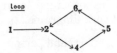

Events have not been clearly ordered. Successor events must be done before a precedent event can be done. The solution for a loop is to reorder the events in a more logical sequence with better determination of preceding events.

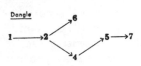

There is no successor event for event number 6. Therefore, event number 6 does not attach itself to the rest of the network diagram. As 6 stands now, it is not required for the completion of the program. Solution is to reevaluate the preceding events to locate a successor event. If 6 is not needed, it should be dropped.

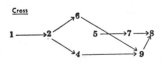

This may be more mechanical than a problem with the program. The network diagram should be redrawn to eliminate the cross.

Source: Reprinted with permission from M.F. Arnold, ed., *Health Program Implementation Through PERT* (San Francisco: American Public Health Association, 1966) pp. 36-37. © 1966, American Public Health Association.

Exhibit 6-21C Steps in Developing a PERT Network

1. Specification of final event	A final event indicates the conclusion of the activity. No more action should take place after the final event. Furthermore, the final event should be tangible and physical, such as "diabetes clinic opened" or "immunizations given to 75 percent of the children."
2. Determination of precedent events	Working backward from the final event, simply list all the other events that have to take place prior to the final event. Do not worry about the order of events now but just list every activity that must take place to lead up to the final event. In the diabetes clinic example, events might include hiring staff, renovating the facility, securing a budget, training staff, publicity and information activities, and printing forms. Activities may be added by experts or consultants as the list is circulated for comments and suggestions.
3. Ordering precedent events and diagraming the network	Take the list of events prepared in step 2 and start to arrange the events in a logical sequence starting with the final event (determined in step 1) and work backward to the beginning event, which will be step 1. As you rewrite the events, to the left of each event write the number indicating the order in which these events must occur. Now you have a sequence listing of the events to the left of the events.
	To the right of each event write the number of the event or events that must come immediately before the event in question if that event is to take place. At this point, consider only the event immediately preceding the specific event under question (see the example in Exhibit 6-22). Note that there is some interdependence relative to several events such as # 10, 13, 24, and 25. Taking

Exhibit 6-21C Continued

	the sequenced events, a network of flow diagram can be prepared (see Exhibit 6-23).
4. Determination of activity time	This step is concerned with how much time it will take to move from one event to another (Exhibit 6-24). Here it is vital to have expert knowledge about all the activities required to reach the next event. Since there will be differences between the planners as to the amount of time required to perform the activities, a mathematical formula is used as follows:

$$t_e = \frac{a + 4m + b}{6},$$

	where t_e is time estimate; m is normal time, a is minimum time, and b is maximum time.
5. Determine critical path	By selecting the priority events, the critical path of the PERT network can be determined. This is usually marked by a heavier line tracing the events from initiation to the final event. Without the events taking place in the critical path as noted, the final event cannot take place.
6. Complete program	Initiate the activities, follow the network diagram, monitor the events, make adjustments as required, and reach the final event.

Source: Reprinted with permission from M.F. Arnold, ed., *Health Program Implementation Through PERT* (San Francisco: American Public Health Association, 1966) pp. 36–37. © 1966, American Public Health Association.

---

prepare resolutions for the difficulties. However, gaming simulations used by health planners differ radically from those played solely with a computer. Most often, the health planners' gaming simulation will use human participants; therefore, the technique is open to all man's frailties. Despite this constraint, the gaming simulation can be a valuable technique in planning for implementation.

Gaming simulations come in a variety of shapes and sizes with a broad spectrum of purposes. However, a number of common structural

Exhibit 6-22 Ordering Precedent Events

Program: Augment DPT-Polio immunization services to lower socioeconomic groups in the county.

Final Event: 50 percent of the preschool children in lower socioeconomic groups in the county immunized against DPT-Polio.

Sequence No.	Event	Preceding Event
27	Final event (outcome)	25, 26
26	Vaccine made available to private physicians	17
25	Outside clinic sites opened	18, 19, 20, 24
24	Health dept. hours expanded	22, 23
23	Medical supplies obtained	14
22	Home visits organized	21
21	Mobile teams established (Dr., nurse, health educator, clerk)	16
20	Volunteers recruited and oriented	13
19	Support of community organizations obtained	13
18	Mass media support obtained	13
17	Support of private physicians secured	13
16	Educational materials produced	15
15	Priorities established for previously identified target groups	13
14	General departments oriented	13
13	Program personnel trained	11, 12
12	Office supplies and equipment obtained	10
11	Personnel recruited	10
10	Board of supervisors approval secured	9
9	County budget submitted	8
8	County budget prepared	7
7	County budget discussed with county administration	6
6	Project application approved by state health department	5

Exhibit 6-22 Continued

5	Application for funds submitted	4
4	Application for funds prepared	3
3	Plan developed	2
2	Decision made to apply for federal grant	1
1	Meeting held to consider program	0

Source: Reprinted with permission from M.F. Arnold, ed., *Health Program Implementation Through PERT* (San Francisco: American Public Health Association, 1966) pp. 36–37. © 1966, American Public Health Association.

components can be found in most that are a central part of the technique. Key components are emphasized in the following requirements:

- participants cast in *roles*;
- *interactions* between those participants in their roles;
- *rules* governing the interaction between the participants while playing their roles;
- *goal(s)* with respect to which the interactions occur; and
- a *criterion* for determining the attainment of the goal, which also indicates the end of the game or simulation.

A game has also been defined as any contest (play) among adversaries (players) operating under constraints (rules) for an objective (winning). A simulation is a representation of reality in which participants assume roles that are assigned to them, and through a series of scheduled meetings they attempt to define the nature and extent of the problem and the goals of the community for dealing with that problem. Both the requirements and the definitions embrace the same principles, which require vital elements in the system to be identified and created in a manner that represents a simplified slice of reality.

Roles refer to the identities the participants are asked to assume for the duration of the gaming simulation. Planners must provide the participants with enough of a description of the role that the player can really assume the part. Players must be cautioned to maintain their role at all times and not revert to their real-life situation. Exhibit 6-26A depicts the role of a blood banker in the hemophilia Blood Money game[22] (Exhibit 6-26). Appendix B details a community drug education game; the role of a psychiatrist is outlined for a participant.

Interactions are the vital part of the gaming simulation because the planner is looking to learn how the real world participants will react in

(Text continues on page 298.)

Exhibit 6-23 Diagramming the PERT Network

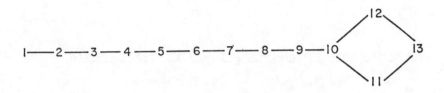

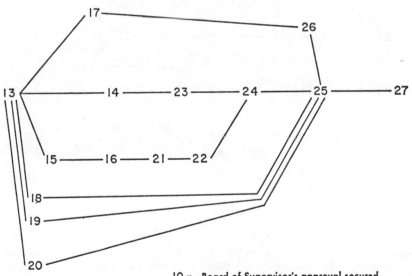

10 –. Board of Supervisor's approval secured

13 – Program personnel trained

25– Outside clinic sites opened

Source: Reprinted with permission from M.F. Arnold, ed., *Health Program Implementation Through PERT (San Francisco: American Public Health Association, 1966), p. 38.* © 1966, American Public Health Association.

Exhibit 6-24 PERT Network for Immunization Program with Activity Time Noted

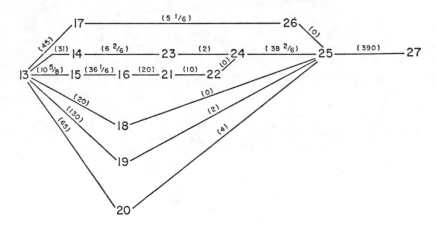

Exhibit 6-25 PERT Network for Development of Open Heart Surgery Unit

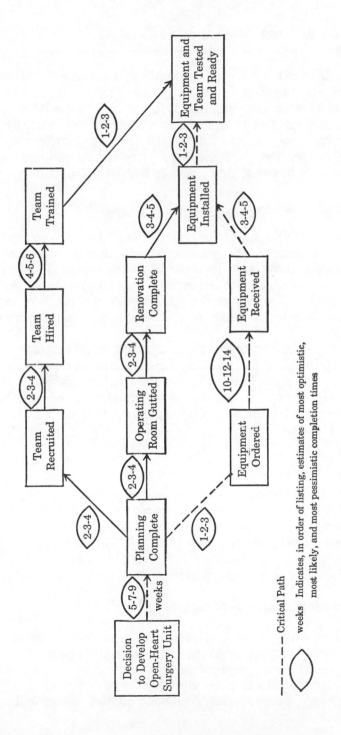

Source: B.B. Longest, Jr., *Management Practices for the Health Professional* (Reston, Va.: Reston Publishing Company, 1976), p. 101. Reprinted with permission. © 1976, Reston Publishing Co.

Exhibit 6-26 Blood Money Gaming Simulation

BLOOD MONEY is a gaming-simulation, but as is often the case, we shall refer to it in the following pages in simplified terms as a "game." It should be clear, however, that it is a game of a special sort, promising not only the fun of typical game play, but the learning possible from active involvement with a model of a segment of reality. It combines, therefore, the playfulness of a game and the seriousness of daily life. We attempt to use the former to illuminate the latter.

B. What's in This Game: Subject and Purpose

BLOOD MONEY simulates on an abstract level the general character of the experience of the hemophiliac and those who provide him with care and blood. It is designed to convey a general understanding of issues and problems in hemophilia care so players can more fully comprehend the worlds of the patient and of those working in the health care sector when these are described in subsequent talks or readings.

In some ways, play of this game, like play of others, is fun. In other ways BLOOD MONEY is not as enjoyable, since it models or simulates experiences that are frustrating and difficult for those who live them in real life. In any case, it has proven an interesting and valuable learning experience for those who have participated, and we are sure you will find it so as well.

C. Who Can Play?

While the specific disease around which the game is built is hemophilia, those who have participated in early runs have suggested that there are many general elements of the patient and care systems in the game that pertain to other diseases. Thus it provides a learning vehicle for those whose concern is not with hemophilia per se, but with the nature, operation, and dilemmas of the health care delivery system.

Appropriate audiences of players include:

1. Those who deal with hemophiliacs and desire a greater understanding of their problems and perspectives—e.g.:
   a. medical and paramedical staff;
   b. secretarial and other staff members;
   c. clinic, hospital, and blood bank administrators and staff;

Exhibit 6-26 Continued

    d. parents and other relatives of hemophiliacs; and

    e. employers, teachers, school administrators, etc.

2. Those who will be dealing with patients—i.e., those in training for or anticipating any of the roles above, such as medical and nursing students.

3. Others interested in understanding hemophilia—e.g.:

    a. blood donors or potential donors, and

    b. other citizens.

4. Students of health—i.e., those interested in problems of the delivery of health care services or elements of the "sick role:"

    a. upper elementary school, junior high school, and senior high school students studying these questions;

    b. college and graduate school students in sociology, psychology, health, etc., courses; and

    c. psychologists and psychiatrists interested in the relationships between physical and mental illness.

5. Policy makers:

    a. local officials,

    b. state and national health care administrators, and

    c. state and national representatives and administrators charged with the development or passage of health care legislation.

The game remains exactly the same for play with these disparate groups. Differences in the experience and knowledge of the participants is brought to bear in the differential character of the postplay discussion-critique and in the follow-up materials presented. It should be noted that the game is *not* designed to be played by persons with hemophilia, although we have, on occasion, invited them to participate by playing the roles of those in charge of delivery of care, while "real life" doctors and others in the delivery system played patients.

D. Number of Players

The game is played optimally with a group of 24–28. As will be described later, however, groups of 20–23 or of 29–35 can be accommodated.

E. Running the Game—Personnel Needed

Two operators are required to run the game. Both should be familiar with it from a thorough reading of this manual. It is strongly recommended that an assistant be recruited to take over some of the respon-

Exhibit 6-26 Continued

sibilities of Operator No. 2. This assistant need not understand the game in its entirety nor be aware of the underlying assumptions of the model. He or she can be "trained" in five minutes, and thus one of the players can be recruited to play this role if numbers permit.

F. Time Requirement

The context of use will vary depending upon the audience (players). For students, it will comprise part of a larger educational program, and be run within normal or extended class periods. For others, it will most often be used as a self-contained program of approximately two and a half hours duration.

The following indicates approximate times needed for play:

1. Introduction: 15 minutes;
2. Play of two rounds: 1 hour 30 minutes;
3. Discussion: minimum 30 minutes;
4. Follow up: as much time as desired, or via printed material that can be taken home and read.

Although it would be best to include all steps in the same time period, it is possible to schedule steps 1 and 2 for one day (one class) and hold the discussion and follow-up soon thereafter (the next class).

G. Space Requirement

One large room is required for play of the game. The furniture must be movable. A number of chairs and approximately seven small tables are needed. A chart for room setup is provided later in the manual.

H. Materials Requirement

The game has been constructed to consist of standard materials that can be easily located and cheaply purchased. All paper materials needed (e.g., role descriptions and charts) are provided in this manual. The number of copies of each page you will need to photocopy is indicated at the top of the page. All purchased materials and most of the paper materials are reusable. Players may, however, occasionally write on the paper materials and you may have to reproduce more for subsequent runs of the game.

Source: C.S. Greenblat and J.H. Gagnon, *Blood Money: A Gaming-Simulation of the Problems of Hemophilia and Health Care Delivery Systems* (Washington, D.C.: U.S. Government Printing Office, 1976).

Exhibit 6-26A Role Sheet

BLOOD BANKERS

Goals: You are in charge of the very limited supply of available blood and are responsible for disseminating it. The blood is represented by *red* chips. You will get new supplies from Operator #2 at the beginning of each round, but the amount of chips will vary depending on the number of donors to the system as a whole (beyond your control) and on your efficiency in dissemination and collection of payment. Inefficiency will lead to cuts in supplies.

You operate one blood bank together and should make joint decisions and divide the work. At least one of you should be present at the bank at all times. Your joint goal is to operate the bank as well as possible to serve the community.

Charges: Yours is a nonprofit operation. Although the blood has been donated, there have been considerable administrative costs incurred in its collection, analysis, storage, treatment, etc., resulting in the necessity to charge for each unit. The basic (and minimum) charge is 2 white chips for each unit of blood (each red chip). The check on your efficiency will be to ascertain whether you have collected twice as many white chips as the number of red chips you have distributed, or have arrangements to collect them soon. You will have to set up your own accounting system.

Welfare agents may ask for proof that their clients have received blood.

Dissemination: Patients should be given blood *only* upon presentation of a prescription from a doctor. These prescriptions should be on yellow papers and must be written with green felt markers and signed by the doctor.

If, at any time, you feel you do not have enough blood on hand to fill the prescription that a citizen presents to you, you may give the patient *less* than is prescribed or send the citizen back to the doctor for a reduced prescription. You should understand, however, that the amount of blood prescribed is *critical* to the further health of these citizens, and that they are in need of getting it in the *right amount* and *very soon* after an attack if they are to avoid extensive further disability.

Source: C.S. Greenblat and J.H. Gagnon, *Blood Money: A Gaming-Simulation of the Problems of Hemophilia and Health Care Delivery Systems* (Washington, D.C.: U.S. Government Printing Office, 1976).

Exhibit 6-26B Senario Material

HEW NEWS

U.S. DEPARTMENT OF HEALTH, EDUCATION, AND WELFARE

PRESS RELEASE   National Institutes of Health
Monday, March 10, 1975   William E. Sanders (301) 496-5343

WASHINGTON, D.C.—Congress today overwhelmingly approved
an all-inclusive Catastrophic Disease National Health Insurance Act.
In a carefully orchestrated move by Senate and House leaders, the
compromise bill, which had gone to a conference committee to resolve
differences, was introduced and passed by the two Houses in the same
day. Leaders of both Houses stated that the large congressional majority assures the President will sign the new compromise bill into law, or
face a certain veto override.

Never again, said the bill's supporters, will Americans be made to
suffer financially from debilitating disease. All U.S. citizens and residents will be covered under the Catastrophic Disease Health Insurance
program.

NEW PAYROLL TAX

The new program will be financed by a 3.5% tax on employers'
payrolls, a 1% tax on employees, and 2.5% on the self-employed up to
$20,000, with the remainder coming from general revenues. All
monies collected are to be paid into the National Catastrophic Health
Insurance Fund. The Fund will be administered by the newly created
Catastrophic Disease Health Insurance Board established under the
Department of Health, Education, and Welfare.

The Board will be advised by the new Catastrophic Disease Health
Insurance Council composed of a representative group of·consumers,
providers, health organization personnel, and other interested parties.

MEDICARE AND MEDICAID STAY

Both the Medicare and Medicaid programs that provide preventive
and catastrophic benefits will remain intact, except that the same
benefits established under the Catastrophic Disease National Health
Insurance Act will be extended to include these programs. It is likely
that Federal and/or State representatives involved in administering
these programs will sit on the Catastrophic Health Insurance Council.

Exhibit 6-26B Continued

BENEFITS

The Act provides that the first $500 spent annually on medical care must be borne by the family or individual suffering from the disease. Thereafter, the government will pay for necessary disease-related treatment—all physician care, hospital days, outpatient care, nursing home stays, supportive services, rehabilitation needs, psychiatric care, inpatient and outpatient drugs including blood and blood products, and prosthetic devices. The program does not cover health needs unrelated to the disease.

REIMBURSEMENT

Reimbursement will be similar to the current Medicare program. The physician bills the patient who files a claim for the reasonable cost allowed by Medicare. Under the Catastrophic Disease program, reasonable cost can be determined by the Catastrophic Disease Health Insurance Board in advisement with the Catastrophic Disease Health Insurance Council.

$25 MILLION FOR PLANNING

The actual start-up date for the Catastrophic Disease National Health Insurance program will be January 1, 1977. Until then, the Act calls for the expenditure of $25 million over a two-year period to plan in detail how the program will work. It is hoped that with adequate planning the program will run smoothly once it is implemented.

Instructions on Questions To Be Addressed and Statements To Be Prepared by Players

Keeping in mind the role you are playing, there are three questions you need to consider with respect to the news you have just heard. At the end of 45 minutes, we need from each group a detailed statement about these three questions to be presented to the group as a whole for its discussion and debate. Following that there will be a short period for reformulations in light of what others have said; and, finally, a brief discussion of these reformulations will take place before we move to the next event.

The questions all have reference to the *first year following the event* and are as follows:

Exhibit 6-26B Continued

1. How will this event affect you?
2. What will you do or try to do because of it? (i.e., How will you alter your behavior, operations, etc.?)
3. What should others in the system do about it? (Product, Care, Payment, and Research and Education interests)

Please try to be as specific as you can in responding to these questions. We hope you will work to define the common elements of your responses through discussion in each group, but minority reports on any dimensions are perfectly appropriate where there is dissent.

Let me also note that we are placing an observer at each table to help collect more detailed reports than you will be able to make in the open discussion. These people will not be interfering in the discussions.

SESSION II
April 24, 1975

I. Instructions of Players

Today's events are a continuation of the events that occurred in the game you participated in last month. For those of you who were not here then, you represent yourself and your type of interest or constituency.

To bring you up to date and to remind everyone of what has occurred before, I will read a summary of events that have happened to medical benefits for hemophilia. As you know, on March 10, 1975, Congress passed the all inclusive Catastrophic Disease National Health Insurance Act. The Act provided for full coverage of hemophilia and all hemophilia-related health needs once the patient or his family paid for the first $500 of care. The program financed by a tax on employer's payrolls and a smaller tax on the self-employed and employees, with the remainder coming from general revenues paid into a Trust Fund. It is administrated through the Department of Health, Education, and Welfare by the Catastrophic Disease Health Insurance Board, which is advised by the Catastrophic Disease Health Insurance Council composed of a representative group of consumers, providers, health organization personnel, and other interested parties. The Act was put into effect in January 1977, following a two-year planning period.

Once the program began, many more hemophiliacs sought care than had been expected. In fact, 13,000 hemophilic patients previously unknown to the system came for treatment. Half of these patients were

Exhibit 6-26B Continued

moderate hemophiliacs who wanted more adequate and frequent treatment. The other half were severe hemophiliacs suffering the chronic effects of hemophilia. These severe hemophiliacs as a group were older, poorer, less skilled, and mainly rural people who had severe disabilities and were seeking adequate treatment for the first time.

Both the moderate and the severe hemophiliac stressed the hemophilia care system very directly. The older, severe group required a great deal of orthopedic surgery, dental care, and psychological and vocational rehabilitation. The moderate patients, like the severe patients, required full diagnostic work-ups and, in the beginning, considerable monitoring of their disease.

The influx of these 13,000 additional hemophiliacs into the system was felt by Congress during the third year of the Catastrophic Disease Health Insurance Program. Congress became alarmed over the amount of money that was going to pay for hemophilia treatment in proportion to the rest of its health care dollar. Rather than changing the payment mechanism or controlling the quality of treatment, Congress decided that the government would continue to pay either to the patient or the patient's doctor a fixed upper limit of $5,000 per hemophilic patient in any given year.

II. Presentation of Scenario 2

Now, with this in mind, I will read the first "News Bulletin."

15 HEMOPHILIA CENTERS TO BE ESTABLISHED

Responding to pressure to improve care within the $5,000 limit set for each hemophiliac, Congress has authorized the Department of Health, Education, and Welfare to establish 15 comprehensive care centers across the United States. Each center will offer comprehensive care, have a complete diagnosis unit able to do both diagnostic tests and genetic testing, and will engage in research, education, and training.

Forty-five million dollars has been appropriated by Congress to establish the 15 centers. Each center will cost approximately $3 million to build. Operating expenses will be funded in part by government money—the first $5,000 of care each hemophiliac receives under Catastrophic National Health Insurance. Ten percent of the income obtained by each center must be spent on research. Each center is free to decide how much of its budget it wishes to allocate for education and training.

Attendance at these centers will be voluntary; neither the patient nor the doctor will have to use the services provided at these centers. The doctor-patient relationship, if it is satisfactory to both parties, would not be disturbed.

Each center will have a patient population of approximately 2,500 hemophiliacs. The 2,500 patient population figure is based on the known number of hemophiliacs seeking care: 38,500. Thus, if 2,500 patients all require the government allotted benefit of $5,000 per hemophiliac, the center's total operating budget would be $12.5 million. For all 15 centers, the budget would be approximately $187.5 million.

The number and location of hemophilia centers in a region were determined on the basis of the known geographical distribution of hemophiliacs. Within certain limits, individual hemophiliacs will be able to attend the facility nearest to them. The 15 cities chosen are Seattle, Washington; Los Angeles, California; Denver, Colorado; Minneapolis, Minnesota; Kansas City, Kansas; Houston, Texas; Chicago, Illinois; Ann Arbor, Michigan; Nashville, Tennessee; Rochester, New York; Pittsburgh, Pennsylvania; Chapel Hill, North Carolina; Atlanta, Georgia; New York City, New York; and Boston, Massachusetts.

---

1. Group Statements by Participants to the Establishment of 15 Regional Centers
a. Care Sector Report

We have problems because, supposedly, we have $15.5 million for each of these hemophilia centers, but we do not really have this money because the patient has the ultimate decision on where to spend his money. This is a great challenge: How can we build these new facilities when these facilities may never be utilized? The patient may choose not to use our services, then where are we? What is required is an ongoing operating budget to allow the center to operate before it has a full complement of patients.

In order to create an operational budget, we recommend initiating a requirement for a yearly comprehensive examination for all hemophiliacs to be given only at the center. This yearly examination would become the qualification for support by the center for that year or this examination report would be sent to a private physician. The private physician, once he received this report, could treat this hemophilic patient for a year.

Considering the staff and the laboratory facilities that are needed for a thorough evaluation, $500 is not an unreasonable fee. This fee is not excessive once it is realized that the evaluation is being conducted by the best people available. After all, the physician will be writing a clear-cut evaluation of the patient's status and making recommendations for care during the following year. This initial $500 examination is not unprecedented; it is similar in principle to having support coming only through qualified programs.

Now, coming to grips with the actual money to build. The proposed National Hemophilia Commission should be charged with finding sites for these 15 comprehensive centers. These sites should be selected on the basis of patient flow, accessibility, and the availability of expert staff. Selection, moreover, should be on the basis of competition. There may be great competition among those cities that have been chosen, for instance, in New York.

Source: C.S. Greenblat and J.H. Gagnon, *Blood Money: A Gaming-Simulation of the Problems of Hemophilia and Health Care Delivery Systems* (Washington, D.C.: U.S. Government Printing Office, 1976).

the staged situation. By creating the role for each participant, the health planner provides human diversity and, it is hoped, represents all the participants and their viewpoints. By providing a scenario for the players, the health planner describes the overall environment in which the players act out their roles. In the Blood Money gaming simulation the participants use a dart board, barter exchange, and a scenario (Exhibit 6-26B) that employs a news release from the federal government. In the drug education game, a front page story and an editorial from the local newspaper are used to set the stage (Appendix B).

Rules and/or guidelines are usually presented to the players as instructions for the gaming simulation. In some situations, the rules detail what the players are allowed to do, and in other games the rules state what the players cannot do and leave the field open for all other actions. Health planners may wish to use both techniques. To stimulate interactions, the planner may wish to set rules that restrict the players to a specific situation and concentration upon a narrow goal; the broader guidelines could be used for a more open gaming simulation where the health planner may be seeking to identify all the ramifications.

Goals can be stated as objectives in the rules or can be incorporated in the role profiles given to each player. An objective might be to arrange for equitable distribution of supplies of blood to hemophiliacs, while the player's role profile might instruct him to gain control over all the hospital beds in the area. Sometimes the goal is stated in terms of what must be achieved to "win" the game. Exhibit 6-26 explains the subject and purpose of the Blood Money gaming simulation. Appendix B does the same for the drug education game.

Criteria for ending the gaming simulation can be when somebody "wins," or an artificial time limit can be imposed—the game ends with whatever resolution has taken place. Exhibit 6-26 and Appendix B both indicate that time limits are being used.

Gaming simulations are particularly relevant in health planning because of the legal mandates to include consumers and providers in the planning process, with the consumers in the majority. To achieve the desired objectives, health planners must be prepared for the human interactions that will take place regarding the implementation of activities. Therefore, it would be prudent to try to anticipate any possible deviations from the proposed implementation process and to prepare for the barriers that may arise within the professional community as well as among the general public. A gaming simulation can provide the health planner with an imitation of the real world working on the activity and suggesting solutions and approaches to achieve cooperation and effective participation toward the desired goals.

Illustrative abstracts from the two gaming simulations already mentioned, the drug education simulation game and the Blood Money
hemophilia game, will indicate concretely how the use of a gaming
simulation fits into the promotion of implementation strategies. To
direct attention to pertinent techniques, each abstract will be listed
with highlights (Exhibit 6-26C and Appendix B).

IMPLEMENTATION AND SOCIOPOLITICAL INTERACTION

Up to this point consideration of implementation has been confined
to the rational, scientific approach to putting decisions into the action
phase. However, the real world does not always abide by rational logic,
and the health planner must be aware of social and political interactions that influence any implementation program. As previously
noted, the gaming simulation can be used as a technique to prepare the
planner for the human factors that arise in setting a project into motion.

L. Fontana and A. Beckerman[23] contend that the major interest
groups in the health sector are the "professionals," represented most
significantly by physicians in group or private practice; the "corporate
sector," represented by hospitals and nursing homes, medical schools,
insurance companies, drug companies, and public health agencies; and
the "consumers." These divisions within the health care area will obviously lead to disagreement when it comes to implementation activities.
Yet, the rules of the game are structured to reach a decision that
conflicting interest groups can accept without suffering any serious
damage.

However, the point is made that the inherent inequality of bargaining power within the interest groups is often not considered in efforts
at representation.[24,25] Politicians, for example, are more inclined to
respond to the demands of special interest groups rather than the actual needs of the entire population. Carrying this concept further, a
study of prior health planning efforts and the structure of the new
Health Systems Agencies led to the forecast that the HSAs will have
little impact on the health care crisis because the HSAs fail to take into
account the dynamics of the health sector. In addition, the researchers
believed that "health planning as presently instituted has been in the
basic interest of the health providers . . . it is mistaken to believe that
health planning is inevitably in the public interest." It was pointed out

Exhibit 6-26C Blood Money and Implementation Activities

What's in this game— subject and purpose	Aims to experience how the hemophiliac gets his care and blood.
Who can play?	Identifies the participants and indicates represen- tativeness.
Number of players	
Running the game— personnel needed	Gives manpower requirements.
Time requirement	Sets sequence of meetings by time periods.
Space requirement	
Materials requirement	
Blood bankers	This is the role profile for the player. Note the goals, the cost charges, and the dissemination of the blood supplies.
Press release from HEW	This is the technique used to set up the scenario in which the game takes place.
Instructions on questions to be addressed and state- ments to be prepared	This moves the players into a consideration of the implementation of various activities.
Session II— instruction of players	Adds to scenario background for the next session.
Scenario 2	This directs the players into another set of circum- stances. The technique of adding additional information to scenarios can be used to redirect the players to focus upon another implementation problem.

Source: C.S. Greenblat and J.H. Gagnon, *Blood Money: A Gaming-Simulation of the Problems of Hemophilia and Health Care Delivery Systems* (Washington, D.C.: U.S. Government Printing Office, 1976).

that the HSA should not be considered a neutral device despite the representation of different segments of the health care sector.[26] A study of health planning in eight model cities projects strongly suggested that providers dominated the decisions in every city.[27] Another analysis[28] concluded that it was unlikely that the HSAs would generate radical changes in the health care system. Rather, the HSA is more likely "to provide an institutional forum for legitimizing existing patterns of power distribution and to accede as slowly as they can to those irresistible exogenous forces that would have produced major change in any event."

To counter this idea, a hospital administrator noted in *Hospitals*, the journal of the American Hospital Association, that planning should address society's needs, and operations should be consonant with the greater social consciousness.[29]

In view of the legislative mandate to have a majority of consumers on the boards of HSAs, the sociopolitical interactions that could affect implementation activities can be increased as the professionals and the corporate sectors work with the nonprofessional consumer. In a report on a training program for consumers in policy-making roles in health care projects,[30] the consumers generally criticized professionals for using complicated, technical language to express simple points. One board member said, "Doctors can rattle on for hours; if you try to ask a simple question, they just take it and go on and on." This type of attitude will seriously affect implementation of a program. However, a basic question raised by professionals concerns whether the public really knows what it wants. Two conflicting points of view have been stated in this respect. One holds that the public, be they consumers, patients, or clients, is unknowing and cannot diagnose their own needs or discriminate among the range of possibilities for meeting them. The other view contends that the consumer is the best judge of his own welfare.[31] In a balance sheet style, the conflict can be presented as shown:

Unknowing	*Best Judge*
Man is ignorant	Man is wise
Protectionism prevails	A free market exists
Man is potentially altruistic	Man is primarily self-interested
Physicians seek out patients	Patients go to the physicians

Fuel for conflicts about implementation activities are evident in this balance sheet of viewpoints.

A ladder of citizen participation developed by S.R. Arnstein[32] illustrates some of the techniques utilized in planning situations, wherein professionals worked with the consumers. Note the choices of style and alternatives offered.

Ladder of Participation

8	Citizen control	
7	Delegated power	→ Degrees of citizen power
6	Partnership	
5	Placation	
4	Consultation	→ Degrees of tokenism
3	Informing	
2	Therapy	→ Nonparticipation
1	Manipulation	

Source: S.R. Arnstein, "A Ladder of Citizen Participation." Reprinted by permission of the *Journal of the American Institute of Planners,* vol. 35, July, 1969.

In planning for the implementation of an activity where the cooperation of the consumer is desired, the level of participation can be crucial in success or failure. As C.B. Galiher and her associates noted, "What is clear is that the health professional needs the consumer to achieve a relevant and responsive health care system."[33]

Given the discussion of the roles of the providers and the consumers relative to health planning implementation, specific attention can be devoted to what the planner must be alert to in the interactional stages. Exhibit 6-27 illustrates the group and community interaction in the planning and implementation processes. Questions for consideration in relating the community structure to health action and the implications of these structures demonstrate the need for the health planner to discover the community power structure. Sources of influence should be kept in mind as the planner mounts the implementation activity and has need of assistance. Then, consideration must be given to the constrictions on health planning implementation of activities. Public versus private interests must be recognized and faced in a manner that does not wreck all program possibility. Still, it is evident that activities do get implemented and programs do come into being. What moves an idea from being significant and important to being urgent

Exhibit 6-27 Group and Community Interaction in the Planning and Implementation Processes

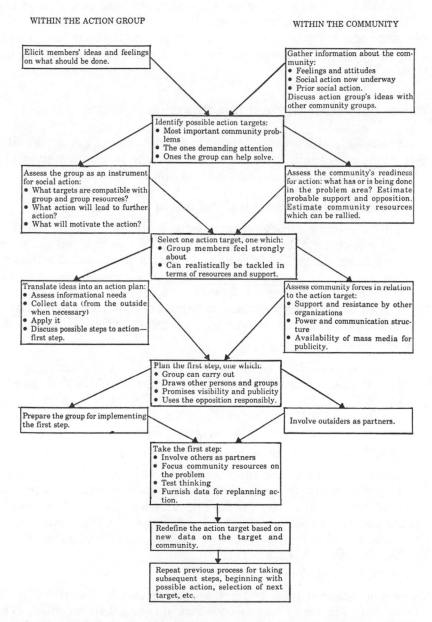

WITHIN THE ACTION GROUP

WITHIN THE COMMUNITY

Elicit members' ideas and feelings on what should be done.

Gather information about the community:
- Feelings and attitudes
- Social action now underway
- Prior social action.
Discuss action group's ideas with other community groups.

Identify possible action targets:
- Most important community problems
- The ones demanding attention
- Ones the group can help solve.

Assess the group as an instrument for social action:
- What targets are compatible with group and group resources?
- What action will lead to further action?
- What will motivate the action?

Assess the community's readiness for action: what has or is being done in the problem area? Estimate probable support and opposition. Estimate community resources which can be rallied.

Select one action target, one which:
- Group members feel strongly about
- Can realistically be tackled in terms of resources and support.

Translate ideas into an action plan:
- Assess informational needs
- Collect data (from the outside when necessary)
- Apply it
- Discuss possible steps to action—first step.

Assess community forces in relation to the action target:
- Support and resistance by other organizations
- Power and communication structure
- Availability of mass media for publicity.

Plan the first step, one which:
- Group can carry out
- Draws other persons and groups
- Promises visibility and publicity
- Uses the opposition responsibly.

Prepare the group for implementing the first step.

Involve outsiders as partners.

Take the first step:
- Involve others as partners
- Focus community resources on the problem
- Test thinking
- Furnish data for replanning action.

Redefine the action target based on new data on the target and community.

Repeat previous process for taking subsequent steps, beginning with possible action, selection of next target, etc.

Source: Sigrid G. Deeds, *A Guidebook for Family Planning Education* (Columbia, Md.: Westinghouse Population Center, 1973), p. 85.

and immediate? Do health planners have a part to play in making a suggested activity urgent?

The following are examples and illustrations of community structure problems, influence sources, constrictions, and determinations of significance and urgency. Some techniques and methods are suggested, and others are implied, for meeting these factors in implementing activities.

Community Structure and Health Action

Actions for health must be related to the structure of the community. Situations cited below are examples of how the community structure could interact with the implementation of a health activity.

- Is health a major problem of concern to the community?

  Public opinion surveys demonstrate that health is not the first concern of the public. Crime control, public safety, and the economy have all ranked higher than health problems. Community leaders tend to place health concerns on a lower level and do not press for many activities. Of course, a possible epidemic or other health threat does mobilize the community, but this is a passing interest and does not remain too long after the threat disappears.

- Why upset the status quo?

  Community leaders tend to avoid conflicts that can affect their own power base. A status quo mentality keeps activities that may be controversial from being implemented. Things have worked reasonably well without this new activity, and the community shows no desire to push something new or different.

- What's the role of business and banking leaders?

  Any activity involving the expenditure of sums of money appears to be dominated by community people associated with industry and with banks. Voluntary health organizations look to these people for advice and for professional help. Generally, these community leaders tend to be conservatives when it comes to implementing a new health activity.

- Is there a payoff for political leaders?

  Payoff does not refer to graft but to whether it is worthwhile for political leaders to become involved. As one politician noted, "The do-gooders will vote for me regardless. Those anti people will vote against me. Why should I antagonize them?" Obviously, the political leaders could be strong influences in the legislative and regulatory aspects of any implementation activity.

• What's the influence of the professionals?

Professionals base their influence upon their narrow technical expertise. Community leaders may request advice on that aspect but not on political or social implications. Professionals are often treated more as expert consultants than participants.

Implications for Health Planners

What does this analysis of the community structure and health action mean to the health planner? What are the implications for implementation? Clearly, the health planner has to identify the community leaders and work with them. Activities will be much easier to implement with the active cooperation of the community structure.

Community leaders can be identified by reputation, by official position and by decision-making ability.

A reputation technique uses one leader to identify others in the community. Then, those named by the first are also asked to identify other leaders, and so on. Eventually the names that appear most often emerge as the agreed upon community leaders by consensus. To use this technique, the health planner could start with a local politician, the president of a large industry in the community, or a bank president.

Decision-making community leaders may be more difficult to identify because these individuals often prefer to remain out of the limelight. Community leaders having the real influence could be political party chairmen or bosses, extremely wealthy individuals, so-called power brokers, socially prominent people, or aides to some of these decision makers. The cooperation of these political forces would make any implementation project infinitely smoother.

Assuming that the community leaders can be identified, how does the health planner motivate the obvious community leaders to participate in the implementation activity? Rational approaches may not really stimulate the community leaders to participate. Tradeoffs may be the situation arising most frequently. What can the health planner do for the community leader in return for active participation? E. C. Banfield[34] noted in his book on political influence that a variety of ways exists to influence people:

• Obligation—the individual feels obligated to participate because it is morally right or personally a duty.

- Friendship—individuals participate because a friend asked them to do so.
- Selling—the individual is responsive to a selling pitch.
- Coercion—the individual is politely blackmailed into activity.
- Rational persuasion—the power of the data and the weight of the presentation persuades the individual.
- Inducement—either positive or negative inducement is used to bring the individual over to your side.

All these incentives must be tailored to fit the specific community leader in the particular situation. The same message does not move all people with equal force.

Sources of Influence

Sources of influence that can be vital to an implementation activity are listed below.

- Money/credit—it is easy to buy what you need if you have the resources.
- Control of jobs—people that feel threatened with the loss of their jobs will be inclined to vote with you.
- Control of information—without all the facts, people may move in the direction desired based on the available information only.
- Social standing—some people are influenced by those whom they consider to be in the social elite.
- Ethnic solidarity—some individuals may feel compelled to participate because they want to help one of their own.
- Legality/constitutionality—the power of the law to urge people to cooperate, usually backed up by sanctions of some type.
- Personal (human) energy—Sheer work and ability to stick with the problem may influence others over time.
- Knowledge/expertise—people can be influenced by people whose intellectual ability they admire and respect.
- Popularity/esteem/charisma—That something extra that cannot be defined, but it charms people into cooperating.

Constrictions on Health Planning Implementation

Most health planners will have to deal with the conflicting self-interests of various individuals and organizations as the planning of implementation activities gets underway. At this point, there may be some thought about the public interest versus the private interest.

- Public interests are served if the decision furthers the ends of the whole public rather than the ends of some specific sector.
- Private and special interests are served by decisions that further the ends of some part of the public at the expense of the ends of the larger public.

Health planners might assume, perhaps naively, that individuals and organizations have the public interest in mind in decisions that revolve around implementation activities. However, a consideration of the types of ends that people could be favoring point out the continuum of real life situations that may constrict the health planner's implementation project. Participants may hold views that are[35]

1. community regarding rather than self-regarding,
2. stable rather than transitory,
3. general rather than particular in reference,
4. pertain to the role of citizen rather than to some private role,
5. common or statistically frequent rather than idiosyncratic or infrequent, or
6. logically or morally justified rather than emotionally or not justified.

Sources of conflict can easily arise in situations where these values are represented at random among those who are needed to cooperate in the implementation program. Some might wish to emphasize coordination over competition. Others might favor their own particular constituency over the general public. Still others might concentrate on cost containment over the environmental impact. In any case, the conflict can be bitter and impose severe constraints on the final implementation effort. Some of the more common restrictions imposed upon the health planner are illustrated below:

- Powerful interest groups strongly represent their adherents to make sure that their area of interest is not encroached in any implementation activity. If a voluntary health organization feels that education of the public is their domain, they will resist any activity that will have others engaging in education of the public about their specific disease. In many instances, the voluntary health agency will have its educational campaign directly linked to its fund-raising drive. Therefore, an implementation activity that intrudes in the educational area threatens their lifeline of donations. Since many of these powerful interest groups have boards of directors with highly placed individuals serving on them, considerable pressure can be brought to bear on influencing the decisions.

- Rapid action may be deferred because of the need to seek a consensus and to avoid conflicts. It takes time and effort to win people over to accept a least common denominator where everybody gains something and nobody loses too much. In the example about education, one agreement that did take place allowed the voluntary health agency to cosponsor all the educational activities with the name of the agency standing out boldly in any educational endeavor. Actually, this compromise probably favored the voluntary health organization since they were so solidly connected with the educational effort by the public anyhow. Many people assumed that the voluntary health agency was the prime power behind the implementation effort.
- Lack of consensus as to purpose tends to result in oiling the wheel that squeaks the most first. Health planners become so tied up in efforts to maintain the status quo that there is a failure to deal with root causes in implementation activities. With divergent viewpoints, the end result might be the pouring of old wine into new bottles to collect grant funds or other funding.
- Insufficient authority to implement activities can quickly force the health planner to a dead stop. This lack of authority could be related to legal powers, to political influence, to a lack of money or manpower, or to a lack of status in the health care community. Can a public health planner have enough authority to move private physicians into participating? One has only to read of the history of the comprehensive health planning agencies (CHPs) to garner a rather extensive listing of difficulties of this nature.
- Confusion concerning health planning models can also constrain implementation efforts of health planners. All the reasonable, logical data in the world might not persuade the individual who knows from "the seat of his pants" how to run an implementation program. Although planners can use many of the techniques presented in this book or more sophisticated technology, there is no universal agreement on what is the best method. Planning is not an exact science. Nevertheless, planning methods and techniques are constantly being developed, reviewed, and reevaluated; and the health planner must take and use the good and discard the methods that do not work in his particular situation.

WHAT MAKES AN IMPLEMENTATION ACTIVITY SIGNIFICANT OR URGENT?

Data and analysis may suggest a host of implementation activities for the health planner to undertake in the community. In the chapter on priorities, the rationale for making decisions was emphasized. Yet, the health planner also has to realize that sociopolitical interactions will come to bear on the decisions as well as any weighting procedure or other priority determination mechanism.

Many activities will fall into the category of being significant health problems that ought to be attacked. Fewer will be classified in the category needing urgent attention. This does not mean that the significant problems are any less important, but that the urgent problems can be less important statistically or logically but higher on the scale sociopolitically.

An implementation activity can be significant for the following reasons:

- People affected—a large silent majority may make the activity numerically important as their lives are affected. There may only be a small number of people affected, but they may be the vocal few that make the activity significant.
- Facilities—if the facility being affected by the activity is on Main Street, it may be a significant program. However, if the facility is "out of sight" then it is "out of mind" and not as important.
- Costs—the higher the cost, the more significant the implementation activity becomes. Questions of tax monies and accountability color the significance.
- Risks/losses—if the activity falls into an all or nothing situation regarding implementation, the activity can engender more importance than if the risk were small.
- Social disruption—the more social disruption that the implementation activity causes, the more significant the project. If the activity escapes the public interest with a yawn rather than a riot, it will remain important but not urgent.
- Effects/benefits—if the implementation activity calls for a high powered rifle to kill a mouse, the activity will not be significant enough to stir action while still retaining its importance.
- Participants—the identity of the participants involved in implementation planning can bring significance to the activity with the weight of their names, their social position, or their connections.

To move an implementation activity from the significant category to the urgent category requiring immediate attention raises the consideration of the following factors:

- Mass communication—all types of mass media provide extensive coverage of the proposed activity and keep the project in the limelight until action is taken to meet the urgent need.

- Crisis labeling—simply labeling the activity as an answer to a crisis situation prompts action. A self-fulfilling prophecy situation occurs. Government officials urging fluoridation of the water supply to prevent dental decay arouses a strong public outcry from those who feel that their freedom of choice is being impinged. Calling something urgent makes it so.
- Pressure (flak)—individuals and organizations maintain constant pressure through letters, phone calls, personal talks, and even picketing, sleep-ins, and boycotts until the urgent situation is rectified. Letters to the editor and strong complaints also create flak.
- Moral values—an appeal to deeply held moral values can create an urgent situation. Welfare recipients stealing the city blind and driving Cadillacs arouses a strong public cry to do something about those people who do not work and sponge off others who do. Moral values are offended and demand action.
- Power—power brokers in smoke-filled back rooms decide that something is urgent, and the activity is implemented quickly.
- Influence—individuals who have the ability to get others to think, feel, or act as they wish influence the decisions that create the urgency.

Many of the human interaction situations that have been discussed have been incorporated into a health planning game that simulates policy-making scenarios. This health planning game was developed by the Columbia University School of Public Health.[36]

TECHNIQUES FOR MEETINGS, GROUPINGS, AND PRESENTATIONS

It is possible that some implementation activities, particularly those with heavy sociopolitical overtone, might involve the use of task forces, study groups, ad hoc committees, or formal presentations to professionals and lay groups. Health planners should be aware of the basic styles and the relation between the intended purpose and the technique. Planners might consider this sequence of questions:

1. What specific objective has to be accomplished?
2. What type of meeting, grouping, or presentation is called for?
3. What subgroupings are needed to achieve the objective?

4. What presentation methods should be used?
5. How can the audience or participants become more involved?

A majority of the meeting styles are listed in Exhibit 6-28 by the purpose, the type, and relevant features of that technique. Although there might not be universal agreement on the exact terminology, the general concept of each method is fairly well accepted.

With the advent of the Health Systems Agencies, it is quite probable that health planners will have numerous situations where an implementation activity will be the calling together of experts in committees to develop areawide plans. These methods and techniques can be adapted to meet the mandates of participation, sociopolitical interaction, representation, and the production of the final product—the recommendations. Most planners probably know the methods and techniques, but a listing highlighting the purposes and the features can serve as a quick and easy reference.

Exhibit 6-28 Meetings, Groupings, and Presentation Techniques

TYPE OF MEETING

If This Is Your Purpose ▼	This Type ▼	Has These Features ▼

WORK CONFERENCE

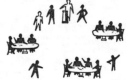

To plan, get facts, solve organization and member problems

- ▼ general sessions and face-to-face groups (15 or less)
- ▼ usually high participation
- ▼ provides more flexible means for doing organization's work

WORKSHOP

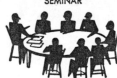

To train each other to gain new knowledge, skills or insights into problems

- ▼ general sessions and face-to-face groups
- ▼ participonts are also "trainers"
- ▼ trainers can be brought in, too

SEMINAR

To share experience among "experts"

- ▼ usually one face-to-face group
- ▼ discussion leader also provides expert information

INSTITUTE

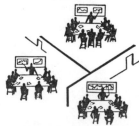

To train in one or several subjects

- ▼ general sessions and face-to-face groups
- ▼ staff provides most of training resources

KINDS OF GROUPINGS

| If This Is Your Purpose ▼ | This Kind ▼ | Has These Features ▼ |

GENERAL SESSION

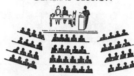

To give orientation or information to total group, transact official business

▼ includes total meeting group
▼ useful for demonstrations, speeches, lectures, films
▼ can be subdivided for limited face-to-face group activities

SPECIAL INTEREST GROUPS

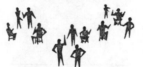

To consider special interests of various members by means of exchange of opinions, experience, and ideas

EXAMPLE:
'Let's plan our golf tournament.'
'How can we get more members interested?'
'Can we get an expert on this subject to address us?'

▼ composed of those interested in subject
▼ usually no action required, but findings may be reported
▼ size varies widely; best if kept small

ORIENTATION GROUPS

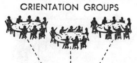

To help new members get acquainted, explain conference mechanics and plan of operation

EXAMPLES:
"What about getting mail?
"Where can we go after hours?
"What's the schedule?

▼ mixed membership from total group
▼ member of planning staff as resource on all questions and to help them get acquainted
▼ exists for brief period at start of conference only

PRESENTATION METHODS

SPEAKER WITH VISUALS

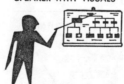

To present complex technical info, such as organization structure, processes, etc.

▼ more thorough and more certain communication but slower and more costly
▼ usually creates greater interest than speaker only

SYMPOSIUM

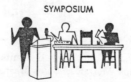

To present information from several points of view

▼ two or more speakers—each usually makes short talk
▼ speakers can help audience set full understanding of specific subject
▼ chairman summarizes and directs questions
▼ audience usually does not participate verbally

If This Is Your Purpose ▼	This Method ▼	Has These Features ▼
To present information, often controversial, from several points of view	**PANEL** 	▼ panel participates—each states views and holds discussion with one another ▼ panel members usually rehearse briefly ▼ discussion is guided by moderator ▼ questions and commentary with audience
To develop several opposing sides of an issue	**FORUM** 	▼ two or more speakers take opposing sides on an issue; address audience rather than each other ▼ moderator summarizes points of view and leads discussion ▼ audience usually limited to asking questions
To help audience analyze individual or group action in "natural" 'setting	**SITUATION PRESENTATION** 	▼ members of group present role play, vignette or case-study (example: showing problems of coordination in staff meeting) ▼ commentator may call attention to specific points as play progresses ▼ audience gains a common experience for discussion afterwards
To dramatize the outer or inner forces that clash in a human situation	**CONFLICT PRESENTATION** 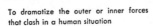 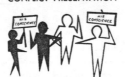	▼ members of group present role play or staged skits ▼ "ghost voice" or "alter ego" talks out loud to show inner thoughts of each character (example: outside pressures on two people in conflict) ▼ audience gains insights into problems through emotional appeal
To demonstrate techniques or skills and show relative effectiveness	**SKILL PRESENTATION** 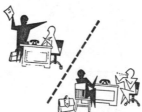	▼ members of group (or live actors) demonstrate several ways of handling a situation (example: ways to sell difficult customer) ▼ audience observes, discusses advantages and disadvantages of various approaches

Source: Reprinted with permission from Hugh Gyllenhaal, "For the Modern Meeting Planner: Guide to Styles, Groups, Methods," *Sales Meetings* 7(January 4, 1957): 19.

REFERENCES

1. J.G. Bruhn, "Planning for Social Change: Dilemmas in Health Planning," *American Journal of Public Health* 63 (July 1973): 602.

2. *Ibid.*

3. R.H. Murray, "Muddling Through Isn't Enough," *Journal of the American Medical Association* 234 (October 20, 1975): 287.

4. S.E. Salasin and H.R. Davis, "A Practical Model for Planned Change," paper presented at the annual meeting of the American Public Health Association, Atlantic City, N.J., November 13, 1972. Also cited in this paper: E.M. Glaser and H.L. Ross, "Increasing the Utilization of Applied Research Results," final report to the National Institute of Mental Health, Grant No. 5 R12 MH09250-02 (Los Angeles: Human Interaction Research Institute, 1971).

5. *Ibid.*

6. D.H. Gustafson, G.L. Rowse, N.J. Howes and R.S. Shukla, "Opportunities for Improvement in Health Systems Engineering," *Inquiry* 14 (March 1977): 87.

7. G.A. Goldberg, "Implementing University Hospital Ambulatory Care Evaluation," *Journal of Medical Education* 50 (May 1975): 435.

8. J.T. Gentry, A.D. Kaluzny and J.E. Veney, "A Comparative Analysis of Factors Influencing the Implementation of Family Planning Services in the United States," *American Journal of Public Health* 64 (April 1974): 376.

9. A.D. Kaluzny and J.E. Veney, "Types of Change and Hospital Planning Strategies," *American Journal of Health Planning* 1, no. 3 (January 1977): 13.

10. *Ibid.*

11. A. Etzioni, *A Comparative Analysis of Complex Organizations* (Glencoe, New York: The Free Press, 1961), pp. 130-141.

12. J.J. McGuire, "Delivering People Care Amid Change," *Journal of the Medical Society of New Jersey* 72 (June 1975): 473.

13. H.H. Sapolsky, "A Solution to the 'Health Crisis'," *Policy Analysis* 3, no. 1 (Winter 1977): 115.

14. M.F. Doody, "Will Providers Change the System?" *Hospitals* 50 (April 1, 1976): 51.

15. National Heart, Lung and Blood Institute. *Handbook for Improving High Blood Pressure Control in the Community* (Washington, D.C.: U.S. Government Printing Office, 1977), p. 36.

16. S.G. Deeds, *A Guidebook for Family Planning Education* (Columbia, Md.: Westinghouse Population Center, 1973), p. 40.

17. American Hospital Association, *The Practice of Planning in Health Care Institutions* (Chicago: AHA, 1973), p. 56-57.

18. H.P. Terrell, "Flow Chart for Optimum Office Efficiency," *Patient Care* 11, no. 13 (July 15, 1977): 165.

19. N. Hirschhorn, J. Lamstein and R. O'Connor, *Problem-Action Guidelines for Basic Health Care: A Tool for Extending Effective Services Through Auxiliary Health Workers* (Cambridge, Mass.: Management Sciences for Health, 1974).

20. G. Stuehler, Jr., "Organizing Organized Medicine Through a Planning and Development Framework (PADFRAME)," *Journal of the American Medical Association* 237 (April 11, 1977): 1589.

21. E.T. Alsaker, "The Basic Technique: Network Analysis," *PERT: A New Management Planning and Control Technique,* by G.N. Stilian *et al.* (New York: American Management Association, 1962), p. 37.

22. C.S. Greenblat and J.H. Gagnon, *Blood Money: A Gaming-Simulation of the Problems of Hemophilia and Health Care Delivery Systems* (Washington, D.C.: U.S. Government Printing Office, 1976).

23. L. Fontana and A. Beckerman, "Interest Groups and Community Health Planning: Cooperation or Cooptation?", paper presented at annual meeting of the American Sociological Association, New York, August 1976.

24. D.F. Mazziotti, "Underlying Assumptions of Advocacy Planning: Pluralism and Reform," *Journal of the American Institute of Planners* 40 (January 1974): 38.

25. P. Clavel, "Planners and Citizen Boards: Some Applications of Social Theory to the Problem of Plan Implementation," *Journal of the American Institute of Planners* 34, no. 3 (May 1968): 130.

26. Fontana and Beckerman, *op. cit.*

27. C. W. Douglass, "Consumer Influence in Health Planning in the Urban Ghetto," *Inquiry* 12 (June 1975): 157.

28. B.C. Vladeck, "Interest-Group Representation and the HSAs: Health Planning and Political Theory," *American Journal of Public Health* 67 (January 1977): 23.

29. E.L. McClendon, "Societal, Organizational Concerns Should be addressed in Planning," *Hospitals* 49 (December 1, 1975): 35.

30. L. Meisner, A. Parker, L. Austin, C. Orr and M.L. Ortega, "A Training Program for Consumers in Policy-Making Roles in Health Care Projects," (Berkeley: School of Public Health, University of California at Berkeley, May 1970).

31. W.C. Richardson and D. Newhauser, "First Question in Health Planning: Does the Public Know What It Wants, or Not?", *Modern Hospital,* 110 (May 1968): 115.

32. S.R. Arnstein, "A Ladder of Citizen Participation," *Journal of the American Institute of Planners* 35 (July 1969): 216.

33. C.B. Galiher, J. Needleman and A.J. Rolfe, "Consumer Participation," *HSMHA Health Reports* 86 (February 1971): 99.

34. E.C. Banfield, *Political Influence. A New Theory of Urban Politics* (Glencoe, New York: The Free Press, 1961), pp. 3-6.

35. M. Meyerson and E.C. Banfield, *Politics, Planning and the Public Interest* (Glencoe, New York: The Free Press, 1955), pp. 322-329.

36. N.M. Clark and M. Pinckett-Heller, "The Health Planning Game: A Simulation in Policy Making," paper presented at the annual meeting of the American Public Health Association, Washington, D.C., November 1977. (Prototype Health Planning Game available from N.M. Clark at Columbia University School of Public Health, 21 Audubon Avenue, New York, N.Y. 10032. $15 plus $1.50 postage and handling).

Chapter 7

Evaluation

An evaluation usually signals the conclusion of a program or project, but it can also mark the beginning of a new cycle of planning. Recommendations and suggestions emanating from the evaluation activity should be utilized for future programs. For an evaluation to be successful, there has to be a direct connection to the specified objectives of the project. The more clearly the objectives are stated, the easier the evaluation will be to conduct.

This chapter will discuss and illustrate evaluation definitions, purposes of evaluation, steps in evaluation, classifications and categories of evaluation, components and elements of measurement, measurement techniques, and problems in evaluation.

In the early 1900s, E.A. Codman of the Massachusetts General Hospital became interested in discovering the outcomes of medical care. Codman wanted to know the relationship between what happened in the hospital and the future health of the patient. In an article on the product of a hospital, Codman stated:

> We must formulate some method of hospital report showing as nearly as possible what are the results of treatment obtained at different institutions. This report must be made out and published by each hospital in a uniform manner, so that comparison will be possible. With such a report as a starting point, those interested can begin to ask questions as to management and efficiency.[1]

However, Codman's efforts were not met with resounding support from the hospitals. This situation points out the need to secure backing from those who are most directly concerned with the evaluation.

Another example involves the evaluation of an ambulatory medical care delivery system.[2] An innovative system was designed to increase access to medical care. Entering patients were screened through a paramedically staffed triage unit that separated patients into three basic health status groups: the well and worried well (68 percent of the patients), the asymptomatic sick (4 percent), and the sick (28 percent). Then, the patients were matched with the appropriate services. Examination of the charts of more than 4,000 patients who either entered the new system or the traditional system revealed the following:

1. the new system increased physician accessibility to new patients by a factor of 20,
2. the new system reduced waiting time for new appointments from six to eight weeks to a day or two,
3. the new system saved physician time and costs for entry work-up by 70 to 80 percent,
4. the new system reduced total resources used throughout the year by $32,500 per 1,000 entrants, and
5. the new system was very satisfactory to patients and generally satisfactory to staff.

This example illustrates a project that appears to be most successful in all aspects. Yet, the question of staff satisfaction does raise an issue of potential additional investigation. Therefore, even with a rewarding concluding evaluation, the process of health planning begins again if the new system is really to meet the needs of the patients as well as the staff.

An argument that is sometimes raised regarding the value of evaluation relates to interpretation. Consider the classic glass of water. Is it half full or half empty? Such is another overwhelming consideration in evaluation: the interpretation of data. As the oft-used maxim goes, "Statistics don't lie, but liars use statistics!"

Evaluation can become a political battle as has been noted by some prominent researchers.[3] This idea has been summed up by V.E. Weckwerth[4] and probably coincides with the views of many others:

1. There is no *one* way to do evaluation.
2. There is no generic logical structure that will assure a unique "right method of choice."
3. Evaluation ultimately involves judgment and will remain so, as long as no ultimate criterion exists for a monotonic ordering of priorities.

4. The crucial element in evaluation is simply who has the power, the influence, and authority to decide.

Although this assessment clearly points out potential human frailties, evaluation is still undertaken within a scientific halo and, perhaps, with aims of objectivity. The element of who has the right to evaluate is crucial; "who" could refer to the consumer, the provider, or to some other body annointed to do evaluation. Specifically, "who" could be line administrators, trained researchers on staff, management consultant firms, peer groups of professionals, consumer advocates, or anybody with knowledge about the program.

In discussing the evaluative research design, E.A. Suchman[5] also reinforces the points made by Weckwerth:

1. It seems to us futile to argue whether a certain design is "scientific." The design is the plan of study and, as such, is present in all studies. It is not a case of scientific or not scientific, but rather one of good or less good design.
2. The proof of hypotheses is never definitive. The best one can hope to do is to make more or less plausible a series of alternative hypotheses.
3. There is no such thing as a single "correct" design. Hypotheses can be studied by different methods using different designs.
4. All research design represents a compromise dictated by the many practical considerations that go into social research.
5. A research design is not a highly specific plan to be followed without deviation, but a series of guideposts to keep one headed in the right direction.

EVALUATION BOUNDARIES

In view of the vagaries of the evaluation, it might be worthwhile to reflect on the definitions of the method and the questions that evaluation seeks to answer.

One definition combines expressive words with examples[6]:

we may simply indicate the range of variation by defining evaluation as the determination (whether based on opinions, records, or subjective or objective data)

of the results (whether desirable or undesirable; transient or permanent; immediate or delayed)

| attained by some activity | (whether a program or part of a program; a drug or a therapy; an ongoing or a one-shot approach) |
| designed to accomplish some valued goal or objective | (whether ultimate, intermediate, or immediate effort of performance; long or short range). |

Clearly, this definition wants to know if the activity is related to the objective that was set forth. Furthermore, the results can fall either way on the scale.

Other definitions support the basic ingredients identified in the above definition. The dictionary notes that evaluation determines or fixes a value, or examines and judges. An American Public Health Association definition calls evaluation the process of determining value or the amount of success in achieving predetermined objectives. G. James[7] stated that program evaluation is the measurement of success in reaching a stated objective. R.H. Brook[8] noted that evaluation measures the extent to which a program achieves its goal, the relative impact of key program variables, and the role of the program contrasted to external variables.

This last definition of evaluation expands the area of concern a bit and brings into view characteristics relating to focus, methodology, and the function of evaluation. J.S. Wholey and his associates[9] also take this point of view in discussing federal evaluation policy with their definition:

> Evaluation (1) assesses the effectiveness of an on-going program in achieving its objectives, (2) relies on the principles of research design to distinguish a program's effects from those of other forces working in a situation, and (3) aims at program improvement through a modification of current operations.

Generally, all the definitions of evaluation relate to the measurement of the results of some activity with the added sophistication of attempting to separate out the variables achieving the anticipated results.

Another mechanism for defining evaluation boundaries does so through the technique of listing questions that an evaluation should answer. The American Public Health Association lists the following five questions:[10]

- How important was the problem toward which the program was directed?
- How much of the problem was solved?
- How effectively did the activities attain their objectives?
- What was the cost in resources of attaining objectives? Was the attainment to cost ratio satisfactory?
- What desirable and undesirable side effects occurred?

Most experts will agree about the questions to be asked in any sound evaluation. An evaluation might not answer all the questions; it is not always possible to do so. Experts tend to disagree about the best means of answering the questions and about what constitutes an adequate response.

E. Herzog[11] listed the following questions for evaluation of efforts to bring about psychosocial change in individuals:

- What is the purpose of the evaluation? (What is to be achieved by doing it?)
- What kind of change is desired?
- By what means is change to be brought about?
- How trustworthy are the categories and measures employed?
- At what point is change to be measured?
- How fairly do the individuals studied represent the group discussed?
- What is the evidence that the changes observed are due to the means employed?
- What is the meaning of the changes found?
- Were there unexpected consequences?

The interrelationship of these questions is apparent. It has also been pointed out that, at times, as much benefit can be secured from the working out of the right questions as from the proposed activity. In addition, satisfaction can be achieved in installments because the evaluation need not wait until the end to learn about the replies to all the questions but can use data from individual questions as the information is secured.

This evolves to the concept of an evaluation process. Within this process, evaluation can occur at any point and usually does. A strong relationship can be noted between evaluation and program planning and operation. A possibility for conflict exists between administrators and evaluators for this reason. The evaluation process has been diagrammed by Elinson:[12]

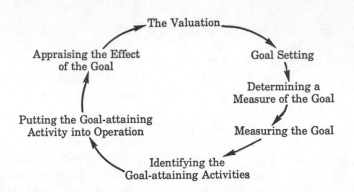

An example can be illustrated:

The Valuation	It is good to live a long time.
Goal Setting	Fewer people should develop coronary disease.
Determining a Measure of the Goal	Baseline mortality statistics by demographics.
Measuring the Goal	Current and past mortality statistics by demographic characteristics.
Identifying the Goal-attaining Activities	Choose from alternatives the conception of early detection centers for coronary disease.
Putting the Goal-attaining Activity into Operation	Establish detection centers in the community and motivate people to come in for an exam.
Appraising the Effect of the Goal	Have the detection centers reduced the mortality from coronary disease?
The Valuation	Was the activity worthwhile? Should it be continued?

Visualization of the evaluation process as a circle stemming from and returning to the formation of values places emphasis on the values in any evaluation effort. At the conclusion of the evaluation effort a new value might arise, or an old one might be modified or reaffirmed. In the example above, the old value, "It is good to live a long time," might be modified to, "It is good to live until 100 if you remain healthy, but if you can't remain healthy it's better not to live past 80."

Any evaluation effort must consider the vested interests that impinge upon the desirable or undesirable results. Conflicting viewpoints must be faced if the results of the evaluation are to stand up to the critics protecting their vested interests.

PURPOSES OF EVALUATION

Evaluation is an inherent part of everyday living as well as a part of all program activities, whether in the health care delivery system or in the manufacture of consumer products. It is vital that health planners understand why the evaluation effort is being undertaken; this understanding must be agreed to by administrators and other decision makers. Without this understanding, the evaluation will have no useful purpose except as an exercise.

Federal legislation has legally mandated the evaluation of the quality of health care. Health Maintenance Organizations (HMOs), Professional Standards Review Organizations (PSROs), and Health Systems Agencies (HSAs) are all engaged in the evaluation of health care. Some critics of the legislation creating these agencies state that the purpose of the evaluation of the quality of health care was to control cost, with quality running second. Consideration of these two elements—cost and quality—can certainly lead to different objectives of the evaluation activity. If cost were uppermost, there could be a tendency to evaluate with the idea of providing only those services deemed necessary to meet whatever standards are appropriate. If quality were uppermost, there could be a tendency to provide services that go beyond the basic minimum and seek to meet optimal standards for the preservation of life. Of course, there is also a relationship between the purposes of evaluation and the values considered of highest priority, as noted in the discussion of the evaluation process cycle.

Considering the variation in values, the following listing notes the major purposes attributed to evaluation:[13]

1. Evaluation can determine whether the objectives of a program are being met. Both the rate of progress and the level of attainment can be measured.
2. Evaluation can pinpoint the strengths and weaknesses of a program and suggest modifications to capitalize upon effective aspects.

3. Evaluation can compare the efficiency and adequacy of various programs and methods aimed at the same objective.
4. Evaluation can monitor standards of performance and provide quality controls.
5. Evaluation aids in the determination of measurable objectives by requiring definitions in operational terms.
6. Evaluation can develop new approaches and procedures as well as new projects for future programs.
7. Evaluation can provide checks on the possibility of negative side effects and alert the staff to the need for alterations.
8. Evaluation can indicate the generalization of an activity to other populations with suggested modifications.
9. Evaluation can recommend priorities among alternative programs in terms of the best utilization of limited resources.
10. Evaluation can add to the base of scientific knowledge and suggest hypotheses for future investigation.
11. Evaluation can test the effectiveness of different organizational structures and health care delivery systems.
12. Evaluation can meet the demand of public accountability by providing justification for continuing or discontinuing programs.
13. Evaluation can boost staff morale by involving them in the examination of their efforts and by setting goals and standards for measurement.
14. Evaluation can foster a critical attitude among staff, increase inter-communication, and result in increased coordination.

However, still dwelling on the role of values in evaluation, it should be noted that not everybody desires an honest evaluation. There are those who use evaluation as a window dressing or to meet the requirements of the law in name only. The purpose of the evaluation for these persons is not program improvement. Evaluation of ongoing, operational activities can fall prey under such circumstances to an overlay of administrative considerations that could lead to pseudo-evaluation. These have been identified as the following:[14]

1. *Eyewash.*   Selection of only the aspects of a program that "look good." Evaluation is limited to those parts that appear successful. This evaluation justifies a weak or bad program through the deliberate choice of the activities that look good.
2. *Whitewash.*   This evaluation seeks to cover up failure or errors by avoiding any objective assessment. An evaluation technique

used here solicits "testimonials" to create a diversion from the failure.

3. *Submarine.* Evaluation aims to "torpedo" or destroy a program, regardless of its worth. Thus, the purpose is to sink the program along with its administrators in clashes over power or prestige among directors or other administrators.

4. *Posture.* Here, prestige is developed by using evaluation as a gesture of objectivity and the assumption of a pose of scientific research. Hence, evaluation becomes a sign of professional status and looks good to the public.

5. *Postponement.* Evaluation is used as an excuse to gain time and delay action by noting the need to seek facts. By the time the evaluation is completed, the crisis will have subsided.

6. *Substitution.* Failure in a vital part of the program can be clouded over by shifting attention to an evaluation of another part of the program where success can be discussed and defended.

These are only some of the ways that the purposes of evaluation can be subverted to meet the needs of a crafty administrator. However, the health planner and evaluator have also to consider their role in assisting an administrator who obviously requires their aid in carrying out the spurious evaluation.

Generally, the two major aspects of the evaluation are to increase the effectiveness of program administration and to provide an essential element of any program activity. Thus, evaluation is an essential part of scientific program management. If operational programs are dedicated to the achievement of desired objectives rather than to the maintenance of the status quo, there will be a constant purposeful utilization of evaluation.

STEPS IN EVALUATION

Keeping in mind that there is no one right way to conduct an evaluation, a series of steps can be considered essential. The steps do not necessarily have to take place in the order noted. However, there does appear to be a more rational flow in the evaluation process if the steps can be followed in sequence. The following six steps are considered vital:[15]

1. identification of the goals to be evaluated,
2. analysis of the problems with which the activity must cope,
3. description and standardization of the activity,

4. measurement of the degree of change that takes place,
5. determination of whether the observed change is due to the activity or to some other cause, and
6. some indication of the durability of the effects.

Clearly, these steps create a scientific approach to evaluation. They have been cited in prior sections of this book and will be discussed in later sections of this chapter. Yet, this approach does not undermine evaluation of a much simpler order, which might not go through the steps noted. It could still be valuable to the program purpose.

Taking more of a managerial perspective,[16] another series of steps has been formulated:

1. formulation of the objectives;
2. specifications of the measures of performance;
3. development of the model, plans, and programs;
4. measurement of results;
5. determination of explanation of degree of success; and
6. recommendations for appropriate actions in view of the variance between the predetermined objectives and the actual results.

Steps 1, 2, and 3 are labeled as the process of planning; steps 4, 5, and 6 as program evaluation; and steps 3, 4, and 5 as management control. A reasonable amount of agreement can be observed between the two listings of steps.

Another method of listing evaluation steps cites four steps with examples of what each step means[17]:

1. Set goals	Definitions in operational terms
	Explicit criteria with behavior and standards noted
2. Data collection	Establish procedures for collection of data
	Develop required tools, questionnaires, etc.
	Set procedures for data collection with set time period
	Store the data on cards, tape, etc.
3. Analysis	Quantitative through statistics, modes, frequencies, etc.
	Qualitative through verbal descriptions, log books, interviews, etc.
	Tests for significance and conclusions
4. Recycle	On basis of data from step 3, adjust the program

Actually, all three lists of evaluation steps have a great deal in common. Health planners might also wish to create their own sequence of steps, adapting portions of these or other listings. In any event, the sequence will still have to contain the identification of goals and/or objectives, the specification of the program and/or activity, the determination of the measurement techniques, the actual collection of hard and/or soft data, the analysis, and the recommendations and/or conclusions.

Regardless of the sequence of steps taken in the evaluation process, there are some general rules that should be observed. E. Herzog[18] noted these "do's" and "don'ts" as she compiled the following realistic set of evaluation guidelines:

- Do bring in the evaluator early. Allow the evaluator to become fully involved. Waiting until the end of the project to employ an evaluator indicates lack of value attached to the evaluation.
- Do pre-evaluative investigation. It's worthwhile to secure a grass roots feeling for what's happening.
- Do engage in systematic study and exploration. This is an evaluation prerequisite. There is no need to reinvent the wheel; history is well known for repeating itself with regularity.
- Do include other disciplines in the evaluation effort. Statisticians, sociologists, social workers, nurses, and others can add to the evaluation with their diversity.
- Do coordinate efforts. This saves time, effort, and wear and tear on staff members.

- Don't use sophisticated evaluative techniques if other alternatives serve as well. Seek the simple approach first.
- Don't use existing case records as your only source of data for evaluation. An obvious bias occurs in this method; the reservations must be stated.
- Don't undertake evaluation unless adequate resources are available. Efforts will be wasted on gerrymandered evaluations.
- Don't undertake lopsided evaluations. It is not necessary to use a high-powered rifle to kill an ant.
- Don't underestimate unpretentious evaluation techniques. Sometimes, a simple yes or no questionnaire is powerful. Merely asking patients "why" can be most revealing.
- Don't believe in the fantasy of a neat, precise, utterly objective science in evaluation. Reliability and validity can be questionable on numerous occasions, as well as other variables.
- Don't overvalue loosely used terms in evaluation activities. Jargon can cloud a study and its results.

CLASSIFICATIONS AND CATEGORIES OF EVALUATION

Classifications and categories of evaluation deal with the various components of the success or failure of programs. In particular, the evaluation classifications define the type of measure to be used in judging an activity. A major distinction that consistently appears in the literature relates to the difference between effort and effect. Effort notes the amount of dollars spent on a program, the personnel involved, the facilities utilized, the number of specimens obtained, or the number of patient visits. Effect deals with the change in health status such as mortality or morbidity, the improvement of specific physical ailments, and the ability to carry on the activities of daily living. There is a great difference between establishing a program and determining whether that program does any good. It is also much easier to evaluate an activity in terms of effort than effect. The additional factor of efficiency also crops up frequently. Efficiency adds the measurement of how well and at what cost the program was conducted, as compared with alternative activities. These three are the most commonly documented categories of evaluation: effort, effect, and efficiency.

One of the more frequently used evaluation classifications was developed by Suchman.[19] It comprises five components: effort, performance, adequacy, efficiency, and process. These components are defined along with examples of questions answered by each component and concrete examples applied to program activities in Exhibit 7-1. To demonstrate the integration of the five elements, the example of a bird in flight is given as the first example for each component. To connect all the components in the bird example results in the consideration of the number of times the bird flapped its wings (effort), how far the bird flew (performance), how far the bird flew relative to the total distance (adequacy), could the bird have flown alternative routes or in air currents to get there faster (efficiency), and what principles of aerodynamics could improve the flight (process).

An example of the application of this five-component classification to the evaluation of a tuberculosis x-ray screening program (Exhibit 7-2) demonstrates the questions to be answered from all five components relative to a single health activity. In addition, the example notes the immediate objectives and the two assumptions underlying the objectives. Health planners should be able to proceed through the example and respond to the questions to gather a feeling for the scope and content of an evaluation utilizing this five-category classification. At times, this classification scheme has been used with different words substituted for three of the five components as noted: performance = effectiveness; adequacy = impact; and efficiency = cost effectiveness. In

Exhibit 7-1 Five Categories of Evaluation

Category	Questions Answered	Examples
Effort The criterion of success is the quantity and quality of activity that takes place; it is an assessment of input (workload) without regard to output.	What did you do? How well did you do it?	Number of times a bird flaps wings without any determination of how far did bird flies. 100,000 chest x-rays of children admitted to kindergarten to discover TB. Counting number of home health care visits with no relation to recovery. Counting people attending clinics and not the cure rate.
Performance This is a performance criterion measuring the results of effort rather than the effort itself; it requires a clear statement of objectives.	Did any change occur? How much was accomplished relative to an immediate objective? Was the change the one intended?	How far did the bird fly? How many cases of TB were found? Relating the number of home visits to reduced hospitalization demands. Relating the number of people attending clinics to reduced morbidity and mortality.
Adequacy The criterion of success is the degree to which effective performance is adequate to the total amount of need.	What portion of the target was achieved? How much progress toward a goal was recorded?	How far did the bird fly in terms of where he had to go? Of the people estimated to have TB and not know it, did the program discover 80 percent of the unknowns? An impact of 10 percent resulted in home visits to 500 people.
Efficiency This criterion is concerned with the evaluation of alternative methods in terms of costs; it represents a ratio between effort and impact.	Does it work? Is there any better way to attain the same results?	Could the bird have arrived at his destination more efficiently by some other means than flying the way he did? Did he take advantage of air currents? Did he fly too high or not high enough? Compared with x-rays, the skin test was more cost effective for children. Lesser trained personnel could make home visits more cost-effective.
Process This is an analysis of the process whereby a program produces the result it does; it is descriptive and diagnostic and looks for unanticipated negative and positive side effects.	What social changes are sought? What are the social communication channels? What are the social barriers? Who are the community leaders?	Learn about the anatomy of the bird and principles of flight to relate to the effort, effectiveness, impact, and cost effectiveness. Parents, particularly mothers, need to be motivated to get their children tested. Appeal to their concept of what good mothers should do for their children. Health care providers need to be informed about home health care and its ability to deliver quality care under general supervision.

330   BASIC HEALTH PLANNING METHODS

Exhibit 7-2 Evaluation of a Tuberculosis Program

Immediate Objectives
A. Provision of appropriate x-ray facilities for general hospitals and encouragement of the use of existing facilities for the x-raying of all adult admissions. As a more practical early objective we may seek to obtain the cooperation of 50 percent of our hospitals and expect them to x-ray 80 percent of
their adult admissions.
   (1) Assumptions
      a. Patients coming to hospitals constitute a group of high enough risk
         to justify giving them special attention. Also that it is easier to reach
         these groups in hospitals than elsewhere. This assumption requires
         constant proof in view of the changing picture of tuberculosis and
         the improvement in the efficiency of x-ray programs for the general
         adult population.
      b. Screening for tuberculosis by use of x-ray involves assumptions as to
         the validity and reliability of this technique.
   (2) Categories of Evaluation
      a. *Effort* Number of films taken, proportion of all hospitals partici-
         pating in survey, proportion of admissions in participating hospitals
         actually x-rayed. Proportion of screened positives followed up with
         additional examinations.
      b. *Performance* Yield of new confirmed cases in hospitals in rural
         areas, small and large cities. Yield of other pathology. Yield for each
         age-sex group of hospital admissions.
      c. *Adequacy* Total cases screened in terms of total potential: (1) in
         participating hospitals, and (2) all hospitals in the area. Total new
         cases found in terms of total unknown cases estimated in the area.
      d. *Efficiency* Considering the total number of new cases confirmed
         per film taken:
         (1) Would the x-raying of other groups have been more productive of
         new cases?
         (2) Was the confirmation rate so low that the program is inefficient?
         (3) Are the right age groups being x-rayed to uncover new cases?
         (4) Are hospitals using the equipment sufficiently to justify the ex-
         pense of the program?
         (5) Are a sufficient number of the cases discovered new cases, or are
         they persons already known?
         (6) Could the cases have been discovered with less effort through
         any other method?
      e. *Process* Under what conditions and in what situations does hospi-
         tal x-raying proceed most effectively? Why? Among which groups?
         Are there any unintended negative consequences to patient? Do
         x-rays reveal any other conditions?

Source: G. James, "Outline for the Evaluation of Tuberculosis Programs," mimeographed (Akron, Ohio: Department of Health, undated).

either case, the scheme still retains its characteristics as noted in Exhibit 7-2.

IMPACT AND PROCESS EVALUATION

Evaluation categories of impact and process evaluation essentially deal with outcomes and interactions, respectively. These two categories put the emphasis on style and feelings for data analysis. Process evaluation focuses upon the feelings of the people involved in the activity, the nuances of human behavior, and the understanding of what's happening. Impact evaluation tends to be hard nosed—seeking solid statistics, objective observations, and a definitive answer to the end goals of the activity. A comparison of these two classifications indicates the questions answered, the method used, and the information garnered relative to an example regarding emergency room utilization (Exhibit 7-3).

FOUR TYPES OF EVALUATION BASED ON OEO's DISTINCTION

Four major types of evaluation were denoted in a study of federal evaluation policy by the Office of Economic Opportunity (OEO). These four types were based, in part, on distinctions made when the OEO was responsible for programs such as Head Start, Upward Bound, Job Corps, and VISTA. In the definitions of the four evaluation categories—program impact evaluation, program strategy evaluation, project evaluation, and project rating—a distinction is noted between program and project.

A federal program refers to the provision of federal funds and administrative direction to accomplish a prescribed set of objectives through the conduct of specified activities. Typically, the federal money goes to intermediaries rather than to final recipients of services.

A project refers to the implementation level of a program, the level where resources are used to produce an end product that directly contributes to the objectives of the program. Therefore, a national Head Start program provided money and management aid, while the local Head Start projects conducted projects providing direct services to the public. Four types of evaluation followed:[20]

- *Program impact evaluation* An assessment of the overall effectiveness of a national program in meeting its objectives or of the relative effectiveness of two or more programs in meeting common

Exhibit 7-3 Comparison of Impact and Process Evaluation

	Process Evaluation	Impact Evaluation
Answers the question:	How to implement?	Should you implement?
Method:	Documentation and description. Asks what is going on, what are the problems.	Systematic observation. Emphasizes design and analysis to determine causality.
Site selection:	Selects sites to *maximize* variation along important dimensions.	Selects sites to *minimize* variation along important dimensions.
Example:	Evaluate the Experimental Medical System Policy (EMS): This policy is designed to reduce community mortality rates (unattended deaths in public and private places) and disability rates by creating a system of linkages between emergency room and communication systems, upgrading ambulance equipment, training ambulance and emergency room personnel, and implementing consumer health education programs.	
Information obtained from two types of evaluation:	How is political and legal cooperation obtained? How is a system set up? (technical and personnel questions)	To what extent is there a reduction in mortality and disability due to the operation of the EMS program?
	What new facilities are set up? What do they cost? How are new training programs developed? Who has responsibility for what?	What is the impact of the EMS program on costs of emergency care?

Source: N.R. Roos, "Evaluating Health Programs: Where Do We Find the Data?", *Journal of Community Health* 1 (1975):39. Reprinted with permission. © 1975 Human Sciences Press, New York, New York.

objectives. This type of evaluation assists policy makers in reaching decisions about program funding levels or in deciding on redirections of a program. Impact evaluation relies on the specification and measurement of appropriate output variables and the use of comparison groups. Environmental and process data usually are not essential.

- *Program strategy evaluation* An assessment of the relative effectiveness of different techniques used in a national program. This type of evaluation informs program managers about the relative effectiveness of the various strategies and/or methods utilized by the projects supported by the national program. These data are then passed on to other projects for adoption. Strategy evaluation depends on definition and measurement of appropriate environmental, input, process, and output variables selected on the basis of suitable analytic models.

- *Project evaluation* An assessment of the effectiveness of an individual project in achieving its stated objectives. This form of evaluation is often required by many federal programs and is carried out by project staff members or consultants. This type of evaluation allows project directors to monitor their efforts and to make modifications of the project as the data are analyzed. Project evaluation requires measurement of the output variables as well as the use of suitable comparison groups. Sometimes, project evaluations simply compare data with performance objectives or baseline conditions because this is more feasible. Comparison groups are omitted, and this can cloud the cause and effect result of the project intervention.
- *Project rating* An assessment of the relative effectiveness of different local projects in achieving program objectives. This type of evaluation provides program managers with information on the relative success of local projects operating within a national program. Project rating depends on definition and measurement of environmental variables and relatively inexpensive output measures, such as short term impact.

A MATRIX FOR EVALUATION OF PREVENTIVE HEALTH PROGRAMS

Preventive health programs have not received as much attention as therapeutic activities with regard to evaluation. A National Conference on Preventive Medicine appointed a task force to consider the question of quality control and the evaluation of preventive health services. In their report in 1974, this task force[21] took the following position:

> there should be assessment of the adequacy of the prevalence of preventive health programs and providers and that the objectives and standards of performance of a program or a provider should be clearly enumerated. Such standards and objectives should then be periodically and systematically evaluated to assure that goals are met. Concomitantly, there should be continued application of quality controls and evaluation of

standards to assure that the most effective modalities are employed to impact on the nation's health. In order to assure that these objectives are obtained, a public commitment supported by adequate program policies and funding is required.

To illustrate the type of evaluation required, a matrix for evaluation was developed by the task force. This matrix includes a definition of primary and secondary prevention with examples from each related to program objectives; structure and organization; and clinical, laboratory, and health education modalities.

A second part of the matrix identifies the evaluation elements and illustrates related examples from primary and·secondary prevention. Evaluation elements in this classification matrix include the penetration rate, cost efficiency, structure and organization, process measures (clinical, laboratory, health education), and program result measures (reduction of incidence, health status). An examination of Exhibit 7-4 indicates clearly what is meant by each of these evaluation elements. However, it will be necessary to set standards and objectives for each of the areas identified in the matrix.

After a perusal of this classification technique, it will help to see the model actually applied to a health program. In the example in Exhibit 7-5, family planning is considered as a preventive health activity. Definitions of the problem from primary and secondary prevention viewpoints are given, as well as facts about the nature of the problem and a summary. Then, the evaluation elements from the matrix are applied. The example illustrates data needed for each evaluation element and applicable methods and results. In addition, ·a general reference list and specific references referred to in the evaluation are also noted. As with many of the other classification categories, numerous similarities can be observed and points of concordance are more frequent than dissimilarities.

WORDS USED IN CLASSIFICATION CATEGORIES

To provide a panorama of evaluation categories and classifications, several additional schemes will be listed for comparison purposes. This will serve to show the agreements as well as to allow for the adaptation of a set of classifications that the health planner might wish to create for a specific purpose by borrowing a pinch from here and a dash from there.

In a discussion of evaluation in public health practice, James[22] listed the following elements in an evaluation schema:

Exhibit 7-4 Matrix for Evaluation

PREVENTIVE MEDICINE IS THAT BRANCH OF MEDICINE WHICH HAS PRIMARY INTEREST IN:

SECONDARY PREVENTION	PRIMARY PREVENTION
SLOWING THE PROGRESS OF DISEASE AND CONSERVING MAXIMAL FUNCTION[a]	PREVENTING PHYSICAL, MENTAL AND EMOTIONAL DISEASE AND INJURY IN CONTRAST TO TREATING THE SICK AND INJURED

ELEMENTS OF A PREVENTIVE HEALTH PROGRAM (PERSONAL AND ENVIRONMENTAL HEALTH)

Element	Example from Secondary Prevention	Example from Primary Prevention
Program Objective	Early detection of disease, maximize health status, prevention of complications	Environmental hazards, behavior modification, reduction of protection from communicable disease
Structure and Organization	Private physician, nurse practitioner	Health Department, school system, voluntary agency, group practice
Clinical Modality	Adequate data base, appropriate therapy	Immunizations
Laboratory Modality	Monitoring of blood sugars, BUNs	Pap smears, lead levels, hemoglobins, chest x-rays
Health Education Modality	Compliance with medication regime, weight reduction	Smoking, accident prevention

EVALUATION OF PREVENTIVE HEALTH PROGRAMS (PERSONAL AND ENVIRONMENTAL HEALTH)

Evaluation Element	Example from Secondary Prevention	Example from Primary Prevention
Penetration Rate	Proportion of target population with disease or condition under ongoing care	Proportion of target population reached
Cost Efficiency	Unit cost per newly discovered case, per case of controlled disease	Unit cost for immunization, fluoridation
Structure and Organization	Facilities, staff, organization, financing, integration of programs; provider range of therapeutic services, follow-up	Facilities, staff, organization, financing, integration of programs; identification and analysis of primary preventive program
Process Measures Clinical	Review of clinical performance by implicit/explicit criteria, tracers	Adequate maintenance of immunizations

Exhibit 7-4 Continued

Evaluation Element	Example from Secondary Prevention	Example from Primary Prevention
Laboratory	Appropriate studies performed	Assessment of quality controls and accuracy of studies
Health Education	Behavioral modification, patient compliance	Knowledge by the population, behavioral modification, accuracy and appeal of material and techniques
Program Result Measures		
Reduction of Incidence	Reduction of complications of disease or condition	Reduction of disease or condition
Health Status	Maximization of individual health status	Decreased mortality or morbidity, decreased work days lost

[a] American College of Preventive Medicine's definition of Preventive Medicine.

Source: Task Force Report, *Quality Control and Evaluation of Preventive Health Services* (New York: Prodist, 1976), pp. 106-107. Reprinted with permission. © 1976 Prodist, a division of Neale Watson Academic Publications, Inc.

- Effort—compare to national standards.
- Performance—what are the outcomes?
- Adequacy—what percent of the problem was solved?
- Efficiency—could the same result be achieved at lower cost?

Deniston and his associates[23] commented on program evaluation. They enumerated the following components:

- Appropriateness—the relative impact of the program.
- Adequacy—degree to which the program eliminates the problem.
- Effectiveness—measure of the extent the program achieves its goal.
- Efficiency—ratio between input and output.

Six interdependent elements in any evaluation undertaking were identified by Weckwerth.[24] He called them the generic structure of evaluation and necessarily a part of the process of evaluation:

Context   (what, where, when, and who).
Content   (program elements being or intended to be provided and why).
Process   (how care is organized and delivered).
Output   (how many times did the bird flap its wings).
Outcome   (did the bird fly?).
Benefit   (how high and far, with what resources).

Exhibit 7-5 Evaluation Study Example

Subject: Family Planning Programs

Primary Prevention. Preventing unwanted pregnancies by contraceptive methods.

Secondary Prevention. Provision of clinic and support services for: (1) unwanted pregnancies (abortion or prenatal care); (2) wanted pregnancies (infertility services and prenatal care).

Nature of the Problem. It was estimated in 1973 that 1.9 million low-income and 1.8 million marginal income women at risk were still apparently without access to effective modern methods of contraception [141] even though the overall crude birthrate declined by more than 41 percent and the general fertility rate declined by 44 percent [142] between the years 1957 and 1973. The Secretary of HEW has given major credit for this decline to the federal family planning efforts. "By reducing unwanted births, the program has been cost effective, saving more than two dollars for every dollar spent."

Summary. Major evaluation enforts in family planning have been directed at the areas of penetration rate, cost effectiveness, effectiveness of the methods employed, and the obvious outcome in terms of fewer pregnancies. There is, however, a dearth of evaluation of quality of clinical process and performance.

General References

A.A. Campbell, "The Role of Family Planning in the Reduction of Poverty," *Journal of Marriage and the Family* 30:236, 1968.

Patricia K. Chokel and Janet T. Dingle, "Using Standard Data for Program Evaluation in Cleveland," *Family Planning Perspectives* 4:216, 1973.

Hector Correa, Vestal W. Parrish, Jr., and Joseph D. Beasley, "A Three-Year Longitudinal Evaluation of the Costs of a Family Planning Program," *American Journal of Public Health* 12:1647, 1972.

Committee on Terminology of the National Family Planning Forum, "A Family Planning Glossary," *Family Planning Perspectives,* 3:34, 1972.

Charles R. Dean, "Staffing Patterns and Clinic Efficiency," *Family Planning Perspectives,* 4:35, 1970.

Steven Polgar and Frederick S. Jaffe, "Evaluation and Record-keeping for the U.S. Family Planning Services," *Public Health Reports,* 8:639, 1968.

Steven Polgar, O. Ornati, and J.G. Dryfoos, "How to Estimate Unmet Need for Family Planning in Your Community," *American Journal of Public Health,* 56:917, 1966

Exhibit 7-5 Continued

Michael J. Reardon et al. "Real Costs of Delivering Family Planning Services—Implications for Management," *American Journal of Public Health,* 9:860, 1974.

M. Tayback, "Evaluation of Family Planning Programs," Paper presented at the Institute in Administration of New Programs in Maternal and Child Health, University of California, Berkeley, January 19, 1966.

Evaluation of Family Planning Programs

Evaluation Element: Penetration Rate

Example of Data Needed and/or Applicable Methods and Results: In the United States, in 1973, it was estimated that 5.6 million low-income and an additional 3.4 million marginal income women needed family planning services. Of these, 65 percent received services from either organized programs or private physicians.[1]

Evaluation Element: Cost Efficiency

Example of Data Needed and/or Applicable Methods and Results: The National Analyst study collected cost data on 45 family planning projects for the program year of 1968–1969 utilizing cost line items and service categories for collection and analysis of the cost data. It was dete.mined that "the per patient cost to the average project for the year 1968–1969 was about $76. If the total operating cost of the 45 projects for the same year was divided by the total number of women seen at least once during the year, an annual unit cost per patient was about $53."[2]

Evaluation Element: Structure and Organization

Example of Data Needed and/or Applicable Methods and Results: In addition to a review of the facilities, scope of services, administrative organization, etc., evaluation of staffing patterns and patient/staff ratios can be carried out. One example of this is Perkins's Patient/Staff Index.[3] By using this particular evaluative measure, it was found that clinics whose staffs were fully utilized during a session reported a higher patient/staff index than clinics which were either over-staffed or under-utilized. It was also found that clinics which report an unusually high index potentially were not providing adequate individual patient care or were requiring existing staff to process too many patients during a single session.

Evaluation Element: Process Modalities—Clinical, Laboratory, and X-ray

Example of Data Needed and/or Applicable Methods and Results: Family planning care standards and criteria have been established by such groups as the ACOG and Maternal and Infant Care-Family Planning Programs. However, there has not been extensive evaluation of care against these standards and criteria.

Evaluation Element: Process Modalities—Health Education

Example of Data Needed and/or Applicable Methods and Results: Planned Parenthood of Buffalo was involved in the production of TV spots and in the follow-up studies of their effectiveness. Each set of TV spots carried a different phone number to call for information, to be able to measure the general responses as well as to find out which spot was most appealing. The effectiveness was judged significant in that 51 percent or approximately every other person who called during the two month period, made and kept an appointment.[4]

Evaluation Element: Program Results—Reduction of Incidence

Example of Data Needed and/or Applicable Methods and Results: Determination of reduction of incidence of pregnancies requires data collection and analysis of birth rate changes, etc., utilizing such sources as census data, birth certificates, hospital delivery figures. For example, in Atlanta, Georgia, a study was done to see if there was any effect from the family planning program at Grady Memorial Hospital. The clinic enrollment had doubled from 1963 to 1968 and during this same period, births at the hospital declined from 7,125 a year to 5,935—a decrease of 17 percent.[5]

Evaluation Element: Program Results—Health Status

Example of Data Needed and/or Applicable Methods and Results: Though implications have been made concerning the effect/benefit of family planning on such areas as housing

Exhibit 7-5 Continued

availability, poverty levels, numbers within the educational systems and an increased female work force[6] as well as improved marital adjustment and less child abuse, little evaluative research has been carried out in this area.

[1] Marsha Corey, "The State of Organized Family Planning Programs in the United States, 1973," *Family Planning Perspectives* 1:15, 1974.

[2] Gerald Sparer, Louise Okada, and Stanley Tillinghast, "How Much Do Family Planning Programs Cost?", *Family Planning Perspectives* 2:100, 1973.

[3] Gordon W. Perkins, "Measuring Clinic Performance," *Family Planning Perspectives* 1:37, 1969.

[4] Jean Hutchinson, "Using TV to Recruit Family Planning Patients," *Family Planning Perspectives* 2:8, 1970.

[5] Carl W. Taylor et al., "Assessment of a Family Planning Program: Contraceptive Services and Fertility in Atlanta, Georgia," *Family Planning Perspectives* 2:25, 1970.

[6] James A. Sweet, "Differentials in the Rate of Fertility Decline 1960-1970," *Family Planning Perspectives* 2:103, 1974.

Source: Task Force Report, *Quality Control and Evaluation of Preventive Health Services* (New York: Prodist, 1976), pp. 149-151. Reprinted with permission. © 1976 Prodist, a division of Neale Watson Academic Publications, Inc.

Clearly, context, content, and process combine in many ways to produce the output, the outcome, and the benefits.

Weckwerth also enumerated the five As of evaluation. These are listed with comments alongside to illustrate the interdependency among the components:

Acceptability	These first four are a dependent sequence.
Accessibility	Services can be deemed appropriate, yet be un-
Appropriateness	available. Or they can be available, yet not ac-
Availability	cessible. Or services can be appropriate, and
and	available and accessible, but still not acceptable
Accountability	to either or both the providers or the consumers. However, accountability overrides the four A's since it is the essence of the moral contractual agreement made between the seeker when he seeks and the server when he serves.

Clearly, all the classifications and categories of evaluation demonstrate that just as there is no single right way to do evaluation, there is surely no single classification or category that is mutually exclusive of all the others. Rather, it is obvious that much borrowing and interexchange of ideas and concepts have taken place. It is probable that this trend will continue in future evaluation classifications. Health planners would do well to closely examine the schemes already noted or others that may be relevant and pick and choose, or adopt wholly an existing classification. It is not necessary to reinvent the wheel.

MEASUREMENT TYPOLOGIES IN EVALUATION

Although a classification or category schematic will point out the information needed to conduct the evaluation, the need exists to translate the classifications into collectable numbers. However, the numbers do not necessarily have to be attached to a frequency distribution or a counting procedure. At times, qualitative data can be transformed into quantitative data by assigning number weights to the respective qualities based on a priority assignment. Therefore, satisfied could be 1, dissatisfied 2, and neutral 0. However, measurements should adhere to generally appropriate qualities to render the evaluation worthwhile. Health measurements should be:[25]

1. objective;
2. repeatable by different observers and at different times;
3. efficient in terms of clear and mutually exclusive divisions, undistorted scale, and broad range of values to be recorded;
4. as simple, generally available, easily performed, and inexpensive as possible; accurate in sensitivity and specificity; and
5. tested in a pilot study to determine the four qualities already listed.

Obviously, not all measurements can adhere to those characteristics. However, if the health planner can keep to a reasonably close approximation, it might be possible to avoid intense criticism of the evaluation.

Some of the most common evaluation measurements fall into the grouping of five "D"s: death, disease, disability, discomfort, and dissatisfaction.[26,27] Each of these will be listed with more detail and a noting of problems connected with each measurement.

1. *Death*   Statistics are usually readily available on deaths and, with analysis, on premature death. However, the population base may be uncertain and there may be incomplete records.
2. *Disease*   These measures are based on departures from physiologic or functional norms appropriate to age and sex and include acute, chronic, self-terminating, and incurable conditions. Indicates the severity of the threat to survival but does not include the measurements of disability or discomfort. Problems with the data relate to the clinical determinations and the other variables involved in causation.
3. *Disability*   Measures note the inability to carry out customary roles and perform customary duties including the loss of produc-

tivity. Acute and chronic disability is counted along with the degree of impairment and the number of days of disability. The relationship of disability to the individual's social role raises questions as does the judgment distinctions between handicapped or disabled persons.

4. *Discomfort* In both acute and chronic forms, measurements regard the degree of severity as well as the proportion of days involved. Includes scientific measures as well as subjective. Since discomfort is usually self-reported, subjectivity is a problem. In addition, other variables of a sociocultural nature influence reporting of discomfort.

5. *Dissatisfaction* Measures cover a broad spectrum of factors relating to physical, intellectual, emotional, and social aspects such as the physician's attitude and the cost of care. Both degree and intensity should be recorded. Yet, these data will be mostly subjective and tainted by other variables.

Measurements of disease are becoming more and more vital as federal legislation and a general upsurge in consumer advocates press for greater improvement in the quality of health care. Professional Standards Review Organizations evaluate care rendered to inpatients and determine whether governmental funds can pay for services rendered. Medical societies advocate required continuing medical education for their physician members. With this heightened interest, health planners can consider an additional expansion of the disease category with the following measures of morbidity:

- tissue alterations confirmed by pathology reports;
- functional alterations recorded by measuring equipment, such as EKGs;
- physical or mental conditions determined by clinical diagnosis by physicians;
- physical or mental disease as reported by the individuals;
- observable symptoms such as rash, swelling, or sores; and
- unobservable symptoms such as headache, guilt, tiredness, or itch.

Again, the more objective the measure, the more respected will be the evaluation. If objective tests are available, they would be the preferred measurement of disease. However, the "curing" aspect of health care is only a part of the picture. A "caring" aspect can be just as important in the total health care and is a vital part of the evaluation. Objective measurements in this area are difficult to achieve. This "caring" factor becomes even more critical when the additional fact is added that much more disease is linked to life style than to actual biological invasion of the body. In any event, research is required to define the objective measurements that can be used to codify the "art of medicine."

Generally, many types of measurements in evaluation activities could be utilized including rankings, ratings, counting, sampling, surveys, records of all types, case studies, field investigations, and even experimental research. Outcome, tracer, criteria, and process are words often associated with the evaluation of the quality of health care. However, the following simplified version of types may prove utilitarian and adjustable:

Measurements in evaluation may be made through:

- *Testing* Either in written or oral form, a test can be administered to measure the subject's knowledge, attitudes, or behavior. Obviously, responses to attitude and behavior questions only indicate a mental process and might not truly reflect the individual's attitude or behavior.
- *Interviews* Measurements can be taken through the use of surveys, depth interviews, opinion polls, group interviews, one-to-one interviews, and expert opinion interviews. In addition, the interviewer can add additional data on environmental factors and intonations. Interviewer bias has to be considered, as well as the point that respondents tend to want to give the answers that they think the interviewer wishes to receive.
- *Reports* These measurements include all types of medical care records and charts, as well as descriptive material such as annual reports and special studies. Statistical data on file from a variety of sources would be measurement fodder in this category. Of course, health planners must be aware that not everything that is written down is absolutely factual.
- *Observations* On-site observations are included here as trained evaluators monitor an activity and prepare reports. Checklists and guides are used to assure objectivity and to pinpoint the required observations. This measurement technique can truly evaluate behavior, as the behavior can be noted with either a yes or a no.
- *Samples* If the health care activity actually involves the production of some product, that product can be collected and evaluated. Questionnaires used in a project could be reviewed by opinion polling experts to determine their worth.

One of the more commonly used measurements in health care evaluation deals with the division of the evaluation into three components:

structure, process, and outcome.[28] Structural measurements include data about facilities and equipment, organizational patterns, financing mechanisms, staffing patterns, and personnel qualifications and experience. Generally, structure components deal with resources. Process measurements include information about provider/physician encounters and the health care system process. These deal mainly with the curing aspects of health care. Outcome measures include individual and population mortality and morbidity, individual physical functioning, and provider and patient satisfaction. Health status is the major concern of the outcome evaluations (Exhibit 7-6). Yet, even in this type of measurement, disagreements arise as to where specific components belong in the structure/process/outcome breakdown. R. Greene[29] lists sources of data, with the least expensive method first and the most expensive last. In addition, the methods are then sorted out using the structure/process/outcome classifications. This listing was modified by Greene from an Institute of Medicine report on quality assessment and is reproduced in Exhibit 7-7.

Data Sources

Routinely reported data about population, resources, and organizations are gathered by health agencies and commonly note information such as the number of hospital beds in a community or the physician to patient ratio. These data are readily available, inexpensively obtained, and describe the structure existing in the area in detail.

Hospital discharge abstracts contain the minimal basic data set needed by all agencies interested in patient admissions. These abstracts are used for billing and claim purposes and for management control. Standardized terminology is used, and computerization can be achieved easily. Both process and outcome measurements are cited. However, there will be limited data about any single admission due to the volume of abstracts recorded.

Claims forms are those used to bill a patient or third party payer for services rendered. These forms have information about the patient, drugs, hospital days, clinic visits, procedural charges, and utilization of special facilities. Similar forms from physicians can be matched with institutional claim forms. Institutions and providers often use different terminology for identical services, making comparisons difficult. There is a movement to supercede existing claims forms by uniform hospital discharge abstracts and ambulatory encounter forms. These claim forms provide a little process data and immediate outcome information.

Prescriptions may be kept on file by pharmacists, institutions, and third party payers and are readily available for evaluation purposes.

Exhibit 7-6 Examples of Components of a Structure, Process,
Outcome Evaluation Measurement

Structure Components	Process Components	Outcome Components
Facilities	Provider/patient encounters	Mortality
Equipment		Morbidity
Organization patterns	Health care system process	Individual physical functioning
Funding	Desirable health practices	
Staffing	Technical aspects of care	Provider satisfaction
Personnel qualifications	"Art" aspects of care	Consumer satisfaction
Personnel experience		Community satisfaction
Environmental quality		Wellness level
Risk factors		Tests and vital signs relative to norms
(Resources)	(Curing process)	(Health status)

Generally, the prescription does not have the diagnosis or the generic drug name but does have patient and provider identification. Prescriptions are documents generated in an ambulatory encounter that give incomplete information about the process of health care.

Encounter forms provide data about ambulatory visits. As noted, there is a movement to standardize the terminology and the forms as with the uniform hospital abstract. The combining of successive visits into an account of "an episode of illness" will provide process and limited immediate outcome data. Since this information can be handled by a computer, evaluation will be inexpensive and easily available.

Source-oriented medical records contain notations from physicians, nurses, consultants, laboratory reports, and contributions from other professionals. These records are sometimes difficult to use because of the masses of data that are poorly organized, incomplete, and possibly inaccurate. Information relates process data and immediate outcome material. However, the sheer volume makes measurement laborious. An abstracting service is provided by the Professional Activity Study (PAS) of the Commission on Professional and Hospital Activities, which covers 1,700 hospitals in the United States and Canada.

Problem-oriented medical records utilize a system developed by L.L. Weed[30] that has all providers using the same pages with the information grouped by the patient's problems with flow sheets used for serially recorded data. These records emphasize noting the logic of health care decisions and allow for the progress to be readily traced through the record. A record of this nature highlights the medical care process

Exhibit 7-7 Relationship Between Evaluation Data and Classification of Data By Structure, Process, or Outcome

Method of Collection	Type of Data Structure	Process	Outcome
Routinely reported data about population, resources and organizations	X		
Hospital discharge abstract		X	X
Claims form		X	
Prescription		X	
Encounter form		X	X
Source-oriented medical record		X	X
Problem-oriented medical record		X	X
Direct observation of physicians	X	X	
Simulation techniques	X	X	
Patient interview		X	X
Patient re-examination and testing			X
Population survey		X	X

Note: Methods of collection ranked roughly by *cost* of collection: least expensive at top, most expensive at bottom.

X = These types of data can be collected by this method.

Source: R. Greene, *Assuring Quality in Health Care: The State of the Art* (Cambridge, Mass: Ballinger Publishing Co., 1976), p. 45. Reprinted with permission. © 1976 Ballinger Publishing Co.

and gives more detail about outcomes, since more than technical detail is required. Records provide a rich source of evaluation data for analysis if the notes can be organized to focus attention to the specific problems.

Direct observation by physicians is the most viable source of process data since the observation is independent of any record or notation. Behavior can be evaluated on site simultaneously with the event. It is possible that the presence of an observer may influence the behavior or not be agreeable to the patient. Furthermore, the observer's reactions require standardization to achieve reliability. This would be a most valuable evaluation, but it would be time consuming and costly.

Simulation techniques using actors or computers evaluate clinical competence and provide process data. Pseudopatients have been used to discover abuse and fraud in government health care programs such as Medicaid. A caution must be taken in that physicians might not act in the same way with computer or artificial simulations as they do in real life.

Patient interviews may be conducted face-to-face, by telephone, or by self-administered questionnaire. Health outcomes, from the patient's viewpoint, detail functional ability, satisfactions about the process of care, and other details about the health care system. Obviously, the evaluation is colored and one-sided. In addition, these data are expensive to gather, and a poor response rate would make the collected data biased.

Patient reexamination and testing involves the duplication of the care giving process by another professional to verify the outcome. This should be an objective outcome measure but is very expensive because of the duplication.

Population surveys include the collection of data using various methods from a representative sample of the community residents. Information can be secured about the process and the outcome measures either from patients or objectively determined methods. This is the most expensive way to secure evaluation data, and the response rate problem is compounded.

No matter what technique is used to evaluate health care, the ultimate source has to be in the provider/patient or consumer interaction. Generally, the more remote from that interaction, the more transcribing and condensing that takes place, usually resulting in a greater likelihood of misinformation and inaccuracy about the event. Recorded data, in whatever form, reflect the ability of the individual to write as well as the actual ability to provide services to the public. Therefore, it is important to make the distinction between the evaluation of the actual activity as observed and the evaluation of the written or recorded descriptive material about the activity.

FRAMEWORK OF EVALUATION BY LEVEL OF MEASUREMENT AND TARGET AND SERVED POPULATIONS

A framework that encompasses elements of the measurement components already discussed was developed by M. I. Roemer.[31] His schematic follows:

Level of Evaluation	Eligible or Target Population	Patients Actually Served
1. Health status outcomes		
2. Estimated quality of service	///////////////	
3. Quantity of services provided		
4. Attitudes of recipients		
5. Resources made available		///////////////
6. Costs of program		

Health status outcomes would include mortality, morbidity, and measures of the individual's ability to function in everyday activities. However, other variables do affect these measures, and there could be some difficulty collecting data.

Quality of service can be judged by medical record audits, direct observations, and adherence to criteria such as those prepared by PSROs. Inadequate and inaccurate medical records have proved quite troublesome in the quality measures, and observation is open to bias. PSRO and other criteria have been labeled as baseline medicine or minimum quality. Obviously, there is no measurement possible for the target population since no services were rendered there.

Quantity of services provided can be measured by merely counting the personnel, facilities, supplies, etc. that were offered and relating them to the services used by the population. There should be no difficulty here unless the records are filled out incorrectly, lost, or misplaced. Measurements would include utilization rates, numbers of tests made, and all other counts of services and manpower and their relationship.

Attitudes of recipients can be measured through self-administered questionnaires, interviews, or surveys. Measures of satisfaction and humanistic and personal aspects of health care can be recorded. A great deal of subjectivity enters the measurements, and the validity of the responses can be legitimately questioned.

Resources made available relate to the preparation and planning for the services or activities. This would be an inventory of the types of physicians and other manpower employed, a listing of the equipment prepared, and a listing of the facilities involved. Again, this should be no problem. There is no need to measure the resources for patients served since the material was made available for the target population.

Costs of the program would include salaries, rentals, supplies, etc. Budgets should readily supply this information. However, hidden costs might be included in this measurement, such as providing for substitutes within the family to replace care rendered within an institution. These per unit measures could then be comparable with the cost of other units. Items such as the cost per case of measles or the drug cost per case could evolve in this category.

Within each of the ten cells (boxes), evaluation requires the comparison of the measurements of at least the following two entities:

1. measures defined across time, i.e., before and after the activity.
2. measures defined across space, i.e., test and control groups.

EVALUATION OF HOSPITAL PERFORMANCE

System efficiency and patient care are included in this proposal for the measurement of care rendered by a hospital. This evaluation method utilizes the elements of the structure, process, and outcome method noted earlier. In addition, the measures are divided into patient care and administrative measures, as seen in Exhibit 7-8. Note the footnote on the exhibit as to the source of these specific measures as compiled by R.M. Grimes and S.K. Moseley[32] in their approach to an index of hospital performance. In addition, about 30 experts in the field ranked the measures through a Delphi technique. On a weighted basis, four patient care and three administrative care measures led the list as follows:

- Patient care: surgical procedures assessment, expert evaluation of patient care, medical staff qualification, medical audit.
- Administrative care: use of management studies, cost per unit of output, expert evaluation of administrative performance.

While there may be some difficulty with quantifying the measures for actual usage, the following operational definitions reveal the general data requirements.

Exhibit 7-8 Suggested Measures of Hospital Effectiveness

Patient Care Measures	Administrative Measures
STRUCTURAL	
Accreditation	Accreditation
Medical staff qualifications	Administrative staff qualifications
Professional staff qualifications*	Use of employee development
Professional staff training*	programs
Special care unit availability;	Personnel per occupied bed
utilization	Services provided
PROCESS	
Medical staff audit	Use of management studies
Average length of stay	Occupancy rate
Autopsy rate	Management planning activities*
Community involvement*	Community involvement*
OUTCOME	
Patient outcome	Cost per unit of output
Surgical procedures assessment	Man-hours per patient day
Adjusted death rate	Financial stability*
Hospital-acquired infections:	
reported; treated	
Malpractice suits*	
ATTITUDINAL	
Expert evaluation of patient care	Expert evaluation of administrative
	performance
Patient satisfaction	Employee satisfaction
(dissatisfaction)	(dissatisfaction)

*Measures indicated were suggested by panelists during Delphi survey; the remainder were gleaned from health research literature.
Source: R.M. Grimes and S.K. Moseley, "An Approach to an Index of Hospital Performance." Reprinted with permission from *Health Services Research*, Vol. 11, No. 3, Fall 1976, p. 289. Copyright 1976 Hospital Research and Educational Trust, 840 North Lake Shore Drive, Chicago, Illinois 60611.

Patient Care Measures

1. Surgical procedures assessment can be measured by the percentage of surgically removed tissues proved to be normal on examination.

2. Expert evaluation of patient care performance can be secured by requesting hospital administrators to rate the hospitals under review on a scale from poor to excellent.
3. Medical staff qualifications can be judged by the percentage of staff who are board certified.
4. Medical audit can be measured by the existence of a medical audit program and the active support of the physicians at the hospital.
5. Accreditation measures can be secured from the latest Joint Commission on Accreditation of Hospitals (JCAH) report with emphasis on comments relating to medical records, medical staff, emergency room, nursing, and laboratory, with rankings given for major and minor problems.
6. Patient dissatisfaction can be measured by the percentage of patients reporting fair or poor service in discharge questionnaires.
7. Autopsy measures reflect the percentage of patients who were autopsied.
8. Average length of stay means the average number of days of hospitalization per patient.
9. Adjusted death rate refers to the percentage of admitted patients who die in the hospital.

Administrative Measures

1. Use of management studies can be counted during recent years with emphasis on staffing, costs, budgeting, employee turnover, clinic waiting times, purchasing procedures, dietary packaging and distribution, computer applications, blood bank inventory analysis, laboratory utilization, and long range planning.
2. Cost per unit of output includes items such as cost per pound of laundry, cost per unit of floor space, cost per laboratory test performed, and cost per x-ray procedure.
3. Expert evaluation of administrative performance can be measured by a peer group rating of hospital administrators.
4. Accreditation can be measured by looking at the JCAH ratings on administration, dietary, maintenance, accounting, and personnel.
5. Personnel per occupied bed is measured by the ratio of full-time equivalent personnel to occupied beds.
6. Employee dissatisfaction can be measured by the percentage of employee turnover.

7. Nursing hours per patient day is a feasible substitute for all personnel hours per day since records may not be easily on hand for all personnel.
8. Administrative staff qualifications can be based upon educational background, number of years of experience, and membership in professional organizations.
9. Use of employee development programs relates to the percentage of employees who attend job-related training programs including inservice programs.
10. Occupancy rate notes the average occupied beds as a percentage of the total number of beds.

Yet, these measures of a hospital's performance are not dominated by a single evaluation measure but by a part that all play in effectiveness. It should be noted that hospitals scoring high on patient care indexes appear to have a high autopsy rate, an effective medical audit program, longer lengths of stay, a higher percentage of board-certified specialists, fewer dissatisfied patients, and were rated higher by peer groups and by the JCAH. Hospitals scoring high on the administrative measures had better educated staff, more experienced staff, did more management analysis, and had more personnel per occupied bed. Peer groups judged the hospital administration higher, as did the JCAH.

Health planners may find fault with the elements listed in the measures of a hospital's effectiveness, but nevertheless, these measures were selected by a group of experts and can be taken at face value or adapted based on additional information. It might also be possible to refine the definitions of measurement more explicitly as additional data become available. For example, total personnel per occupied bed could be expanded as records reveal who does what for the patient.

In any case, the determination of the components of what constitutes an evaluation of the patient care and the administrative health care aspects of the hospital are worth measuring. This proposal can be taken as a starting point.

METHODOLOGY MATRIX FOR PROFESSIONAL STANDARDS REVIEW

With the passage of federal legislation requiring the establishment of PSROs, the need arose for an evaluation of the medical care received by inpatients paid for by the federal government under various programs such as Medicare and Medicaid. S. Shindell[33] developed the matrix of methodology shown in Exhibit 7-9. This matrix summarizes

Exhibit 7-9 Matrix of Methodology

	PROSPECTIVE	CONCURRENT	RETROSPECTIVE
ESTABLISH STANDARDS	Concensus of Physician Panel on Medical Need: –Outpatient Diagnosis –Ambulatory Procedure	Disease/Age – Specific Length of Stay Norms from: –Data Systems –Third-Party Payers –Foundation – PSRO	Concensus of Physician Panel: –Tissue Review –Death Review –Utilization –Audit
CONDUCT ACTIVITY	Preadmission Screen by: –Nurse Coordinator –Physician Consultant	1. Pre-set Expected Stay 2. Check at Predetermined Date for: –Discharge –Reasons for Extension	Hospital Profile to Select Problems Chart Review by Medical Records, Nurse Coordinator or Other Selective Pattern Review
DOCUMENT ACTIVITY	Admission Abstract: –Identify Patient –Identify Physician –Specific Condition –Contemplated Procedure –Action Taken	Inclusion in Standard Discharge Abstract: –Pre-set Norm –Condition Accounting for Extension	Inclusion of Audit Codes in Discharge Abstract Variations from Accepted Norms
ANALYZE RESULTS	Comparisons: –Admission Rates –Hospital-Hospital –Present-Past –Review Norms	Comparisons: –Actual-Expected Index –Hospital-Hospital –Present-Past –Review Norms	Comparisons: –Degree of Variation –Hospital-Hospital –Present-Past –Review Norms

Source: S. Shindell, "The Elements of Professional Standards Review," *Journal of Legal Medicine* 1 (1973): 34. Reprinted with permission. © 1973 *Journal of Legal Medicine.*

a variety of measurement sources of use in a medical care evaluation system.

Three types of medical reviews are identified across the top; prospective, concurrent, and retrospective. Four activities are listed along the left margin; establish standards, conduct activity, document activity, and analyze results.

Prospective review refers to the evaluation of the hospital admission prior to actual admission to determine if hospital admission is medically necessary. Of course, this refers only to elective hospital admission and not emergencies.

Concurrent medical review takes place while the patient is still occupying the hospital bed and evaluates the continued occupancy of that bed by that patient.

Retrospective medical review occurs after the completion of the hospital stay and deals with the events and the outcomes of the hospital stay.

"Establish standards" refers to the recognized need to use some previously agreed upon guidelines for use in evaluating actual performance. These guidelines must be based on sound medical judgment and be consistent with the needs of the patient.

"Conduct activity" means that the guidelines are now being used by somebody to review medical care. This activity concerns how the evaluation is carried out.

"Document activity" refers to the fact that the physician and others document whatever care is being rendered. The care rendered should be in keeping with currently acceptable therapeutic procedures.

"Analyze results" is the end goal of the entire process; it looks at accomplishments. Comparisons of experiences in different settings and a measurement of benefits are included here. Prior to analysis, objectives should be known so that data can be collected and a determination can be made of whether the objectives have been reached.

A Review of the Process

Prospective review guidelines are based on a consensus among physicians of the rationale for hospital admission. Sample criteria for short stay hospital review have been prepared by the American Medical Association and the specialty medical associations. Generally, the question is whether the procedure could be accomplished on an outpatient basis without a hospital stay. The review can be conducted by a nurse coordinator and/or a physician consultant. A preadmission request form could also be used. In either case, there has to be an authorization for the admission that is based on the established standards. Documentation is clear and notes the identity of the patient and the physician, the specific condition, the contemplated procedure, and the action that was taken. This provides the information required for the analysis. Analysis can compare experience with regard to the predetermined guidelines, can compare experience from hospital to hospital, or can compare experience over a time period in the past and the present.

Concurrent review sets guidelines or standards based on existing available statistics, such as health care data banks, reports from third party payers, or foundation and PSRO reports. From these data, anticipated lengths of stay can be noted for specific conditions and related to age, sex, or other demographic variables. Norms can be selected at 50th percentiles or median stays or average stays. The conduct of concurrent review requires the nurse and/or the physician consultant to indicate the expected discharge date and check for the actual discharge time, or for reasons for an extension of the hospital stay. Documentation takes place routinely if the patient is discharged as expected. An explanation is required where the stay is extended to show the medical evidence for the extension. Analysis is similar to that used in the prospective review. An actual-expected index would indicate the relationship between expected length of stay and the actual stay. A ratio of 1.0 would mean that all stays were as expected. A 1.2 index would mean that there were 20 percent more days used than the expected. This index can be calculated by hospital, by department, by diagnostic category, by physician, by age of the patient, and so on. These ratios can then be used for comparative evaluation.

Retrospective review refers to areas where most of the experience in medical care evaluation has taken place using physician panels and tissue review, death review, utilization review, and medical audit as measures of the quality of care. Here, process and outcome measures are evaluated. Generally, preset standards are used in the reviews. The conduct of activities takes place through chart review and/or specifying diseases to compare against a profile of standards such as PSRO guidelines. A nurse coordinator, with or without consultation with a physician or committee, reviews the materials. Documentation involves the committee reports, with notes about the correction of deficiencies and special audit codes for abstracting. Analysis is similar to the other two review types, with a degree of variation in comparisons used for feedback to the hospital staff. This feedback then becomes the basis for appropriate change in hospital procedures and for continuing medical education.

With this type of evaluation matrix, the activity or project can be examined prior to the onset of a project, during the program, and after the conclusion. Using the four steps of standards cited, the evaluation should have objectives and data to use for the analysis.

This methodology can be adapted to other forms of evaluation, and the steps can be expanded to include additional aspects. Of major importance is the filling in of each cell with the details required to follow through on the actual evaluation. Thus, the matrix serves as a skeleton. This method is another tool that can be used in evaluation if the planner feels comfortable with it.

CHARACTERISTICS OF MEDICAL CARE EVALUATION STUDIES

The subject of medical care evaluations is a kissing cousin to the matrix of methodology for professional standards review. Generally, medical care evaluations are conducted retrospectively and are in-depth assessments of the quality and/or nature of the use of selected health services or programs. A restudy of a medical care evaluation measures the effectiveness of any corrective actions taken as a result of the first evaluation, but not necessarily by repeating the original evaluation. As an example, one could study why certain laboratory tests were not being utilized for specific diagnostic categories and, in the restudy, note any change in their utilization.

Exhibit 7-10 lists the characteristics of medical care evaluations as prepared in the PSRO Program Manual. These factors are stated explicitly and do not require any additional clarification. In addition, Exhibit 7-11 shows the general format for the conduct of a medical care evaluation with nine steps indicated. Again, the steps are evident and indicate the flow of the work.

Usually, the most commonly raised objection to a medical care evaluation is that the study is conducted by staff people from within the organization. Critics state that this is the equivalent of letting the fox guard the chicken house.

REQUIRED EVALUATION MEASURES IN THE HEALTH PLANNING LAW

At several points in the National Health Planning and Resources Act of 1974 (P.L. 93-641), the mandate is given to the Health Systems Agencies and to the secretary of HEW to review health care in terms of acceptability, accessibility, availability, continuity of care, cost, and the quality of care. Cost was given special emphasis in the law because of the high rate of inflation in the medical care services sector. Furthermore, the additional cost was not seemingly resulting in a proportionate return in lowered mortality or morbidity. An argument arises in using these characteristics for evaluation as to the relation between quality of care and cost. Some critics feel that PL 93-641 places cost first and quality second. These six factors in this typology for measurement have obvious interrelationships. The definitions given in Exhibit 7-12 are an effort to provide specific framework for the HSAs when measuring the characteristics.

These six analytic characteristics should take into account the views of the consumers and the community as well as the providers. In consideration of each one of the factors, the interpretation of the variable could be different depending upon the viewpoint.

PL 93-641 directs the HSAs to include goals, objectives, and immediate actions in their Health Systems Plans and their Annual Implementation Plans to deal with these six characteristics as the status of the health care delivery system is evaluated in each of the more than 200 health system areas in the United States.

Exhibit 7-10 General Characteristics of Medical Care Evaluation
Studies

1. They are specifically designed in-depth studies focusing on particular potential problem areas.
2. They are usually of short duration.
3. They may be prompted by cases in which screening parameters have indicated possible instances of substandard quality. Alternatively, they may
   focus on subjectively perceived instances of medical care administrative
   inefficiency or substandard quality.
4. They may be performed by a single hospital, or where common problems
   exist, by a group of hospitals in a coordinated effort.
5. For the most part, they do not deal with an individual patient or practitioner but will require information related to the care provided by a
   number of practitioners to a number of patients.
6. They constitute an important link to the continuing education aspects of the
   PSRO effort. The results of MCE studies should be used by a hospital or
   PSRO in the development of curriculum for and in the monitoring of the
   effectiveness of its continuing education efforts.
7. The results of MCE studies can be used to monitor the effectiveness of
   admission certification and continued stay review and identify areas (diagnoses or physicians) where admission certification and/or continued stay
   should be instituted or intensified.
8. The results of some MCE studies will often identify needed changes in the
   organization and administration of health care delivery. When such is the
   case, the PSRO or hospital should provide this information to those responsible for making such changes and help to assure that necessary action is
   taken.
9. Data necessary for MCE studies may be collected retrospectively and/or by
   the review coordinator during a patient's confinement in the hospital.
   Analysis of the data is done retrospectively.

Source: Section 705.34 *PSRO Program Manual.*

Examples of the type of evaluative measurements that might be
collected for each of the six characteristics include the following:

Acceptability	Patient satisfaction via questionnaire.
	Provider satisfaction.
	Compliance or noncompliance with therapy.
Accessibility	Sociocultural barriers to securing care.
	Use of foreign language material and providers who speak the language.
	Facility reachable by public transportation?

Exhibit 7-11 General Format for Performing a Medical Care
Evaluation Study

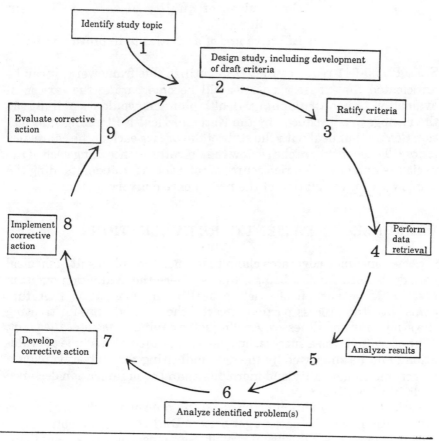

Availability	Enough general hospital beds in area?
	Specialty services available in community.
	Quantity of health personnel of area.
Continuity of care	What referral system exists?
	Is there a record showing all services to a single individual?
	Relations between governmental and private sectors.
Cost	Comparison of charges and actual costs.
	Role of cost in stimulating or deferring care.
	Cost coverage by third party payers for comparison.

Quality   Relationship among structure, process, and out-
                           come factor.
                        Comparison of quality of care at different
                           facilities.
                        Effectiveness of activities to improve quality.

Since PL 93-641 requires that HSAs utilize this framework, it can be
anticipated that these six words will become part of the lexicon of
evaluation in health planning. Health planners would do well to read
the monographs produced by the National Health Planning Information Center that deal with the state of the art for each of the characteristics.[34] These monographs review the literature concerning each of the
variables and provide a rich source of references for understanding the
framework for evaluation of the health care delivery system.

PRINCIPLES OF PATIENT CARE EVALUATION

Some consumer advocates claim that since the end result of medical
care deals with human beings, this is where the evaluation ought to
start. A large portion of existing health care evaluation literature
deals with the process portion of care—the methodolcgy for treating
the symptoms and illnesses. An oft-quoted saying illustrates the point,
"The operation was a success, but the patient died." This type of evaluation could be supported by the data indicating that life style plays a
larger role in mortality and morbidity than the organization designed
to deliver health care.

Patient care evaluation emphasizes the outcome of the health care
intervention. Did the patient get better? Die? Or was the patient disabled? This reverses the usual procedures in medical care evaluations;
outcome is investigated before the process. In other words, find out how
the better outcome developed by following the process and structure of
care for those patients. Also, unlike retrospective review, the data
should not be limited to what is recorded in charts or notes. It would be
unusual for the patient's reasoning to appear in the hospital records.
Yet, from an outcome viewpoint, the thinking of the patient would be
most illuminating. Why didn't the patient take the medicine as ordered? Noncompliance with therapeutic regimen is a vital subject. A
visit to the patient's house may reveal that one-third of the broad
spectrum antibiotic was never used by the mother for the child's strep
throat infection despite the fact that the physician told the mother to
finish the medicine in about ten days. Here, the outcome would not be
what the physician anticipated. This type of data can be secured in

Exhibit 7-12 Suggested Definitions of the Characteristics of the Health Care System

Acceptability	An individual's (or group's) overall assessment of the available medical care. The individual appraises such factors as the convenience, cost, quality, results, and provider attitudes in determining the acceptability of health services.
Accessibility	An individual's (or group's) ability to obtain or use services, given the fact that they are available. It may be measured either in terms of use, which is the definitive verification of access, or in terms of the existence or absence of barriers and obstacles to use.
Availability	A measure of the supply of health services, as correlated with need and distribution, and an indication of the resources able to provide it.
Continuity	A measure of the degree of effective coordination of effort in providing services, regardless of whether care is provided within one setting or within multiple settings. Actual need, preventive care, and single as opposed to continuing treatment are ancillary considerations.
Cost	The expenses incurred in providing or in receiving a service or good. Expenses should be distinguished from charges, which are the prices assigned or the amount billed for a service. Although charges might or might not be the same as costs, or based on them, they are frequently used as a measure of cost.
Quality	A measure of the degree to which health services delivered to a patient, regardless of by whom or in what setting, approximate satisfactory delivery of services as determined by health professionals. Quality is frequently described as having three dimensions: (1) quality of *input resources* (certification and/or training of providers—both manpower and facilities), (2) quality of the *process* of service delivery (use of appropriate procedure for a given condition), and (3) quality of *outcome* of service use (actual improvement in condition or reduction of harmful effects).

interviews, home visits, observations, and questionnaires—not in existing medical charts.

Since patient care evaluations concern people with diverse sociocultural backgrounds, the criteria should be flexible rather than absolute. Differences must be accounted for and related to the outcomes of health care. A. Harwood[35] describes the hot-cold theories of treatment popular among some cultures: a hot disease has to be treated with a cold medicine, and vice versa. Therefore, the providers must be familiar with the classifications of diseases and medicines into their hot or cold categories before being able to evaluate the care received by those patients, linking that care to outcomes. So many variables influence what the patient does or does not do that the evaluation must be flexible enough to accommodate these factors.

In view of the fact that patients and other outsiders might be brought into the evaluation methodology, again being quite different from medical care evaluations, there is a need for support from all quarters. Hospital staff as well as community organizations and individuals need to work together to achieve a worthwhile evaluation of patient care. This can seem threatening to hospital staff members; but if the purpose of improved health care is uppermost, the barriers should be overcome. This cooperation could be eased by including integrated committees early in the patient care evaluation procedures. In addition, these integrated committees could be utilized to assist in the data collection and suggest mechanisms for the appropriate collection. They could even participate in the interviewing or administering of questionnaires. Surely, there must be a commitment to the patient care evaluation concept and not a "What does the patient know?" attitude.

Application of statistical techniques to patient care evaluation should be undertaken with caution. Much of the measurement data is attitudinal. Strict numerical quantification is created by assigning values to prospective responses such as 1 for dissatisfied, 2 for satisfied, and 0 for neutral. Although this assignment of numerical weights allows for statistical analysis, the intensity of a 1 or a 2 is not evident in the scoring, nor is the differential numerically apparent.

Without a mechanism for doing something about any deficiencies discovered during a patient care evaluation, the procedure falls flat. There should be an approach to channel into a hospital and/or community education effort a correction of the gaps in the patient care process. Health planners would do well to include in the active patient care evaluation project those individuals who have the responsibility for implementation of the steps required to correct deficiencies. These individuals could be included on the working committees, on the advisory board, or as consultants—thereby making them part of the evaluation team and perhaps instilling a commitment to the recommendations for change.

Because the patient care evaluation activity itself may be the most potent means of producing change, the procedure must constantly be repeated. Health care providers could react to the investigation by trying to do better even before any results are known. Individuals react to the knowledge of the evaluation procedures and to the presence of investigators. This can be verified if baseline data are collected prior to any study and compared during and after the evaluation. Therefore, even in instances where the health planner does not really anticipate support and cooperation, the evaluation might procede on the assumption that the activity itself could be stimulating changes.

In a patient care evaluation where much of the data must be secured subjectively, it would be worthwhile to pretest instruments designed to collect information. The health planner should check to make sure that the questions are understandable by the respondents and that the responses provide the information sought. Pretesting should be done with patients or staff from another comparable facility so as not to bias the answers from the intended audience. A quick method of pretesting could use five to seven individuals with a similar range of intellectual ability and other variables as in the intended audience. Administer the instrument to the brightest respondent first, and then solicit suggestions for changes. Make modifications in the instrument, and then administer to the next brightest; make changes and administer to the next respondent, and so on down the line. By the time the planner gets to the end of the sample the instrument should be fairly accurate.

A rather adaptable method for developing the instruments can be the use of open-end questions used in an interview form. A small number of these open-end interviews should yield enough data to construct the instruments to use in the pretest phase of the patient care evaluation.

A major distinction in a patient care evaluation is the point of view from which the evaluation proceeds. Rather than being a "medical" care evaluation or a "professional" standards review or other provider type of evaluation, this evaluation starts with the effect on the consumer of health care services.

Exhibit 7-13 details the ten basic principles of patient care evaluation and summarizes much of what has been discussed earlier. In addition, the three case histories of inappropriate patient care evaluation (Exhibit 7-14) illustrate some of those principles. However, the health planner might consider the three case histories without any bias and

Exhibit 7-13 Patient Care Evaluation: Ten Basic Principles

Principle 1: Selectivity must be exercised in determining the aspects of patient care to be evaluated.

Principle 2: Topic areas for patient care evaluation should be selected according to a rational system that recognizes the frequency and severity of patient disability in the absence of treatment and the possibility that appropriate medical intervention may significantly reduce that disability.

Principle 3: Topic areas selected for patient care evaluation should reflect a prior recognition of what is important and where deficiencies are likely to be encountered.

Principle 4: In developing criteria to be applied to evaluated cases, at least in retrospective studies, the usual procedures associated with inquiry in medicine should be reversed; outcomes should be investigated before the process that led to those outcomes is examined.

Principle 5: The availability of data should not determine what data are examined.

Principle 6: Criteria associated with patient care evaluation should be flexible rather than absolute.

Principle 7: Active support must be enlisted in all phases of the medical audit program within a hospital or a community.

Principle 8: Extreme caution should be used in applying statistical techniques to patient care evaluation data.

Principle 9: Except in rare instances, deficiencies in patient care should be channeled into a hospital's educational program and should not have punitive implications.

Principle 10: Because a limited, topic-oriented approach to patient care evaluation cannot be comprehensive by definition, and because the activity itself may be the most potent means of producing change, the procedure must be iterative.

Source: C. Zeleznik, "Patient Care Evaluation: 10 Basic Principles," *Hospital Medical Staff* 2 (January 1973): 8. Reprinted with permission. © 1973 American Hospital Association.

develop any manner of framework, classification, or typology to use in evaluating the given data. As an exercise, the case histories could be examined using any of the methods cited in this section.

SCALES OF MEASUREMENT AND STATISTICAL TESTS

Having discussed the varying levels of measurement and the differing typologies that utilize hard data such as mortality and morbidity

Exhibit 7-14 Case Histories of Inappropriate Patient Care Evaluation

Case History No. 1

In a study of appendectomy, it was learned that a particular physician on the staff of a large metropolitan hospital had a much higher incidence of ruptured appendices in patients he operated on as compared with patients operated on by his peers. This led to a censure of the offending physician and restriction of his privileges. However, it was not recognized that the majority of the physician's patients were referred from the emergency room, which was utilized mostly by a Spanish-speaking clientele from a lower socioeconomic level. Closer examination of the data suggested that the "problem" involved failures in communication between the patients and the staff of the emergency room. This failure involved a language barrier. The physician under examination was not technically inept, and the analysis should not have led to a restriction of privileges. Additionally, there was a failure on the part of the patients to seek early medical attention. Solution to the problem required a change in staffing of the emergency room to make Spanish-speaking personnel always present and an educational program directed to the community. This would require commitments from the community, both financial and otherwise.

Case History No. 2

In a study of infants born with severe respiratory distress syndrome, it was discovered that 33 percent of the infants died. A set of variables believed to be important was selected for analysis. The variables included the following: having a chest x-ray performed as part of diagnostic work-up; monitoring of respiratory rate, retractions, and cyanosis; measurement of the infants' ambient oxygen and their arterial oxygen and the recording of same hourly for the first six hours in the intensive care nursery; and administration of parental fluids. Such variables are considered to be process variables. Statistical analysis of the complete set of data showed a very low correlation between compliance with the process criteria and the mortality of the infants in the study. The correlation was, in fact, zero for several of the criteria and negative for others.

On the other hand, no data were studied relative to the babies' relative risks including, for example; birthweight, Apgar score, or the number of maternal prenatal visits to the physician. In many cases, no doubt, these items reflected problems of education and the socioeconomic status of the mothers. Presumably, some corrective measures were available to the obstetricians who should have been involved in the study. However, since the health status of the mother and the quality of prenatal care given to her may play an important role in the survival of the newborn, community factors may be what is really important in the ultimate control of this problem. It is difficult to see how the study as conceived would have led to a recognition of this possibility.

Exhibit 7-14 Continued

Case History No. 3

In a study of patients having undergone cholecystectomy in a community hospital, it was discovered that some 13 percent had postoperative complications such as a collection of pus and bile in the subhepatic area. It was also learned that only half of the patients had a drain inserted during surgery. This was a violation of the criteria set by the audit committee which required that at least 85 percent of the patients should have this procedure. Further inquiry disclosed that half of the entire series were the patients of one surgeon. Moreover, it was noted that he did not usually follow the prescribed procedure. The audit committee was prepared to impose sanctions upon the offending individual. However, closer examination of the records disclosed that of the 48 patients operated upon by this individual, 12 did in fact have the prescribed procedure. None of the patients without the procedure had complications, whereas seven of the patients with the procedure had complications. The length of stay for the patients without the procedure was shorter and within defined limits, whereas those with the procedure exceeded maximum limits in most cases. Further investigation revealed that all of the patients not receiving the prescribed procedure were under 50 years of age. This suggested that the surgeon in question was utilizing judgment relative to when he would employ the procedure and that his judgment was quite good. Statistical analysis of the series disclosed that a greater portion of outcome variance relative to these complications were accounted for by patient age, weight, and status of health than any other variables (18%). Reduction in the complication rate might be addressed through emphasis upon the patient factor in this case rather than through the physician factor.

Source: J.S. Gonnella, and C. Zeleznik, "Factors Involved in Comprehensive Patient Care Evaluation," *Medical Care* 12: (1974): 932. Reprinted with permission. © 1974 J.B. Lippincott Co.

---

and soft data such as attitudes, it is appropriate to distinguish the scales of measurements. Data can usually be divided into four categories: nominal, ordinal, interval, and ratio scales. Exhibit 7-15 defines the relations, gives examples of appropriate statistics and appropriate statistical tests, as well as an example of the data each scale can measure.

Nominal scales classify data in nonoverlapping classifications that are equivalent to each other. Measuring hair color would call for categories of brown, black, red, or blonde without any distinction between the hair. Only the specific quality is counted. Standard nomenclature used in the international classification of diseases is a nominal scale since the specific quality being measured is disease and there is no measurement difference between the diseases. This is the lowest order

Exhibit 7-15 Four Levels of Measurement and the Statistics
Appropriate to Each Level

Scale	Defining Relations	Examples of Appropriate Statistics	Appropriate Statistical Tests	Examples of Measures
Nominal	(1) Equivalence	Mode Frequency Contingency coefficient		Hair—brown/black/ red
Ordinal	(1) Equivalence (2) Greater than	Median Percentile Spearman r_s Kendall τ Kendall W	Nonparametric statistical tests	Disease—mild/moder- ate/severe
Interval	(1) Equivalence (2) Greater than (3) Known ratio of any two intervals	Mean Standard deviation Pearson product- moment correlation Multiple product- moment correlation		Temperature scales
Ratio	(1) Equivalence (2) Greater than (3) Known ratio of any two intervals (4) Known ratio of any two scale values	Geometric mean Coefficient of variation	Nonparametric and parametric statistical tests	Pulse, height, weight measures

Source: S. Siegel. *Nonparametric Statistics for the Behavioral Sciences.* (New York: McGraw-Hill, 1956), p. 30. Reprinted with permission. © 1956 McGraw-Hill Book Company.

measurement scale and equals a frequency count; no relationship counts among the variables.

Ordinal scales add to the equivalence the distinction of an ordered set of relationships among the data with degrees of difference measured. Patients can be cured, improved, unchanged or worsened. Disease can be severe, moderate, or mild. People can be over six feet tall or under six feet tall. The variable is still equivalent, but the ordinal scale adds the ability to relate the measurements.

Interval scales add to the equivalence and the ordered set of relationships as an operationally defined distance between the rankings. Examples of interval scales are the Celsius and Fahrenheit temperature scales in which the units between adjacent degrees are equal.

Both these scales have arbitrary starting points; there is no absolute zero as in the Kelvin scale. Therefore, it would be incorrect to say that 40 degrees is twice as hot as 20 degrees. In health care evaluation, it is rare to find an interval scale that is not also a ratio scale since the measurement has to be related to a base value. Attitude measurements are, therefore, also difficult to classify within an interval scale because of the inability to equate the intervals between the measures. Is a "one" in patient satisfaction two units lower than a "three" in patient satisfaction?

Ratio scales have all the qualities of the other three plus the ability to relate the data to an absolute zero. Pulse, visual, and auditory acuity are examples of ratio scales in health care. Height and weight measurements also illustrate ratio scales that have equal intervals and clearly indicate that a person six feet tall is twice as tall as someone three feet tall. Ratio measurements allow for the use of sophisticated testing of data.

Health planners should be aware of the distinction among the scales and of the limitations of their data when the evaluation is proposed. To try to force nominal data into complicated statistical testing would hardly be appropriate. If health planners are not familiar enough with the methods to undertake their own development of scales and statistical testing, a consultant should be utilized early in the planning project.

EVALUATION RESEARCH DESIGNS

Health planners might wish to conduct evaluations that are actually research designs. This decision should be made early in the planning process to allow for a direct relationship among the objectives and the research design for the evaluation. Adding in an evaluation research design after the activity has started tends to raise questions about biases and the real value of the evaluation.

Evaluation research designs may be pre-experimental, true experimental, or quasi-experimental as shown in Exhibit 7-16. Each evaluation has some comments noted in the exhibit.[36]

One-shot case studies have no baseline data and no control group for comparison purposes. This type of evaluation yields "testimonial" evidence that the project was a success. Administrators are merely reassured that the clients liked the services. Essentially, a project is initiated, and the evaluation measures the response.

One-group, pretest–posttest studies introduce a baseline measurement of the group prior to the new activity. Problems can arise with

Exhibit 7-16 Variations in Evaluation Research Designs[a]

Pre-Experimental Designs:

1. One-Shot Case Study   X   O
   (weakest but most common evaluation research design)

2. One-Group, Pre-Test/Post-Test Design. . . . . O_1 X O_2
   (does not permit one to attribute changes to the program being evaluated)

3. The Static Group Comparison . . . .   X O_1
   (affords no way of knowing that the two groups were equivalent *before* the program) O_2

True Experimental Designs (particularly applicable to field experiments and to experimental demonstration projects):

4. Pre-Test/Post-Test, Control Group Design . . . .
   R O_1 X O_2
   R O_3 O_4

5. Solomon Four–Group Design . . . .
   (controls and measures both the experimental effect and the possible interaction effects of the measuring process itself)
   R O_1 X O_2
   R O_3 O_4
   R   X O_5
   R O_6

6. Post-Test Only, Control Group Design . . . .
   R   X O_1
   R O_2

7. Comparison of Alternative Program Strategies . . . .
   R O_1 X_1 O_2
   R O_3 X_2 O_4
   R O_5 X_3 O_6
   R O_7 O_8

Quasi-Experimental Designs:

8. Nonequivalent Comparison Group Design . . . .
   O_1 X O_2
   O_3 O_4
   (well worth using in many instances in which Designs 4, 5, and 6 are impossible)

9. Comparison of Alternative Program Strategies, Comparison of Local Projects . . . .
   O_1 X_1 O_2
   O_3 X_2 O_4
   O_5 X_3 O_6
   O_7 O_8

10. Time-Series Design . . . . O_1 O_2 O_3 O_4 X O_5 O_6 O_7 O_8

11. Multiple Time-Series Design . . . . O_1 O_2 O_3 O_4 X O_5 O_6 O_7 O_8
    (excellent quasi-experimental design, perhaps the best of the more feasible designs) O_9 O_{10} O_{11} O_{12} O_{13} O_{14} O_{15} O_{16}

---

[a]Adapted from Campbell and Stanley (14) and Suchman (142). Campbell and Stanley present a much more extensive list of quasi-experimental designs.

X = exposure to experimental activity
O = observations and measurements of effects taken
R = random assignment to the groups

Source: J.S. Wholey, et al. *Federal Evaluation Policy. Analyzing the Effects of Public Programs* (Washington, D.C.: The Urban Institute, 1970), p. 88.

the fact that the pretest measurement can condition the group for the activity to follow. Extraneous events cannot be controlled for, and time alone can result in a measurement change.

Static group comparison has two groups, with one exposed to the activity and the other not. Two basic questions are whether the two groups were equivalent before the activity, and are the groups matched for demographic characteristics.

Pretest–posttest control group designs have two equivalent groups. Random assignment is made to the respective groups, with measurements before and after the activity. Effectiveness is indicated by the significance of the differences between the measurements $0_2 - 0_1$ and $0_4 - 0_3$. However, the question of sensitizing the groups with the pretest still remains.

Solomon's four group designs meet most objectives since the four groups are randomly chosen—two groups pretested and two not tested. Experimental activity is prepared for one pretested group and one not pretested. Measurements are taken of all four groups after the exposure to the activity. Pretest bias can be noted, and other variables can be controlled. This is a true evaluation research design, but it is expensive.

Using a posttest only, control group designs start with random groups. One group is exposed to the activity with a postmeasurement. This design assumes that the activity produced the results and collects no data about what level existed in the groups prior to the activity.

Comparison of alternative strategies starts with random groups and exposes the groups to different activities, with one control group not exposed to any activity. Measurements are made after the exposure of all the groups. Again, there can be a pretest bias, and it could be a problem to isolate the effects of each separate activity.

Quasi-experimental design number eight is similar to number four without the random groups. Number nine is similar to number seven without random groups.

A time-series design for evaluation takes measurements of the group a number of times prior to and after exposure to the experimental activity. This allows for a comparison over time to see if any changes occurred before the activity, or how long after the activity the changes continued.

A multiple time-series design adds a control group to the earlier time series. This allows for measurements of the control group afterward for comparison to see if the changes remain the same between the two groups.

Generic questions concerned with evaluation research concern the following:

- how to select equivalent experimental and control groups,
- identifying the target group for study,
- securing volunteers as well as a representative group,
- what type of random group population is needed,
- how to divide the population into experimental and control groups,
- how to identify what is producing the change,
- why is the change occurring,
- differences between input and related effects of other causes, and
- what is success, and how is it measured.

A collection of quotations illustrate far better than any additional narrative the complexities of evaluation research and the possibilities for error that health planners should be alert to in evaluation (Exhibit 7-17).

A SAMPLING OF EVALUATION MEASUREMENT INSTRUMENTS

Evaluation measurements can be achieved through the use of numerous techniques and included under the rubric of instruments. Among the instruments used are tests, scales, indicators, indexes, guidelines, criteria standards, norms, and a host of questionnaires. In this section, illustrative examples will be noted, but there will certainly be no attempt to be comprehensive. Compilations do exist in book form to assist the health planner in developing his own testing mechanism for his specific project. More than 600 pages of attitude questionnaires are contained in a book by M.E. Shaw and J.M. Wright.[37] Each attitude scale is explained and information detailed about the reliability, the validity, and the results using each instrument. Another book by L.G. Reeder and his associates[38] contains 500 pages of detail about projects in the health and medical care areas along with descriptions of the instruments, the results, and an explanation about the use of the test instrument.

Illustrations in this section should be used for ideas and adaptation, since most test devices need to be refined for the particular project and should take into account language differences, sociocultural interpretations, health care organizational variations, and other factors unique to the activity to be evaluated. Instruments should be pretested with a target population similar to the one proposed for the activity to correct

Exhibit 7-17 Appropriate Quotations for Evaluation Research

- Under precisely controlled experimental conditions, animals do as they jolly well please. *Harvard Law of Biology.*

- Like boats, some researchers toot loudest when they're in a fog. *Source unknown.*

- Without all the facts, the computer is either stymied or generates erroneous output at lightning-like speeds. *Source unknown.*

- No amount of experimentation can ever prove me right; a single experiment may at any time prove me wrong. *Einstein.*

- "Throw your material together as rapidly as possible and send a note in to the Society for Experimental Biology and Medicine, to be published in the next proceedings."
"But I am not ready to publish! I want to have every loophole plugged up before I announce anything whatever!"
"Nonsense! That attitude is old fashioned. . . ." *Sinclair Lewis in* Arrowsmith.

- Researchers are not to be summarily dismissed as promiscuous collectors of facts or producers of truck loads of confirmatory observations. *Source unknown.*

Source: Charles M. Wylie, ed., *Research in Public Health Administration. Selected Abstracts III and IV*, 1964 and 1965, page 3 in each issue. (Baltimore, Md.: Johns Hopkins University, School of Hygiene and Public Health). © Johns Hopkins University Press.

any bugs in the testing device. In addition, there has to be a detailed plan for the administration of the evaluation testing device or devices, including a timetable and the training of personnel to collect the data.

Testing instruments can be divided up into evaluations of knowledge, attitudes, or behavior. Evaluation of knowledge is probably the most familiar to anybody who ever attended school and had to take an examination. This is the easiest instrument to administer, prepare, and analyze. Exhibit 7-18 illustrates various types of questions that are used to test for knowledge.

Multiple choice questions (1 and 2) give the respondent the opportunity to consider the best choice. Since the correct answer is in view, the memory of the test taker might be jogged into the right answer. Fill-in questions (3 and 4) are a bit more difficult since only the rest of the sentence gives a clue as to the answer. Matching questions (5) allow the respondent to have a bit of memory help and to use the process of

Exhibit 7-18 Evaluation of Knowledge Via Testing

---

1. Blue Cross and Blue Shield are types of: A. private insurance B. health insurance C. state medicine D. socialized medicine E. group medicine.
2. A medical specialist in pregnancy and childbirth is: A. a gynecologist B. an opthalmologist C. a dermatologist D. an obstetrician E. a pediatrician.
3. A lateral curvature of the spine is called _____.
4. The _____ arch extends across the foot back of the toes.
5. Vitamin A   ___Prevention of rickets
   Vitamin D   ___Prevention of pellagra
   Vitamin K   ___Prevention of night blindness
   Niacin   ___Prevention of hemorrhagic disease of the newborn
   Thiamine   ___Prevention of beriberi
6. T or F   The major cause of death in 1900 was chronic diseases.
   T or F   Smallpox vaccination was developed by Pasteur.
   T or F   Koch developed the method of isolating and studying bacteria.
7. Identify the following: Lister, Sabin, Schick, Snow.
8. What are the five commonly known sexually transmitted diseases?
9. Describe some of the most common cardiovascular diseases.
10. List the early signs and symptoms of cancer.

---

trial and error. Some matching questions make it a bit more difficult by having more than the exact number of choices to match. True and false questions (6) allow the test taker to guess with a fairly high probability of being right. Clues in these type questions usually relate to the words such as "never" or "always," which signify the answer cannot be in agreement. Identification questions (7) require the respondent to write brief descriptions. No clue is given to allow for a memory jog to assist the test taker. This type of probe is useful when the evaluation requires the participant to know some facts by rote. Recall questions (8 and 10) ask for facts outright to be written down from memory. The question can ask for the information as a list, or by the number of facts required or as an enumeration without a set number. This is also a question that ranks among the more difficult because the clues are few, if any, and guessing is almost completely eliminated. These recall questions could be used to evaluate the patient's grasp of basics that are considered vital to his health, such as a diet or drug regimen. Essay type questions (9) allow respondents to put together whatever information they might have into a narrative. It is more time consuming to use and requires the preparation of a model answer for grading. However, the essay does allow the respondent to organize the data, and the test judges the ability to connect facts logically into a rational explanation. Some persons who do poorly with objective tests find the essay type provides them with an opportunity to display their knowledge.

MEASURING ATTITUDES

Evaluating the attitudes of the participants is obviously a problematic procedure. How can the health planner be sure that the attitudes expressed are really true ones? An answer to that problem is not simple and requires the consideration of responses to attitude questions along with additional data about the individual. Nevertheless, health planners might wish to evaluate the public's attitude toward a new clinic, or an appointment system to replace a first-come first-served system. Results from an attitude questionnaire can give some indication of the receptiveness to the idea by the consumers.

Attitudes can be evaluated by paper and pencil tests, interviews, observations, and facial expressions. The patient satisfaction questionnaire in Exhibit 7-19 illustrates the type of questions that can be used. Patients were to respond by indicating one of five choices to each statement: strongly agree/agree/uncertain/disagree/strongly disagree. These attitudinal questions can be regrouped for analysis by their generic application, such as physicians/hospital/drugs/costs and insurance. Then, the health planner can analyze attitudes about various aspects of the health care system. Sometimes, if the attitude questionnaire is long enough, the same attitude can be questioned again to see if the respondent repeats the same answer. If the two responses are different, a question could be raised about the truth of the answer or the validity of the question.

Two simple questions could reveal a great deal about a project or activity. For instance, people could be asked:

1. What did you like about the medical care you received here?
2. What didn't you like about the medical care you received here?

Information again could be grouped generically to indicate points at which health services might be improved. This type of question does not tell the intensity of the like or dislike unless there is an additional probe that asks patients to rank their likes and dislikes from most to least, or some variation of that procedure that gives the planner an idea of the strength of the attitude.

Environment also plays a role in collecting evaluation data about attitudes. If the questionnaire is administered in the health facility,

Exhibit 7-19 Patient Satisfaction Questionnaire

For each statement, the respondent is asked to choose whether they strongly agree/agree/uncertain/disagree/strongly disagree

1. Parking is a problem when you have to get medical care.
2. Doctors aren't as thorough as they should be.
3. If I have a medical question, I can reach someone for help without any problem.
4. The fees doctors charge are too high.
5. Without proof that you can pay, it's almost impossible to get admitted to the hospital.
6. I'm very satisfied with the medical care I receive.
7. Doctors always tell their patients what to expect during treatment.
8. In an emergency, it's very hard to get medical care quickly.
9. Most people are encouraged to get a yearly exam when they go for medical care.
10. The care I have received from doctors in the last few years is just about perfect.
11. Sometimes doctors taks unnecessary risks in treating their patients.
12. The amount charged for medical care services is reasonable.
13. Doctors are very careful to check everything when examining their patients.
14. There are enough family doctors around here.
15. I think my doctor's office has everything needed to provide complete medical care.
16. It's hard to get an appointment for medical care right away.
17. Medical insurance coverage should pay for more expenses than it does.
18. I hardly ever see the same doctor when I go for medical care.
19. Doctors act like they are doing their patients a favor by treating them.
20. Doctors always avoid unnecessary patient expenses.
21. Places where you can get medical care are very conveniently located.
22. Doctors cause people to worry a lot because they don't explain medical problems to patients.
23. Most people receive medical care that could be better.
24. Doctors ask what foods patients eat and explain why certain foods are best.
25. My doctor's office lacks some things needed to provide complete medical care.
26. The medical problems I've had in the past are ignored when I seek care for a new medical problem.
27. Doctors respect their patients' feelings.
28. If more than one family member needs medical care, we have to go to different doctors.
29. Office hours when you can get medical care are good for most people.
30. There are enough doctors in this area who specialize.
31. I think you can get medical care easily even if you don't have money with you.
32. Doctors let their patients tell them everything that the patient thinks is important.
33. Doctors don't advise patients about ways to avoid illness or injury.
34. There are things about the medical care I receive that could be better.
35. There are enough hospitals in this area.
36. Doctors hardly even explain the patient's medical problems to him.
37. I am happy with the coverage provided by medical insurance plans.

Source: J.E. Ware, Jr., M.K. Snyder and W.R. Wright. *Development and Validation of Scales to Measure Patient Satisfaction with Health Care Services.* Volume 1 (Carbondale, Ill.: Prepared for the National Center for Health Services Research by the Southern Illinois University School of Medicine, 1976), p. 75.

patients could be reluctant to respond truthfully. Patients might wish to please the staff and give them answers that they think the staff wants to hear. In addition, patients would not wish to endanger their medical care relationship since they expect to be back at the facility for medical care another time, or on an ongoing basis. Thus, anonymously answered attitude questionnaires stand a better chance of eliciting a true response. In addition, the choice of self-administered or administered by a staff person questionnaires could influence the responses. If the self-administered attitude test takes place in the facility, the patient might feel that the staff could tell whose questionnaire is whose, even if anonymously filled in. If the self-administered questionnaire is taken home and returned by mail, the patient might feel more confident about the confidentiality of the information. Yet, studies have shown that even with mailed-in questionnaires, people checked under the stamp to see if a code number was listed for identification purposes. Obviously, there is no easy or right answer to the choice of environment for the collection of attitude evaluations. However, in any evaluation, the health planner should attempt to assure the respondents that the information is anonymous, that there is no need for personal identification, that the responses will be used to measure the quality and effectiveness of health care, and that truthful answers will lead to necessary changes in the health care delivery system.

EVALUATING BEHAVIOR

When all is said and done, behavior is the single most important factor to measure. Individuals can score high on knowledge evaluations, can reflect the correct attitudes toward their health care, yet still not behave as required by following their diets, taking their pills, and returning for follow-up examinations. Noncompliance has been reported as a consistent problem in health care. Patients often have the knowledge and the correct attitudes but do not follow the physician's orders.

Evaluation of behavior can best be tested by actual observation on the site where the expected behavior is to take place. If the patient with diabetes is to give himself an insulin injection at home, the evaluator should be at the house to watch the patient and check off the procedures as the patient actually gives himself the injection. If patients on a low sodium diet are to prepare their meals and eat at home, the evaluator should check out the meal the patient actually eats. However, the evaluation should take place as part of the regular routine and not be especially staged for the evaluation; the patient should not be alerted to the fact of an evaluation. The evaluation could be unannounced and spontaneous so no preparations could be made in advance. For instance, nurses could visit the homes of children who had strep throat and were given medication with instructions to give the medicine to the child for ten days. Home visits could be scheduled for the eighth day, when the nurse could ask to see the bottle of medicine and measure the amount left.

Behavior evaluated in this manner usually requires a check list to be used by the observer to standardize the data collected. Preparation of the checklist also pinpoints the behavior that the activity was designed to influence. Furthermore, the checklist can indicate what degree or portion of behavior is acceptable.

If behavior cannot be evaluated by direct observation at the locale where it takes place, tests can be administered to have the respondent demonstrate the expected behavior. Patients could be asked to use food models to prepare their three low fat meals for the day. Patients with diabetes could be asked to prepare an injection and demonstrate on an orange. A patient could be asked to produce the medic alert card that he was told to carry at all times. Given a written narrative or vignette, the patient could be asked to tell what he would do to demonstrate the tested behavior. However, in most cases this evaluation of behavior is once removed from the real life situation. The question remains as to whether the patient would really follow the exhibited behavior pattern in the solitude of the home environment (Exhibit 7-20).

At times, the evaluation questionnaire contains all three elements—knowledge, attitude, and behavior. Supposedly, if respondents score high on all three, the chances of their following through with the actual behavior are much greater. Studies indicate that the health care provider who motivates the patient as well as explaining and teaching what has to be done achieves better behavior from the patient.

GUIDELINES, CRITERIA, AND STANDARDS IN EVALUATION

Although guidelines, criteria, and standards are words that are almost interchangeable, some evaluation procedures do define the terms for their own purposes, as in the PSROs. However, dictionary meanings can be used for the moment. Guidelines refer to leading or directing; criteria refer to standards on which a judgment or decision is based; standard refers to something established by authority, custom, or general consent as a model or example. In addition standard, criter-

Exhibit 7-20 Evaluation of Behavior Via Testing

---

1. Demonstrate the correct procedure for testing urine for sugar and ketones.
2. Using these food models, prepare your three meals for the day.
3. Using this orange, prepare and inject insulin into the orange.
4. Show me your medic alert diabetic identification.
5. On this diagram of the body, indicate how you would choose injection sites.
6. Show me how you take care of your feet. Demonstrate washing and drying.

---

ion and yardstick are listed as synonyms. The dictionary meanings infer a direct relationship among the words. Evaluation examples will reflect the dictionary meanings, and the PSRO exception will be explained when that specific PSRO evaluation device is discussed.

An evaluation technique that is often used is to measure an activity against established guidelines, criteria, and/or standards. Usually the guidelines are established by professional peer groups, and the specifics represent a consensus of opinions. Critics note that the guidelines may actually tend to conform to a least common denominator approach to the problem. At times, the guidelines are based on the accepted textbooks in the field and express conservative medical opinion that concurs with the majority of those involved in setting the guidelines. Following through with this line of thought, if the activity does meet established guidelines, there is probably still considerable room for improvement.

P. A. Lembcke[39] developed six elements common to all criteria for use in the medical audit of patients' records. Since so much evaluation is designed to utilize the patient's medical record as the source of data, the elements are worth consideration. Exhibit 7-21 lists and explains each of the six elements. Note that the criteria should be in writing and should leave little room for interpretation. If the criteria can be verified by concrete laboratory tests, x-rays, specific examinations, or other absolute data, all the better. Sometimes, various providers indicate that the criteria are inappropriate for their institution. Therefore, the criteria should be uniform regardless of those variables and achievable within routine operations. Criteria also have to be prepared for each particular disease or condition to be evaluated, along with the closely related aspects of that condition in a totality that can reflect on the pertinent outcome of the medical care rendered to the patient. Lastly, the criteria must conform with agreed upon levels of high quality care and indicate what the providers should be doing to achieve that level of care.

These elements, common to all criteria, should be kept in mind as

Exhibit 7-21 Elements Common to All Criteria

Objectivity	Stated in writing with sufficient precision and detail to make them relatively immune to varying interpretations by different individuals.
Verifiability	So framed that points on which they rest could be verified by laboratory examination, consultation, or documentation.
Uniformity	Independent of such factors as size or location of hospital, qualifications of the physician, or social or economic status of the patient.
Specificity	Specific for each kind of disease or operation to be evaluated, and all significant and closely related diseases or operations in the same patient considered as a unit.
Pertinence	Pertinent to the ultimate aim of the medical care being evaluated, and based on results rather than intentions.
Acceptability	Conforms with generally accepted levels of good quality as set forth in leading textbooks and articles based on scientific study.

Source: P.A. Lembcke, "Medical Auditing by Scientific Methods Illustrated by Major Female Pelvic Surgery," *Journal of the American Medical Association* 162 (October 13, 1956): 646. Reprinted with permission. © 1956, 73 and 77 the American Medical Association.

the health planner develops his own set of guidelines, criteria, and standards to evaluate an activity or program.

As part of a nationwide study on the costs of medical care undertaken in the United States in the 1930s, R. I. Lee and L. W. Jones[40] prepared a publication on the fundamentals of good medical care. They developed "Articles of Faith" that included eight specific statements, as shown in Exhibit 7-22. Note that the general definition and the eight "Articles of Faith" do not relate to a description of good medical care in any specific situation. However, these good faith statements do identify the generic components of good medical care. In each of the eight areas, the evaluator should seek to make judgments concerning the dimension of care rendered to the patient. For example, Article 2 calls attention to the need to emphasize prevention. However, the opportunities for prevention in medical care have to be identified and evaluated. This may vary from situation to situation and in respect to what medical science has to offer. Furthermore, as is evident, prevention has to be considered in competition with other health care

Exhibit 7-22 Articles of Faith

Good medical care is the kind of medicine practiced and taught by the recognized leaders of the medical profession at a given time or period of social, cultural, and professional development in a community or population group. The concept of good medical care that has been employed in this study is based upon certain "Articles of Faith," which can be briefly stated.

1. Good medical care is limited to the practice of rational medicine based on the medical sciences.
2. Good medical care emphasizes prevention.
3. Good medical care requires intelligent cooperation between the lay public and the practitioners of scientific medicine.
4. Good medical care treats the individual as a whole.
5. Good medical care maintains a close and continuing personal relation between physician and patient.
6. Good medical care is coordinated with social welfare work.
7. Good medical care coordinates all types of medical services.
8. Good medical care implies the application of all the necessary services of modern scientific medicine to the needs of all the people.

Source: R.I. Lee and L.W. Jones. *The Fundamentals of Good Medical Care.* Publication No. 22 of the Committee on the Costs of Medical Care (Chicago: University of Chicago Press, 1933). Reprinted with permission. © 1933 University of Chicago Press.

priorities and conflicting professional views on the value of prevention activities. From an operational vantage point, the specifics of Article 2 need much greater refinement to be administratively feasible. Because of its concern for the general public, Article 8 widens the boundaries of good medical care to include the total population served by the total health care system. This statement adds the needs of the people and thereby raises the concept of unmet health care needs in the population as part of overall good medical care.

These "Articles of Faith" present an overall philosophy as a criterion for good medical care. Perhaps, these eight standards are those that can be determined by reading incorporation documents, annual reports, and observing the general tone of what is going on in the hospital.

A. Donabedian[41] took the Lee and Jones formulation and fleshed out the general statements with specifics, as shown in Exhibit 7-23. Although Donabedian's specifics are completely detailed in Exhibit 7-23, a condensed outline is presented here to allow the health planner to compare the specifics with the eight Articles of Faith. Basically, the criteria concentrate on two aspects of care: physician behavior and the client/provider relationship. These two divisions have the following components:

Exhibit 7-23 Guidelines for Physician Behavior and for the Client-Provider Relationship

I. Physician behavior
   A. Technical management of health and illness
      1. Adequacy of diagnosis
         a. Skill and discrimination in obtaining appropriate and complete information using the requisite clinical, laboratory, and other diagnostic techniques
         b. The use of valid information (accurate diagnostic tests) or inferences (e.g., from physical examination)
         c. Sound judgment in evaluating the information obtained
         d. Completeness in evaluating the information obtained
         e. Validity of diagnosis
      2. Adequacy of therapy
         a. Choice of effective and specific therapeutic regimen prescribed with due regard to expected risks arising from therapy and the condition to be treated
         b. Adequate management of pain, discomfort, and distress without undue prejudice to the diagnostic process
         c. Informing the patient about risks and side effects associated with treatment
         d. Maintaining adequate surveillance with the object of reducing risks and maximizing benefits
      3. Parsimony or minimum redundancy in diagnostic and therapeutic procedures (The issue of efficiency in terms of the economic use of resources, although an important factor in the organization of medical care, will not be considered here. The emphasis will be on the logical necessity to have certain items of information and the therapeutic necessity to use certain treatments.)
      4. Full exploitation of medical technology
         a. Maximum effectiveness in applying existing technology; knowledge of the technology and skill in its application
         b. Discrimination in the introduction and utilization of new technology
         c. Discrimination in discarding old methods
      5. Full exploitation of professional and functional differentiation. Recognition by the physician of his own limitations and the use of other specialists and of other professions where the need arises
   B. Socioenvironmental management of health and illness
      1. Attention to social and environmental factors, especially within the family and at work, having relevance to the following:
         a. Identifying and eliminating barriers to seeking and maintaining care
         b. Arriving at the professional definition of need

Exhibit 7-23 Continued

      c. Adjusting the frequency and content of the periodic review of all well persons
      d. Obtaining and evaluating information in the diagnostic process
      e. Planning and recommending treatment
    2. Use of larger social units (usually the family) as the units of care wherever appropriate in terms of:
      a. Therapeutic manipulation of social and environmental factors in the interests of the individual patient
      b. Using the larger unit as an object of care: for example, in considering the family epidemiology of infectious disease and the social impact of long term illness on the family
    3. Use of community resources on behalf of the patient
    4. Attention to broader community interests, for example in the reporting of communicable diseases
  C. Psychological management of health and illness
    1. Attention to psychological and emotional factors in:
      a. Identifying and eliminating barriers to seeking and maintaining care
      b. Arriving at the professional definition of need
      c. Adjusting the frequency and content of the periodic review of well persons
      d. Obtaining and evaluating information in the diagnostic process
      e. Planning and recommending treatment
  D. Integrated management of health and illness
    1. Periodic review of "well" persons with special attention to promotion of mental and physical health, the early detection of physical and emotional deviations, through the use of appropriate screening mechanisms, and the use of appropriate primary preventive techniques for illness, accidents, injury, behavioral and emotional problems, etc.
    2. Using visits for the care of illness as occasions for the management of health
    3. Adequate follow-through on suspected abnormalities or health problems
    4. Identification of "high risk" situations and appropriate adaptation of the amount and content of health management and medical care to such risk
    5. A developmental and anticipatory or interceptive orientation in the management of health and illness with due attention to preventive management. Attention to preventing physical, social, and behavioral breakdown
    6. Attention to rehabilitation and restoration of function
  E. Continuity and coordination in the management of health and illness
    1. Continuity and coordination of care for individual patients through

Exhibit 7-23 Continued

       either the establishment of a personal relationship with one physician or the coordination of care provided by several physicians and/or both mechanisms

  2. Adequacy of the individual patient record and its ready availability as the major tool of coordination and continuity of care

  3. Continuity and coordination of care for several or all members of a family and the availability of family health records to the treating physician

II. The client-provider relationship

It is possible to select a subset of normative goals to define the dimensions of quality in clinical care because there is some congruence.

  A. Some formal attributes of the client-provider relationship

    1. Congruence

      between physician and patient expectations, orientations etc.

    2. Adaptation and flexibility

      The ability of the physician to adapt his approach not only to the expectations of the patient (for greater or less affectivity, for example) but also to the demands of the clinical situation in terms of greater or lesser control, greater or less reciprocation of emotional involvement, and so on

    3. Mutuality

      Gains for both physician and patient

    4. Stability

      A stable relationship between patient and physician

  B. Some attributes of the content of the provider-client relationship

    1. Maintenance of maximum possible client autonomy and freedom of action and movement (especially critical for institutionalized patients)

    2. Maintenance of family and community communication and ties (especially critical for institutionalized patients)

    3. Maximum possible degree of egalitarianism in the client-provider relationship

    4. Maximum possible degree of active client participation through

      a. sharing knowledge concerning the health situation

      b. shared decision making

      c. participation in carrying out therapy

    5. Maintenance of empathy and rapport without undue emotional involvement of the provider

    6. Maintenance of a supportive relationship without encouragement of undue dependency

    7. Maintenance of a neutral, noncondemnatory attitude toward moral and other values of the client

Exhibit 7-23 Continued

    8. Confining provider influence and action within the boundaries of his legitimate social functions
    9. Avoidance of exploitation of the client economically, socially, sexually, etc.
   10. Maintenance of client dignity and individuality
   11. Maintenance of privacy
   12. Maintenance of confidentiality

Source: A. Donabedian. "Promoting Quality Through Evaluating the Process of Patient Care," *Medical Care* 6(1968): 181. Reprinted with permission. © 1968 J.B. Lippincott Co.

  I. Physician behavior
    A. Technical management of health and illness
    B. Socioenvironmental management of health and illness
    C. Psychological management of health and illness
    D. Integrated management of health and illness
    E. Continuity and coordination in the management of health and illness
 II. The client/provider relationship
    A. Formal attributes of the client-provider relationship
    B. Attributes of the content of the provider-client relationship

This division into physician behavior and the client/provider relationship relates to the type of evaluations of health care quality that conclude that consumers desire both technical competence and personal interest, or, as stated in other studies, curing and caring. These specifics identified by Donabedian also can be fit into the structure/process/outcome categories used in the evaluation of health care.

ASSESSMENT CRITERIA IN AN ANALYTIC SYSTEMS FRAMEWORK

Four criteria are used as the basis for the assessment of the level of health care delivery systems in a framework that deals with the planning and evaluation of health services. Assessment criteria of comprehensiveness, quality, continuity, and economy are integrated with a structure, process, and outcome breakdown. Effectiveness and efficiency are also added into the analysis. Exhibit 7-24 gives the definitions and relationships, and Exhibit 7-25 details the operationalization of the assessment categories.

Exhibit 7-24 Planning and Evaluation of Health Services. An
Analytic Systems Framework Utilizing Assessment
Criteria of Comprehensiveness, Quality, Continuity,
and Economy: I. Definitions and Relationships

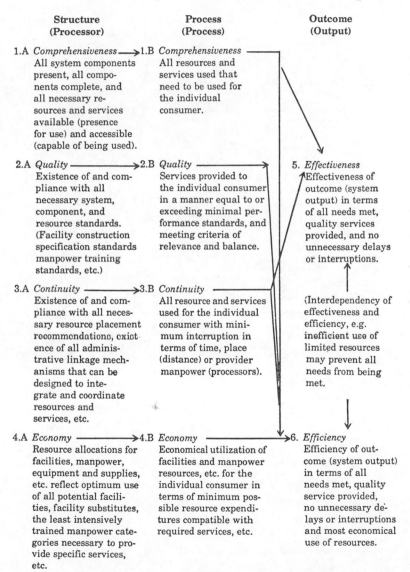

Structure (Processor)	Process (Process)	Outcome (Output)

1.A *Comprehensiveness* ⟶ 1.B *Comprehensiveness*
All system components present, all components complete, and all necessary resources and services available (presence for use) and accessible (capable of being used).
All resources and services used that need to be used for the individual consumer.

2.A *Quality* ⟶ 2.B *Quality* ⟶
Existence of and compliance with all necessary system, component, and resource standards. (Facility construction specification standards manpower training standards, etc.)
Services provided to the individual consumer in a manner equal to or exceeding minimal performance standards, and meeting criteria of relevance and balance.

5. *Effectiveness*
Effectiveness of outcome (system output) in terms of all needs met, quality services provided, and no unnecessary delays or interruptions.

3.A *Continuity* ⟶ 3.B *Continuity*
Existence of and compliance with all necessary resource placement recommendations, existence of all administrative linkage mechanisms that can be designed to integrate and coordinate resources and services, etc.
All resource and services used for the individual consumer with minimum interruption in terms of time, place (distance) or provider manpower (processors).

(Interdependency of effectiveness and efficiency, e.g. inefficient use of limited resources may prevent all needs from being met.

4.A *Economy* ⟶ 4.B *Economy* ⟶ 6. *Efficiency*
Resource allocations for facilities, manpower, equipment and supplies, etc. reflect optimum use of all potential facilities, facility substitutes, the least intensively trained manpower categories necessary to provide specific services, etc.
Economical utilization of facilities and manpower resources, etc. for the individual consumer in terms of minimum possible resource expenditures compatible with required services, etc.
Efficiency of outcome (system output) in terms of all needs met, quality service provided, no unnecessary delays or interruptions and most economical use of resources.

Source: J.T. Gentry. "A More Rational Approach to Health Care Delivery." Reprinted with permission from HOSPITAL PROGRESS, August, 1973. Copyright 1973 The Catholic Hospital Association.

Exhibit 7-25 Planning and Evaluation of Health Services. An Analytic Systems Framework Utilizing Assessment Criteria of Comprehensiveness, Quality, Continuity, and Economy: II. Operationalizing Assessment Categories

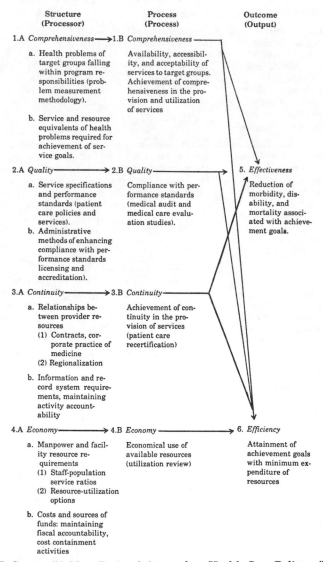

Structure (Processor)	Process (Process)	Outcome (Output)
1.A *Comprehensiveness*⟶1.B *Comprehensiveness*		
a. Health problems of target groups falling within program responsibilities (problem measurement methodology).	Availability, accessibility, and acceptability of services to target groups. Achievement of comprehensiveness in the provision and utilization of services	
b. Service and resource equivalents of health problems required for achievement of service goals.		
2.A *Quality* ⟶ 2.B *Quality*		5. *Effectiveness*
a. Service specifications and performance standards (patient care policies and services).	Compliance with performance standards (medical audit and medical care evaluation studies).	Reduction of morbidity, disability, and mortality associated with achievement goals.
b. Administrative methods of enhancing compliance with performance standards licensing and accreditation).		
3.A *Continuity* ⟶ 3.B *Continuity*		
a. Relationships between provider resources (1) Contracts, corporate practice of medicine (2) Regionalization	Achievement of continuity in the provision of services (patient care recertification)	
b. Information and record system requirements, maintaining activity accountability		
4.A *Economy* ⟶ 4.B *Economy*		6. *Efficiency*
a. Manpower and facility resource requirements (1) Staff-population service ratios (2) Resource-utilization options	Economical use of available resources (utilization review)	Attainment of achievement goals with minimum expenditure of resources
b. Costs and sources of funds: maintaining fiscal accountability, cost containment activities		

Source: J.T. Gentry. "A More Rational Approach to Health Care Delivery." Reprinted with permission from HOSPITAL PROGRESS, August, 1973. Copyright 1973 The Catholic Hospital Association.

Health planners should note that this analytic systems framework contains the six characteristics mandated by the National Health Planning and Resources Development Act (PL 93-641): acceptability, accessibility, availability (cell 1B), continuity (cell 3), cost (cells 4 and 6), and quality (cell 2). Clearly, as has been mentioned previously, evaluation measurement instruments borrow from each other and exchange terminology and concepts. What must be inferred from their long history is that a major barrier has to be related to establishing mechanisms to make these evaluations part of the routine operating procedures and to keep the evaluation mechanisms working smoothly to do what they are designed to do—measure health care outcomes.

Assessment criteria in this analytic system also need to have the specifics added in to make this framework useful in particular instances of evaluation. However, the specifics required here can be related more easily to existing guidelines. Under structure, the licensing and accreditation already exist. Most states have licensing procedures and agencies, and adapt the requirements of the Joint Commission on the Accreditation of Hospitals. Under process, medical audit and medical care evaluation details have already been worked out by professional specialty associations and by some PSROs. Under outcome, morbidity and mortality rates have been determined by most public health departments and by HEW for comparison purposes. These are only examples of the specifics that can be readily plugged into this analytic systems framework with the assessment criteria being translated into existing data sources.

Health planners can use this scheme by taking each cell and asking the questions that have to be answered and the type of data required for the evaluation. In most instances the measurement data will be available to note in each cell for the evaluation. Where the specific measurement is not available, the health planner might have to develop his own based on surveys, projections, other study results, or even educated guesses.

Sometimes the criteria are established by an official agency that provides the numbers to be plugged into an analytic framework. National guidelines for health planning with respect to general hospital beds, obstetrical inpatient services, pediatric inpatient services, neonatal inpatient services, open heart surgery units, cardiac catheterization units, radiation therapy services, computed tomographic scanners, and end-stage renal disease units are illustrated in Exhibit 7-26. In addition to the guidelines, a short discussion explains the rationale behind the selection of a numerical guideline. Critics commented that the proposals were too detailed and would provide less flexibility for

Exhibit 7-26 National Guidelines for Health Planning

AUTHORITY.—Sec. 1501, Public Health Service Act, 88 Stat. 2227 (41 U.S.C. 300k-1).

Subpart A—General Provisions

§ 121.1 Definitions.

Terms used herein shall have the meanings given them in 42 CFR 122.1.

§ 121.2 Purpose and scope.

Section 1501 of the Public Health Service Act requires the Secretary to issue, by regulation, national guidelines for health planning. The guidelines are to include national health planning goals (section 1501(b)(2)) and standards respecting the supply, distribution, and organization of health resources (section 1501(b)(1)). This subpart includes general provisions applicable to such goals and standards; Subpart B of this part sets forth specific national health planning goals; and Subpart C sets forth specific standards respecting the supply, distribution, and organization of health resources.

§ 121.3 Applicability of national guidelines to Health Systems Plans.

Section 1513(b)(2) of the Act requires health systems agencies, in the development of their Health Systems Plans, to give "appropriate consideration" to the national guidelines for health planning. Health Systems Plans must also "take into account" and be "consistent with" the standards respecting the supply, distribution, and organization of health resources set forth in Subpart C of this part.

(a) *Meaning of "consistent with."* A Health Systems Plan will be considered "consistent with" a standard set forth in Subpart C of this part where it: (1) Establishes a goal which is not in excess of the level set forth in the standard where that level is stated as a maximum, or not less than the level set forth in the standard where that level is stated as a minimum, and (2) includes plans which, if implemented, are reasonably calculated to achieve that goal within five years, except where a specific adjustment is justified in accordance with Subpart C of this Part or § 121.6.

(b) *Effective date.* Health Systems Plans established after December 31, 1978, must be consistent with each standard set forth in Subpart C of this part.

§ 121.4 Applicability of national guidelines to State health plans.

Each State's State health plan developed under Title XV of the Act must be "made up of" the Health Systems Plans of the health systems agencies within the State, revised as found necessary by the Statewide Health Coordinating Council to achieve their appropriate coordination with each other or to deal more effectively with Statewide health needs. Section 1524(c)(2)(A) of the Act. Since Health Systems Plans must individually give appropriate consideration to the national guidelines for health planning and take into account and be consistent with the standards respecting the supply, distribution, and organization of health resources, the State health plan will accordingly reflect the guidelines.

Exhibit 7-26 Continued

§ 121.5 Responsibility of health systems agencies.

Subject to the authority of the Statewide Health Coordinating Council to require the revision of Health Systems Plans under section 1524(c)(2)(A) of the Act, each health systems agency is responsible for analyzing the needs and conditions in its health service area and applying the national guidelines for health planning in the development of its Health Systems Plan, including the need for adjustments.

§ 121.6 Adjustments of standards for particular Health Systems Plans.

Subpart C of this part includes provisions for adjustment of individual standards. In addition:

(a) Health systems agencies must make such adjustments as may be necessary:

(1) To take into account special needs and circumstances of Health Maintenance Organizations; and

(2) To take into account services available to local residents from Federal health care facilities.

(b) Whenever a health systems agency concludes, on the basis of a detailed analysis, that development of a Health Systems Plan consistent with one or more of the standards set forth in Subpart C of this part would result in:

(1) Residents of the health service area not having access to necessary health services;

(2) Significantly increased costs of care for a substantial number of patients in the area; or

(3) The denial of care to persons with special needs resulting from moral and ethical values;

and that result cannot be avoided through use of the adjustments specifically provided for in the standard or in paragraph (a) of this section, the agency may include in the Health Systems Plan a special adjustment of the standard or standards which will avoid this result. Whenever a special adjustment is so included, the plan must also contain a detailed justification for the adjustment and documentation of the circumstances that are the basis of the justification. In the case of an adjustment included on the basis of subparagraph (1) or (2) of this paragraph, the plan must further include an analysis indicating whether the need for such an adjustment is permanent. If it is, the supporting rationale must be documented and if it is not, an estimate must be included of how long inclusion of the adjustment will be required along with a detailed justification for that length of time.

(c) Any proposed adjustment under this section and the analyses supporting it must be reviewed by the State health planning and development agency in its preparation or review of the preliminary State health plan under section 1523(a)(2) of the Act and by the Statewide Health Coordinating Council in its preparation or review of the State health plan under section 1524(c)(2) of the Act. On the basis of that review, and consistent with Statewide health needs and the need to coordinate Health Systems Plans as determined by the Statewide Health Coordinating Council, the adjustment may be made part of the State health plan. The Statewide Health Coordinating Council shall report its comments on and disposition of the proposed adjustments to the Secretary under section 1524(c)(1) of the Act.

Subpart B—National Health Planning Goals [Reserved]

Subpart C—Standards Respecting the Appropriate Supply, Distribution, and Organization of Health Resources

§ 121.201 General hospitals—Bed supply.

(a) *Standard.* There should be less than four non-Federal, short-stay hospital beds for each 1,000 persons in a health service area except under extraordinary circumstances. For purposes of this section, short-stay hospital beds include all non-Federal short-stay hospital beds (including general medical/surgical, children's, obstetric, psychiatric, and other short-stay specialized beds). Conditions which may justify adjustments to this ratio for a health service area are:

Exhibit 7-26 Continued

(1) *Age.* Individuals 65 years of age and older have a higher hospital utilization rate—up to four times that of the general population—than any other age group. Bed-population ratios for health service areas in which the percentage of elderly people is significantly higher (more than 12 percent of the population) than the national average may be planned at a higher ratio, based on analyses by the HSA.

(2) *Seasonal population fluctuations.* Large seasonal variations in hospital utilization may justify higher ratios. Plans should reflect vacation and recreation patterns as well as the needs of migrant workers and other factors causing unusual seasonal variations.

(3) *Rural areas.* Hospital care should be accessible within a reasonable period of time. For example, in rural areas in which a majority of the residents would otherwise be more than 30 minutes travel time from a hospital, the HSA may determine, based on analyses, that a bed-population ratio of greater than 4.0 per 1,000 persons may be justified.

(4) *Urban areas.* Large numbers of beds in one part of a Standard Metropolitan Statistical Area (SMSA) may be compensated for by fewer beds in other parts of the SMSA. Health service areas which include a part of an SMSA may plan for bed-population ratios higher than 4.0 per 1,000 persons reflecting existing patterns if there is a joint plan among all HSAs serving the SMSA which provides for less than 4.0 beds per 1,000 persons in the SMSA as a whole.

(5) *Areas with referral hospitals.* In the case of referral institutions which provide a substantial portion of specialty services to individuals not residing in the area, the HSA may exclude from its computation of bed-population ratio the beds utilized by referred patients who reside outside both the SMSA and the HSA in which the facility is located.

(b) *Discussion.* There is general agreement that the number of general hospital beds in the United States is significantly in excess of what is needed and that utilization of acute in-patient care resources is often higher than necessary. Excess bed capacity and use contribute to the high cost of hospital care with little or no health benefits. Empty beds are often filled by patients who could be cared for as well or better in less expensive ways, such as ambulatory care or home care. The Institute of Medicine's Report on "Controlling the Supply of Hospital Beds" in 1976 recommended that the nation should achieve at least a 10 percent reduction in the bed population ratio in the next five years and further significant reductions thereafter. The Institute statement noted: "This would mean a reduction from the current national average of approximately 4.4 non-Federal short-term general hospital beds per 1,000 population to a national average of approximately 4.0 in five years and well below that in the years to follow." Similarly a study reported by Inter-Study of Minneapolis, Minn. the same year concluded that a 10 percent reduction in hospital bed supply would be a desirable and reasonable first step toward reducing excess hospital capacity. As part of the process for determining this standard, the Department reviewed projections in State health facilities planning plans. Such plans have set targets for future hospital bed supply that, on an aggregate nationwide basis, project just under 4.0 beds per thousand. Many States set lower targets. Health Maintenance Organizations and similar groups have shown that high quality care can be provided with less than 3.0 beds per 1,000 population. Thus, 4.0 beds per 1,000 population is a ceiling, not an ideal situation. HSAs are expected to identify the desirable local ratio, working closely with the State Health Planning and Development Agency and the Statewide Health Coordinating Council. It is anticipated that in subsequent plans HSAs will be required to indicate how they will reach a bed-population ratio of less than 3.7 per 1,000 population, except under extraordinary circumstances. HSAs whose areas are now below the 4.0 per 1,000 level are urged to attempt to decrease bed-population ratios below 3.7 per 1,000 population. In areas where Federal medical facilities and Health Maintenance Organizations provide substantial services to local residents, lower ratios

Exhibit 7-26 Continued

should be readily achievable. Population growth must be carefully analyzed; in many cases, this factor alone will bring the area below the target level if no unnecessary additional beds are built. Under some conditions, a higher target ceiling may be justified by the HSA. Travel distance to the nearest hospital is one of the most important factors to be analyzed, especially in rural areas. A planning criteria of 30 minutes has been set, in line with the policies of many local and State health planning agencies around the country. In analyzing ways of reducing bed supply, it should be recognized that greater savings will be achieved when entire facilities are considered. In developing such plans, priority consideration should be given to maintaining and strengthening resources that are emphasizing activities identified as national health priorities in Section 1502 of the Act.

§ 121.202 General Hospitals-Occupancy Rate.

(a) *Standard.* There should be an average annual occupancy rate of at least 80% for all non-Federal, short-stay hospital beds considered together in a health service area, except under extraordinary circumstances. Conditions which may justify an adjustment to this standard for a health service area are:

(1) *Seasonal population fluctuations.* In some areas, the influx of people for vacation or other purposes may require a greater supply of hospital beds than would otherwise be needed. Large seasonal variations in hospital utilization which can be predicted through hospital and health insurance records may justify an average annual occupancy rate lower than 80% based on analyses by the HSA.

(2) *Rural areas.* Lower average annual occupancy rates are usually required by small hospitals to maintain empty beds to accommodate normal fluctuations of admissions. In rural areas with significant numbers of small (fewer than 4,000 admissions per year) hospitals, an average occupancy rate of less than 80% may be justified, based on analyses by the HSA.

(b) *Discussion.* There is substantial evidence that excess capacity and use

contribute significantly to high hospital costs. The 1976 report by the Institute of Medicine, for example, found that "there is a growing concern that the surpluses of hospital beds are contributing significantly to the recent rise of health care costs at a rate well beyond that of general inflation. This concern has not only to do with the cost of maintaining unused hospital bed capacity, but also with the unnecessary and inappropriate uses of hospital beds, especially those in the short-term care category." Occupancy rates currently average about 75% nationwide. Many hospital capacity studies, including those by InterStudy and the Bureau of Hospital Administration of the University of Michigan, indicate that an average hospital occupancy rate exceeding 80% is a reasonable target. In addition, many State and local health planning agencies have established higher occupancy targets. For example, health planning agencies in Illinois, New Jersey, New York, Massachusetts, Michigan and Wisconsin, have recommended occupancy rates higher than 80% for larger hospitals. Higher averages have been advocated, especially for medical-surgical units. While past studies typically apply these rates to individual institutions, the Department, in line with the objectives of community-wide planning, has extended this concept to apply on an area-wide basis. Within local health service areas, hospitals of varying size and circumstances will have varying occupancy rates; a collective rate exceeding 80% on an area-wide basis is a reasonable, achievable goal except in rural areas and when situations present extraordinary circumstances. Increases are to be attained through constrained capacity growth and improved planning and management. It is not, of course, intended that increased rates be achieved through unnecessary hospital admissions or stays.

§ 121.203 Obstetrical Services.

(a) *Standard.* (1) Obstetrical services should be planned on a regional basis with continuing linkages among all obstetrical services and with neonatal services.

Exhibit 7-26 Continued

(2) Hospitals providing care for complicated obstetrical problems (Levels II and III) should have at least 1,500 births annually.

(3) There should be an average annual occupancy rate of at least 75 percent in each obstetrical unit with more than 1,000 births per year.

(b) *Discussion.* The importance of developing regional systems of care for maternal and perinatal health services has been broadly recognized. The Committee on Perinatal Health, representing the American Academy of Family Physicians, American Academy of Pediatrics, American College of Obstetricians and Gynecologists, and the American Medical Association issued a report in 1976, "Toward Improving the Outcome of Pregnancy." The report identified opportunities to reduce rates of maternal, fetal, and neonatal mortality as well as to improve deployment of scarce resources, especially those needed to provide comprehensive services for high-risk patients. The impact on quality of care of both under-utilization and over-utilization was emphasized.

The report states: "A systematized, cohesive regional network including a number of differentiated resources is the approach most likely to achieve the objective. Each component of the regional system must provide the highest quality care, but the degree of complexity of patient needs determines where, and by whom, the care should be provided." Level I hospitals provide services primarily for uncomplicated maternity and newborn cases.

Level II hospitals provide services for uncomplicated cases and for the majority of complicated problems, and certain neonatal services. Level III hospitals are able also to handle all the serious types of illness and abnormalities. Established arrangements should provide for early access of high-risk pregnant women and prompt referrals among levels of care as appropriate. Regional planning should include a cooperative, coordinated network of hospitals, physicians and other health care professionals, providing (1) expert consultation and referral (2) basic and continuing education for health professionals and con-

sumers, (3) transport of selected patients to facilities possessing more specialized maternal and neonatal services, (4) a continuing evaluation of the effectiveness and costs of regionalized programs. In 1972 the American College of Obstetrics and Gynecology identified a minimal target of 1,500 births per year for facilities in communities of 100,000 population or more to provide a full range of obstetrical services in an efficient manner. In 1974, this figure was revised: "The experience of many obstetric departments indicate that the size, equipment, services and personnel adequate to maintain a consistently high standard of ordinary obstetrical care and a reasonably economic operation generally require more than 2,000 deliveries." "Standards for Obstetrical and Gynecological Services," Committee on Professional Standards of the American College of Obstetricians and Gynecologists, 1974.) The Committee on Perinatal Health also identified the 2,000 minimum figure for facilities identified as Level II facilities. In determining the 1,500 target, the Department took into consideration these reports as well as the comments received from the public and from members of the expert advisory panel, particularly the criticism that a 2,000 target was too strict. The 1,500 level is in line with the policies of many local and State health planning agencies and can help assure more economic use of specialized resources. The Department also recognizes that there are substantial differences among facilities which provide different ranges of services and there are circumstances, such as those involving special moral and ethical preferences, which may necessitate the HSA providing an adjustment to this standard. In addition, in order to promote more economical use of resources the Department has established the 75 percent minimum occupancy rate in each obstetrical unit for Level II and III facilities. The 75 percent figure was derived from an analysis of various occupancy rate figures in a number of source documents, whose recommendations range from 50 percent to over 80 percent. The Hill-Burton Program recommended an oc-

Exhibit 7-26 Continued

cupancy level for obstetrical units of at least 75 percent. The Department anticipates that institutions operating at Level II and III will usually be able to exceed this level. In keeping with the national priority set forth in Section 1502 of the Act for the consolidation and coordination of institutional health services, the consolidation of multiple, small obstetrical units with low occupancy rates should be undertaken unless such action is undesirable because of needs to assure ready access and sensitive care.

§ 121.204 Neonatal Special Care Units.

(a) *Standard.* (1) Neonatal services should be planned on a regional basis with continuing linkages with obstetrical services.

(2) The total number of neonatal intensive and intermediate care beds should not exceed 4 per 1,000 live births per year in a defined neonatal service area. An adjustment upward may be justified when the rate of high-risk pregnancies is unusually high, based on analyses by the HSA.

(3) A single neonatal special care unit (Level II or III) should contain a minimum of 15 beds. An adjustment downward may be justified for a Level II unit when travel time to an alternate unit is a serious hardship due to geographic remoteness, based on analyses by the HSA.

(b) *Discussion.* For this standard, the Department has adopted the professionally endorsed concept of regionalization, involving various levels of care. Under this concept, Level III units are staffed and equipped for the intensive care of newborns as well as intermediate and recovery care. Level II units provide intermediate and recovery care as well as some specialized services. Level I units provide recovery care. Neonatal special care is a highly specialized service required by only a very small percentage of infants. The Department believes that four neonatal special care beds for intensive and intermediate care per thousand live births will usually be adequate to meet the needs, taking into account the incidence of high risk pregnancies, the percentage of live births requiring intensive care, and the average length of stay. ("Bed" includes incubators or other heated units for specialized care, and bassinettes.) In addition, the Department has established a minimum of 15 beds per units for Levels II and III as the minimum number necessary to support economical operation for these services. Both standards are supported and recommended by the American Academy of Pediatrics. The American Academy of Pediatrics has noted that "the best care will be given to high risk and seriously ill neonates if intensive care units are developed in a few adequately qualified institutions within a community rather than within many hospitals. Properly conducted, early transfer of these infants to a qualified unit provides better care than do attempts to maintain them in inadequate units." This regionalized approach is reflected in the minimum size standard which is designed to foster the location of specialized units in medical centers which have available special staff, equipment, and consultative services and facilities. Since perinatal centers, which include neonatal units, will serve the patient load resulting from a representative population of more than one million, a defined neonatal service area should be identified by the relevant HSAs in conjunction with the State Agency. Special attention must also be given to ensure adequate communication and transportation systems. Hospitals with such units should have agreements with other facilities to serve referred patients. The regional plan should include a structured ongoing system of review, including assessment of changes in health status indicators.

§ 121.205 Pediatric Inpatient Services— Number of Beds.

(a) *Standard.* There should be a minimum of 20 beds in a pediatric unit in urbanized areas. An adjustment downward may be justified when travel time to an alternate unit exceeds 30 minutes for 10 percent or more of the population, based on analyses of the HSA.

(b) *Discussion.* The 1977 report of the Committee on Implications of Declining Pediatric Hospitalization Rates, for the National Research

Exhibit 7-26 Continued

Council, states that "for a policy of housing children separately to be effective, certain minimum services and facilities are needed, thus requiring bed capacity utilization to make provision for these services and facilities economically feasible." This standard was developed by the Department in this context. Pediatric services should be planned on a regionalized basis with linkages among hospitals and other health agencies to provide comprehensive care.

A number of sources support a minimum unit size of 20 pediatric beds, including planning agencies in California, Massachusetts, Ohio, Pennsylvania, and Wisconsin. Consolidation of pediatric care in units of at least 20 beds in urbanized areas will promote the concentration of nursing and support staff with special pediatric knowledge and skills, the increased training of staff, and the provision of special treatment and other ancillary facilities which meet the special needs of children. (A pediatric inpatient unit is a specific section, ward, wing, hospital or unit devoted primarily to the care of medical and surgical patients less than 18 years old, not including special care for infants.) The criteria of 30 minutes travel time reflects interest in ensuring that children remain close to their homes, family, and friends. Frequent visits to hospitalized children are highly desirable and can be an aid to improvement and recovery. The American Academy of Pediatrics has recommended to its State Chapters that child health plans should provide that primary care for children should be available within 30 minutes. This access standard is consistent with those of many local and State planning agencies such as those in Massachusetts, New York, Pennsylvania, and Wisconsin.

§ 121.206 Pediatric Inpatient Services— Occupancy Rates.

(a) *Standard.* Pediatric units should maintain average annual occupancy rates related to the number of pediatric beds (exclusive of neonatal special care units) in the facility. For a facility with 20–39 pediatric beds, the average annual occupancy rate should be at least 65 percent; for a facility with 40–79 pediatric beds, the rate should be at least 70 percent; for facilities with 80 or more pediatric beds, the rate should be at least 75 percent.

(b) *Discussion.* Variable occupancy rates are designed to reflect the need for smaller units to maintain the capacity to accommodate normal day-to-day fluctuations in admissions and to set aside pediatric beds for particular ages and types of cases. Such scheduling problems are less severe in pediatric units of a greater capacity. Moreover, large units are able to sustain higher occupancy rates because they are frequently associated with regional centers which serve patients needing types of care that can be scheduled on a more flexible basis. It is not intended, of course, to encourage unnecessary admissions or stays to achieve these levels. This standard is identical to that recommended by the American Academy of Pediatrics.

§ 121.207 Open Heart Surgery.

(a) *Standard.* (1) There should be a minimum of 200 open heart procedures performed annually, within three years after initiation, in any institution in which open heart surgery is performed for adults.

(2) There should be a minimum of 100 pediatric heart operations annually, within three years after initiation, in any institution in which pediatric open heart surgery is performed, of which at least 75 should be open heart surgery.

(3) There should be no additional open heart units initiated unless each existing unit in the health service area(s) is operating and is expected to continue to operate at a minimum of 350 open heart surgery cases per year in adult services or 130 pediatric open heart cases in pediatric services.

(b) *Discussion.* Open heart surgery for congenital and acquired heart and coronary artery disease represents a marked advance in patient care. Highly specialized open heart procedures require very costly, highly specialized manpower and facility resources. Thus, every effort should be made to limit duplication and unnecessary resources related to the performance of open heart procedures, while maintaining high quality care. Mini-

Exhibit 7-26 Continued

mum case loads are essential to maintain and strengthen skills. (Open heart surgery procedures are defined as procedures which use a heart-lung by-pass machine to perform the functions of circulation during surgery.) A minimum of 200 adult open heart surgery procedures should be performed annually within an institution to maintain quality of patient care and make most efficient use of resources. This standard is based on recommendations of the Inter Society Commission on Heart Disease Resources. In order to prevent duplication of costly resources which are not fully utilized, the opening of new units should be contingent upon existing units operating, and continuing to operate, at a level of at least 350 procedures per year. The 350 level assumes an average of 7 operations a week, a schedule that in the Department's judgment is feasible in most institutions providing these services. In units that provide services to children, lower targets are indicated because of the special needs involved. The established level for pediatric units is consistent with the recommendation of the Pediatric Cardiology Section of the American Academy of Pediatrics. In determining the utilization target of 130 pediatric open heart cases, the Department used the same ratio as for adult units. In the case of units that provide services to both adults and children, at least 200 open heart procedures should be performed, including 75 for children. Data collection and quality assessment and control activities should be part of all open heart surgery programs.

§ 121.208 Cardiac Catheterization Unit Services.

(a) *Standard.* (1) There should be a minimum of 300 cardiac catheterizations, of which at least 200 should be intracardiac or coronary artery catheterizations, performed annually in any adult cardiac catheterization unit within three years after initiation.

(2) There should be a minimum of 150 pediatric cardiac catheterizations performed annually in any pediatric cardiac catheterization unit within three years after initiation.

(3) There should be no new cardiac catheterization units opened in any fa-

cility not performing open heart surgery.

(4) There should be no additional adult cardiac catheterization units opened unless the number of studies per year in each existing unit in the health service area(s) is greater than 500.

(b) *Discussion.* The modern cardiac catheterization unit requires a highly skilled staff and expensive equipment. Safety and efficacy of laboratory performance requires a case load of adequate size to maintain the skill and efficiency of the staff. In addition, the underutilized unit represents a less efficient use of an expensive resource and frequently reflects unnecessary duplication. Based on recommendations from the Inter-Society Commission on Heart Disease Resources, the Department believes that a minimum level of 300 cardiac catheterizations per year is indicated to achieve economic use of resources. Several State health planning agencies, such as New Jersey, suggested a higher minimum level and the Department will be considering whether a higher level should be established in the future. The Department has also determined the existing units should be performing more than 500 cardiac catheterizations before any new unit is opened. The 500 level is based on an average of two catheterizations a day, a rate that is in the Department's judgment readily achievable in most institutions providing these services and that will foster more effective use of current resources prior to the development of additional resources. More than 600 cardiac procedures are performed annually in some institutions. Pediatric cardiac catheterizations require special facilities and support services. Lower target numbers are presented in these cases because of the special conditions and needs of children. The established levels are consistent with the recommendations of the Section on Cardiology of the American Academy of Pediatrics and the Inter-Society Commission on Heart Disease Resources. The patient studied in the cardiac catheterization unit is frequently recommended for open heart surgery. While acceptable inter-institutional referral

Exhibit 7-26 Continued

patterns exist in some areas, cardiac catheterization units should optimally be located within a facility in which cardiac surgery is performed.

§ 121.209 Radiation Therapy.

(a) *Standard.* (1) A megavoltage radiation therapy unit should serve a population of at least 150,000 persons and treat at least 300 cancer cases annually, within three years after initiation.

(2) There should be no additional megavoltage units opened unless each existing megavoltage unit in the health service area(s) is performing at least 6,000 treatments per year.

(3) Adjustments downward may be justified when travel time to an alternate unit is a serious hardship due to geographic remoteness, based on analyses by the HSA.

(b) *Discussion.* While various types of radiation are indicated and used for tumors with different characteristics, megavoltage equipment is accepted as the most efficacious for treatment of deep-seated tumors. Megavoltage equipment is expensive to purchase, install, and support on a continuing basis. Every effort should thus be made to avoid unnecessary duplication of this costly resource. Established standards should provide needed treatment capabilities while preventing unnecessary duplication of radiation therapy units and underutilization of existing capacity. A unit refers to a single megavoltage machine or energy source. The most common types of units to deliver megavoltage therapy are cobalt 60 and linear accelerators. Treatments are meant to be the same as patient visits. A treatment or visit averages 2.2 fields, according to reports from the American College of Radiology. They also report that about half of new cancer patients require megavoltage radiation therapy, and that many require subsequent courses of treatment. The American College of Radiology has indicated that at least 300 cancer cases annually are a reasonable minimum loan for a megavoltage radiation therapy unit in order to maintain an efficient high quality operation. Based on the information and recommendations of the College, as well as comments received

from the public and from members of the expert advisory panel which reviewed the standard, the Department has set a minimum standard of at least 300 cancer cases per unit per year. In 1974, the Department commissioned a study of the use of radiation therapy units. A committee appointed by the American College of Radiology and the American Society of Therapeutic Radiology to review that study suggested that economical operation of radiation units would call for existing units to do 5,000–8,700 treatments per year. The 7,500 level was included in the September 23, 1977, NPRM. This target would have required units to treat an average of 30 patients per day. Based on comments received from the profession and the general public, the Department has adjusted the standard downwards to 6,000 treatments per year, an average of about 25 patients per day to take into account variations in patient mix and work schedules. Since many institutions meet and exceed these targets, this standard in the Department's judgment represents an attainable, efficient level of operation. The indicated target levels are minimal and should generally be exceeded. Special purpose and extra high energy machines which have limited but important applications may not perform 6,000 treatments per year and should be evaluated individually by HSAs in the development of Health Systems Plans.

§ 121.210 Computed Tomographic Scanners.

(a) *Standard.* (1) A Computed Tomographic Scanner (head and body) should operate at a minimum of 2,500 medically necessary patient procedures per year.

(2) There should be no additional scanners approved unless each existing scanner in the health service area is performing at a rate greater than 2,500 medically necessary patient procedures per year.

(3) There should be no additional scanners approved unless the operators of the proposed equipment will set in place data collection and utilization review systems.

(b) *Discussion.* Because CT scanners are expensive to purchase, maintain

Exhibit 7-26 Continued

and staff, every effort must be made to contain costs while providing an acceptable level of service. Full and appropriate utilization of all existing units, regardless of location, will prevent needless duplication and limit unnecessary increases in health care costs. Estimates and surveys for full utilization of CT scanners range from 1,800 to over 4,000 patient procedures a year. (One patient procedure includes, during a single visit, the initial scan plus any necessary additional scans of the same anatomical region.) The Institute of Medicine, the Office of Technology Assessment and others have carefully reviewed these data and the capabilities of various available units.

The Department has reviewed these analyses as well as the extensive literature that has been developed on CT scanners. In arriving at a standard for the minimum use of these machines, the Department has considered a variety of factors, including the difference in time required for head scans and body scans, variations in patient mix, the special needs of children, time required for maintenance, and staffing requirements. Moreover, the Department considered the actual operating experience of hospitals and institutions reflected in reports on the use of CT scanners. The standard set in the Department's guidelines is intended to assure effective utilization and reasonable cost for CT scanning. These machines are expensive, and therefore must be fully used if excessive costs are to be limited. The Department recognizes that the cost of some machines is declining, particularly those that perform only head scans which require less time. For machines that do predominantly head scans, the standard represents an extremely minimum level appropriate to insure efficient and effective utilization.

For scanners capable of performing both head and body scans, it is imperative that they be effectively used in order to spread the high capital expenditures over as much operating time as possible. As the Institute of Medicine report stated, "The high fixed costs of operating a scanner argue for as high a volume of use as the equipment allows without jeopar-

dizing the quality of care." The Department believes that a 50–55 hour operating week both is consistent with the actual operating experience of many hospitals, and also a reasonable target. Based on reported experience for the time required for both head scans and body scans, the Department estimated that a patient mix of about 60 percent head scans and about 40 percent body scans, making allowance for the other factors identified above, would allow a CT scanner to perform about 2,500 patient procedures per year if it is efficiently used about 50–55 hours per week. This estimate assumes a higher percent of body scans than is currently being performed. If fewer than 40 percent body scans are performed, than 2,500 patient procedures would involve even less than 50–55 hours per week. Basing the standard on a higher percentage of body scans also takes account of current trends toward increased proportions of such scans.

The Department believes that sharing arrangements in the use of CT scanners is desirable, in line with the national health priorities of section 1502. Individual institutions or providers should not acquire new machines until existing capacity is being well utilized. In planning for CT scanners, the HSA should take into consideration special circumstances such as: (1) An institution with more than one scanner where the combined average annual number of procedures is greater than 2,500 per scanner although the unit doing primarily body scans is operating at less than 2,500 patient procedures per year; (2) units which are or will be operating a significant portión of the time under collaborative fixed protocol clinical trials, and (3) units which are, or will be, servicing predominantly seriously sick or pediatric patients. A summary of the data collected on CT scanners should be submitted by the operators to the appropriate HSA to enable it to adequately plan the distribution and use of CT scanners in the area. The data to be collected should include information on utilization and a description of the operations of a utilization review program.

Exhibit 7-26 Continued

§ 121.211 End-Stage Renal Disease (ESRD).

(a) *Standard.* The Health Systems Plans established by HSAs should be consistent with standards and procedures contained in the DHEW regulations governing conditions for coverage of suppliers of end-stage renal disease services, 20 CFR Part 405, Subpart U.

(b) *Discussion.* The ESRD Program was created pursuant to Section 2991 of the Social Security Amendments of 1972 (Pub. L. 92-603), which extends Medicare benefits to any individual who has end-stage renal disease requiring dialysis or transplantation, provided that such individual: (1) Is fully or currently insured or entitled to monthly benefits under Title II of the Social Security Act; or (2) is the spouse or dependent child of an individual so insured or entitled to such monthly benefits. In order for an ESRD facility to qualify for reimbursement under the program, the facility must meet the conditions for coverage of suppliers of end-stage renal disease services as established by regulation. These conditions incorporate standards which relate to the supply, distribution, and organization of ESRD facilities. The standards were developed by the Department of Health, Education, and Welfare and were based on extensive consultation with professionals and other persons knowledgeable in the areas of nephrology and transplant surgery. Because these standards are already published as regulations, they are not republished here. The regulations do not try to encourage any particular type of dialysis setting. It is widely recognized that self-care dialysis can significantly contain costs without impairing the quality of care of the suitably chosen patient. The organization of resources to support self-care dialysis is therefore encouraged to the maximum extent practicable.

[FR Doc. 78-1562 Filed 1-19-78; 8:45 am]

Source: Federal Register, January 20, 1978.

local planning by HSAs, would be difficult to achieve, and might lead to unemployment among hospital workers. However, members of Congress stated that it was time to set numerical standards. Government officials also predicted that the nation would save more than $2 billion annually if the recommendations were achieved.

CRITERIA CHECKLIST

Another type of criteria checklist enumerates the elements to be evaluated, asks simply whether each element is there, and assigns a value to each criterion. Exhibit 7-27 was designed for the evaluation of the structure of a shared health facility, sometimes called a Medicaid mill. Structural elements were divided into separate categories, and they are listed with the percentages assigned to them: general (23 percent), patient flow (2 percent), record system (7 percent), pharmacy (6 percent), radiology (5 percent), ECGs (4 percent), laboratory (9 percent), equipment and supplies (22 percent), physical facilities (17 percent), and examination rooms (5 percent). In addition to the yes/no

Exhibit 7-27 Sample Page From a Criteria Checklist Evaluating Ambulatory Care Facility

Facility # _____ Date of Audit _____	Compliance			
	Yes	No	N/A	Comments

D. Which tests are done on the premises?

Chest____ Barium____ UGI____

IVP____ Skull____ Extremities____

Back X-rays____ Mammography____

VI. E.C.G.'s (Total 4%)

   A. The availability of an E.C.G. machine on the premise at all times. (2%)

   B. E.C.G. machine equipped with 12 leads (2%)

VII. Laboratory (Total 9%)

   *A. If lab on premises (more than CBC & urinalysis) is it licenses by the New York City Health Department?

     If Yes, permit # _____

   B. "Small" lab procedures performed limited to those approved by Bureau of Labs for non licensed labs (Hgb, Hcl, urine) (3%)

   C. Lab specimens labeled to include: (2%)

     1. name or identifying code.
     2. Medicaid # of patient

   D. Routine lab specimen picked up daily when facility is open (4%)

   E.* If commercial lab used, is it licensed by N.Y.C. Dept. of Health

     Name _____

     Address _____

     N.Y.C. Bureau of Lab. # _____

     Expiration Date _____

   F. Routine Lab Work returned in a maximum of _____ days

* 5 point penalty if the answer is no, no credit for a yes answer.

Source: Grateful acknowledgment is given to the New York County Health Services Review Organization (NYCHSRO) for development of these Criteria Checklists (Exhibits 7-27 and 7-28), which are used by NYCHSRO (Manhattan's PSRO) in its review system.

response, the evaluator can add comments or note that the criterion is not applicable (N/A). Furthermore, additional data can be recorded such as permit numbers for radiology, identification of commercial laboratories, last inspection date for fire extinguishers, and the number of patients scheduled for a period of time. Criteria identified with an asterisk receive a five-point penalty if the answer is no and no credit for a yes answer (Exhibit 7-28). This criteria checklist gives highest value weights to four elements in evaluating the structural components of health care facilities, as follows:

- Physician on premise at all times when facility is open for physician care.
- Patients have a primary care physician who is responsible for their medical care.
- Arrangements for assisting patients requiring care during off hours.
- Emergency kit to include seven listed items.

Thirteen items receive a weight of one point, and two receive one-half point each (Exhibit 7-28).

This type of criteria evaluation can be reasonably objective because a majority of the elements can be observed and verified immediately without subjective interpretation.

MODEL SCREENING CRITERIA FOR USE IN PSRO REVIEW

Professional Standards Review Organizations have been established to review medical care received by inpatients that is paid for by government funds, mainly Medicare, Medicaid, and maternal and child health programs. In cooperation with almost all specialty and subspecialty medical associations, the American Medical Association oversaw the development of criteria. About 75 percent of the hospitalizations within each specialty are covered by these standards. In addition, the length of the hospital stay for each diagnosis is also to be calculated by local PSROs and included in the criteria. Norms, criteria, and standards are defined in the *PSRO Program Manual* published by the federal government and relate to these guidelines as follows:

- Norms are "numerical or statistical measures of usual observed performance."
- Criteria are "predetermined elements against which aspects of the quality of a medical services may be compared. They are devel-

Exhibit 7-28 Checklist Items Categorized By Relative Weights for Evaluation of Ambulatory Care Facility

---

5 points (20%)

1. Physicians on premise at all times when facility is open for physician care.
2. Patients have a primary physician who is responsible for their medical care.
3. Arrangements for assisting patients requiring care during off hours.
4. Emergency kit to include: ambu-bags or portable oxygen, airway, sodium bicarbonate, epinephrine, corticosteroids, benadryl, 50 percent glucose and water.

4 points (24%)

1. Designation of an individual (physician or lay administrator) responsible for coordinating and managing facility activities full time.
2. Medical director in facility at least 25 percent of the time.
3. Maintainance of a central daybook for the facility which includes: patient's name, Medicaid number, doctors seen, and referrals.
4. Maintainance of a patient drug use profile for pharmacies in or adjacent to the facility.
5. Routine laboratory specimens picked up daily when facility is open.
6. Current biologicals.

3 points (12%)

1. All practitioners share the same medical records except dentist (centralized system).
2. Identification of x-ray film to include: patient's name or code, data, L/R indication.
3. Small laboratory procedures performed limited to those approved by bureau of laboratories for nonlicensed laboratories (Hgb, Hct, urine).
4. Complete audio and visual privacy during examination.

2 points (30%)

1. Operational appointment system for revisit patients.
2. A sign indicating free choice of pharmacists conspicuously posted in the pharmacy.
3. Radiology equipment currently registered with the local department of health.
4. The availability of an ECG machine on the premise at all times.
5. ECG machine equipped with 12 leads.
6. Laboratory specimens labeled to include: name or code, Medicaid number of patient.
7. Clean refrigerator with proper temperature and storage.
8. Adequate supplies of syringes and needles.
9. Provision for destruction of syringes and needles.
10. Provision for appropriate sterilization of nondisposable equipment is used.
11. Certificate of Occupancy posted.
12. Clean patient toilet facilities with soap, towels, and a functioning sink.
13. No evidence of rodent or vermin infestation.
14. Locked space for syringes and needles.
15. A functioning sink with soap and towels, in or near examination room.

1 point (13%)

1. Thermometer in refrigerator to monitor temperature.
2. Adequate supplies of clinical thermometers.
3. Adult height and weight scales.

Exhibit 7-28 Continued

4. Infant weight scales.
5. Eye chart with mark to identify 20- or 10-foot distances.
6. List of practitioners employed in the facility posted.
7. Lighting sufficient to meet minimum public facility lumination requirements.
8. Ventilation—heat and cooling capacities sufficient to meet minimum public facility ventilation standards.
9. Overall seating capacity sufficient to meet needs of the patients.
10. Storage space area for necessary supplies and equipment.
11. Alternate means of egress.
12. Exits identified.
13. Fire extinguisher available—2.5 gallon water type per 2500 square feet or 1 per floor.

1/2 point (1%)

1. Wall surfaces clean and in good repair.
2. Floor surface clean and in good repair.

---

oped by professionals relying on professional expertise and on the professional literature."

- Standards are "professionally developed expressions of the range of acceptable variation from a norm or criterion."

Exhibit 7-29 presents criteria for screening that embody the above definitions. A reviewer, usually a registered nurse, will compare the record of the patient with the criteria for that diagnosis. Variations from the criteria will be noted, and the attending physician will be asked to explain or a consultant medical reviewer will speak with the attending physician. (Sometimes a variation of this technique will be used.) In the criteria related to critical diagnostic and therapeutic services, screening benchmarks indicate the services that are required (100 percent) and those unwarranted (0 percent). Again deviations may have to be explained by the attending physician.

Length of stay for each diagnostic category will be based upon local hospitalization data as determined by the local PSRO. All other parts of the criteria were agreed on by the professional specialty groups as being the appropriate medical care criteria as of this time. PSRO criteria are to be reviewed and changed periodically as necessary.

INDICATORS AND INDEXES

Although indicators and indexes are sometimes regarded as equivalents, J.A. Solon[42] does distinguish between them. He states that an

Exhibit 7-29 PSRO Guidelines—June 1976.

	June 1976	
	H-ICDA	ICDA-8
Appendicitis	540,540.0	540,540.0
	540.1,542	540.9,541
	543	542,543

I. ADMISSION REVIEW

    A. REASONS FOR ADMISSION

        1. Scheduled for operation (interval appendectomy or drainage of abscess)
        2. Diagnosis or suspicion of acute appendicitis

    B. INITIAL LENGTH OF STAY ASSIGNMENT (see explanation)

II. CONTINUED STAY REVIEW

    A. REASONS FOR EXTENDING THE INITIAL LENGTH OF STAY

        1. Peritonitis or abscess
        2. Persistent high fever (possible septicemia, pneumonia, urinary tract infection)
        3. Wound complication (e.g., hematoma, fistula, infection, dehiscence, nonclosure of incision)
        4. Postoperative bowel obstruction
        5. Presence of concomitant diagnosis (e.g., diabetes, cardiopulmonary disease, thrombophlebitis)

    B. EXTENDED LENGTH OF STAY ASSIGNMENT (see explanation)

III. VALIDATIONS OF:

    A. DIAGNOSIS

        1. Positive tissue report if appendectomy performed

    B. REASONS FOR ADMISSION

    No entry necessary

IV. CRITICAL DIAGNOSTIC AND THERAPEUTIC SERVICES

	Screening Benchmark
A. CBC including differential	100%
B. Appendectomy or drainage of abscess (within 24 hours of admission if under 18 years of age)	100%
C. Rectal examination	100%
D. Urinalysis	100%
E. Administration of laxative	0%

V. DISCHARGE STATUS

    A. Alive
    B. Afebrile (temperature less than 100° F or 37.7° C for more than 24 consecutive hours)
    C. Tolerating diet
    D. Wound healing satisfactorily
    E. Plan for follow-up

Exhibit 7-29 Continued

VI. COMPLICATIONS

    A. PRIMARY DISEASE AND TREATMENT-SPECIFIC COMPLICATIONS

        1. Generalized peritonitis or intraperitoneal abscess
        2. Sepsis
        3. Wound complication (e.g., infection, hematoma, dehiscence)
        4. Postoperative bowel obstruction
        5. Respiratory complication-atelectasis, pneumonia

    B. NONSPECIFIC INDICATORS

        1. Any extension of initial length of stay assignment, if appendix
           not ruptured
        2. Second operation
        3. Blood transfusion

Developed by AMERICAN ACADEMY OF PEDIATRICS, AMERICAN COLLEGE OF SURGEONS,
      and the AMERICAN PEDIATRIC SURGICAL ASSOCIATION.

		June 1976	
Hypertension (Include accelerated, encephalopathy)		H-ICDA 400,438.3	ICDA-8 400,436

I. ADMISSION REVIEW

    A. REASONS FOR ADMISSION

        1. Diastolic blood pressure in excess of 110 mm Hg
        2. Failure to respond to antihypertensive therapy
        3. Neurologic or sensorium abnormalities
        4. Investigate secondary cause of hypertension (e.g., renal disease,
           renal-vascular abnormality, adrenal disease)
        5. Uncontrolled congestive heart failure or renal failure (rising BUN)

    B. INITIAL LENGTH OF STAY ASSIGNMENT (see explanation)

II. CONTINUED STAY REVIEW

    A. REASONS FOR EXTENDING THE INITIAL LENGTH OF STAY

        1. Secondary cause of hypertension discovered (e.g., renal disease,
           renal-vascular abnormality, adrenal disease)
        2. Unresponsive to initial antihypertensive therapy
        3. Neurologic abnormalities
        4. Congestive heart failure
        5. Renal failure (rising BUN or creatinine)

    B. EXTENDED LENGTH OF STAY ASSIGNMENT (see explanation)

III. VALIDATIONS OF:

    A. DIAGNOSIS

        1. Diastolic blood pressure in excess of 90 mm Hg

Exhibit 7-29 Continued

B. REASONS FOR ADMISSION

    1. Historical documentation of failure to respond to antihypertensive therapy
    2. Documentation of neurologic or sensorium abnormalities
    3. Documentation of renal, renal-vascular, or adrenal abnormality

IV. CRITICAL DIAGNOSTIC AND THERAPEUTIC SERVICES

	Screening Benchmark
A. Blood pressure recorded daily, as a minimum	100%
B. BUN or creatinine	100%
C. Electrocardiogram	100%
D. Fundoscopy	100%
E. Radiologic examination of the chest and IVP	100%

V. DISCHARGE STATUS

    A. Antihypertensive therapy (e.g., salt restriction, antihypertensive medication)
    B. Documented plan of follow-up
    C. Resolution of reason for admission

VI. COMPLICATIONS

    A. PRIMARY DISEASE AND TREATMENT-SPECIFIC COMPLICATIONS

        No entry appropriate

    B. NONSPECIFIC INDICATORS

        1. Surgery

Developed by AMERICAN COLLEGE OF CARDIOLOGY.

Source: American Medical Association and Thirty-eight National Medical Specialty and Professional Societies. *Sample Criteria for Short-Stay Hospital Review. Screening Criteria To Assist PSROs in Quality Assurance* (Chicago, Ill.: AMA, 1976), pp. 67-68, 317-318.

---

indicator is an unidimensional measure, and an index is a composite of weighted factors. In this vein, a publication of the National Center for Health Statistics also stated, "a health index is a measure which summarizes data from two or more components and which purports to reflect the health status of an individual or defined group."[43] In addition, the following distinctions were made by Solon:

Indicators	*Indices*
Elements	Composites
Narrow scope	Broad scope
Specific	General
Direct	Derived
More tangible	Less tangible

Clearly, the distinctions highlight the fact that an indicator is a measure of some particular single element or aspect of health care, while the index is a grouping of indicators into a composite.

Following along with this concept, Solon presents a suggested definition of a health status index:

> A quantified, standardized, weighted *composite* of a set of selected indicators of an individual's or a population's health status, which together—on some kind of scale—presumes to give a *broad*-spectrum representation of an individual's or a population's *general* health and wellbeing. (Emphasis added.)

Within this definition, how can health status indices be used in evaluation? Some examples can be listed:

- Populations can be compared.
- Changes over time can be observed.
- Problems can be identified, and their magnitude measured.
- Cause and effect relationships can be suggested.
- Needs can be forecast.
- Priorities for the allocation of resources can be determined.
- Program objectives can be specified numerically.
- Program effectiveness can be measured statistically.
- Social policy and goals can be formulated.
- Patient management can be assessed.
- Medical audits can be compared.
- Research studies can use indices for evaluation.

Additional examples of the uses of health status indices can be reviewed in the publication, *Clearinghouse on Health Indexes; Cumulated Annotations, 1975,* published by the National Center for Health Statistics.[44]

Examples illustrating the use of specific indicators are fairly common in evaluation. Exhibit 7-30 provides comparative data about variations in surgical rates in North America, Britain, and Sweden for six

Exhibit 7-30 Variations in Surgical Rates in North America, Britian, and Sweden

	Saskatchewan	USA	England	Sweden
Removal of tonsils and adenoids	111	60	42	30
Veins ligated or stripped	3	5	10	15
Hernia repair	29	25	23	17
Haemorrhoidectomy	10	13	5	5
Cholecystectomey	16	15	9	26
Hysterectomy	30	31	24	8
All operations	616	626	444	•

Note: Rates for selected surgical operations per 10,000 population in Saskatchewan, USA, England, and Sweden.

Source: R.F. Logan, "Assessment of Sickness and Health in the Community: Needs and Methods," *Medical Care* 2 (1964): 173. Reprinted with permission. © 1964 J.B. Lippincott Co.

common surgical procedures. An examination of these specific indicators might pinpoint problems in the United States in regard to certain surgical operations and suggest policies or the need for additional evaluation.

Another example illustrated in Exhibit 7-31 relates to an evaluation that might consider indicators of days of bed disability, limitation of activity, hospital discharges, hospital days, and of deaths. An individual hospital or group of hospitals in an area could calculate its own ranking and numerical counts for comparison with the data from a national source. This comparison could serve as an indicator of measurement and as an evaluation of activities.

Time trend indicators allow for a comparison over time of specific rates. Exhibit 7-32 shows life expectancy at birth by sex and by sex and race from 1901 to 1971 in the United States. Health planners wishing to assess the statistics for their own community could plot their data and observe the relation to the U.S. time trend. Any number of graphs could be compiled for hosts of specific indicators, against which the health planner could make comparisons.

INDICATORS OF THE QUALITY OF CARE

Although the compilation of some indicators of the quality of care by Donabedian[45] does not give exact numbers, the direction is noted for

Exhibit 7-31 Illustrative Diseases/Conditions Accounting for Ill Health-Ranking of Diseases According to Health Impact, U.S. 1971

Disease/Condition	Days of BM Disability		Limitation of Activity		Hospital Discharges		Hospital Days		Deaths	
	Rank	Days*	Rank	No. Using Limitations*	Rank	Numbers*	Rank	Days*	Rank	Numbers*
Influenza & pneumonia	1	206,241	—	—	2	1,311	11	3,444	4	55
Upper respiratory	2	164,310	16	280	1	1,000	1	17,921	—	—
Heart disease	3	93,137	1	3,954	12	217	9	3,837	1	741
Arthritis	4	57,539	2	3,377	5	695	3	15,273	—	—
Mental disorders	5	41,965	4	1,741	3	1,249	2	17,097	—	—
Fractures & dislocations	6	35,625	—	—	6	646	4	7,795	—	—
Malignant neoplasms	7	32,374	15	374	—	—	—	—	2	333
Impairments of back & spine	8	31,895	3	1,963	—	—	—	—	—	—
Hypertensive without heart involvement	9	27,476	6	1,193	9	314	12	2,780	8	8
Bronchitis	10	27,338	18	180	—	—	—	—	10	5
Asthma	11	25,997	7	1,150	—	—	—	—	12	2
Cerebrovascular disease	12	24,763	10	630	11	264	7	5,128	3	203
Paralysis	13	24,052	9	861	—	—	—	—	—	—
Diabetes	14	23,739	8	966	10	280	10	3,498	5	33
Impairments of lower extremities	15	20,930	5	1,727	—	—	—	—	—	—
Ulcer	16	17,569	14	412	8	492	6	5,245	7	8
Emphysema	17	13,124	11	574	—	—	—	—	6	22
Hernia	18	11,943	12	506	4	726	8	4,805	9	7
Gall bladder	19	11,692	19	81	7	580	5	5,922	11	4
Absence of extremities	20	7,347	17	218	—	—	—	—	—	—
Impairments of upper extremities	21	5,491	13	485	—	—	—	—	—	—

*In Thousands

Note: - means not available.

Source: Unpublished data from the National Center for Health Statistics in *Health Planning and Public Accountability Seminar Workbook* (Germantown, Md.: Aspen Systems Corp., 1976).

Exhibit 7-32 Time Trend Indicators

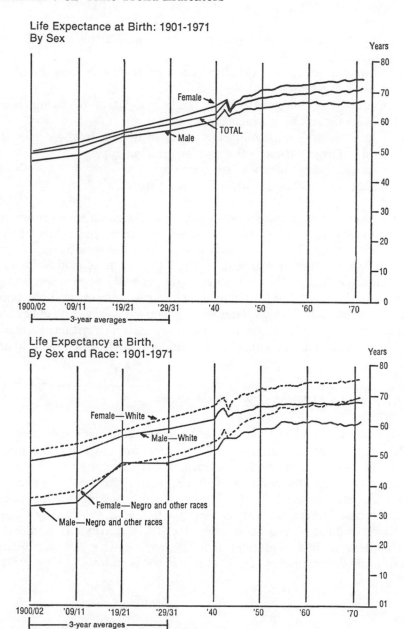

Life Expectance at Birth: 1901-1971
By Sex

Life Expectancy at Birth,
By Sex and Race: 1901-1971

Source: U.S. Department of Commerce, *Social Indicators 1973* (Washington, D.C.: U.S. Government Printing Office, 1973), p. 2.

the health planner who wishes to go this route. These indicators are grouped into the following general headings:

I.   Characteristics of the settings within which the medical care process takes place.
II. Characteristics of provider behavior in the management of health and illness.
III. Other provider behaviors possibly indicative of strength or weakness in the organization of care.
IV. Client behaviors possibly indicative of defects in the organization of care or the client-provider relationship.
V.   Characteristics of use of service.
VI. Characteristics of health and other outcomes.

There is an obvious relationship between the guidelines presented by Donabedian in the section on criteria and these indicators of the quality of care. Exhibit 7-33 clearly enumerates the specific indicators that the health planner can seek out and use to make evaluations of care rendered. Again, the indicators could probably be reordered into the commonly used classifications of structure, process, and outcome without too much difficulty. These could be used as a yes/no checklist or as a comparative indicator with numbers, rates, or ratios attached. In either case, the method provides a solid base upon which to build an evaluation.

HEALTH STATUS INDEX

This formula for a health status index combines specific indicators of health status into a mathematical equation to determine the magnitude of a health problem. For evaluation purposes, the health status index can be calculated before and after an activity to see if any change occurs. Indicators included in the health status index include inpatient days, outpatient days, days of restricted activity, and mortality. Since not all the indicators can be incorporated into a mathematical health status index, the health planner must choose those that are most influential in the determination of the status of the population being evaluated.

Exhibit 7-33 Some Indicators of the Quality of Care

Numerous variables have been used as indicators of the quality of care. The following is meant to give an impression of possible approaches, rather than a complete listing. Selected components of the "medical care process" are used to classify the indicators listed.

I. Characteristic of the settings within which the medical care process takes place

It is assumed that good care is more likely to be provided when the settings are favorable, and that we know what constitutes a "favorable" setting

A. Physical structure, facilities and equipment
   1. Presence or absence of certain facilities and equipment in relation to specific care functions
   2. Space and physical layout in relation to function
B. General organizational features
   1. Ownership and auspices
   2. Profit or nonprofit status
   3. Accreditation, affiliation and residency approval status
   4. Other intrainstitutional functional relationships (for example, as part of a regionalization program)
   5. Group practice, partnerships, "solo" practice
C. Administrative organization
   1. Boards of trustees: their composition and activities
   2. Administrator: qualifications and relationships with board and staff
D. Staff organization
   1. Qualifications: formal degrees, certification, experience, etc.
   2. Number of staff related to work load
   3. Staff organization and policies governing staff activities
      a. Educational functions: maintenance and promotion of staff competence
      b. Control functions: utilization review, various types of audits of staff performance, etc.
E. Fiscal and related aspects of organization
   1. Hospital accommodation
   2. Source of payment of bill and extent of patient participation in payment
F. Geographic factors
   1. Distance, isolation, etc.

II. Characteristics of provider behavior in the management of health and illness

It is assumed that there are acceptable standards of what constitutes "goodness," and that good care makes a difference in terms of health outcomes.

A. Extent to which screening and case-finding activities are carried out
   1. Routine procedures applicable to the older age group: Examples are activities for the detection of glaucoma, diabetes, cervical cancer in women, lower bowel cancer, breast cancer, visual and hearing defects
   2. Screening and case-finding activities related to special-risk situations. Examples are: bleeding from the rectum (sigmoidoscopy); blood in the urine (cystoscopy); indigestion (barium meal and occult blood); hypertension (eyegrounds, urine, catecholamines, etc.)
   3. Follow-up on "red flag" findings with appropriate diagnostic and therapeutic activities. Examples are: bleeding from body orifices; certain abnormal laboratory findings (urine or blood sugar, for example)

Exhibit 7-33 Continued

B. Diagnostic activities
  1. Diagnostic work-up
     a. Frequency of performance of specified test per unit population
     b. Diagnostic work-up for specified disease situations: volume and nature of tests, etc.
  2. Patterns of diagnostic categorization: completeness, exhaustiveness, specificity, etc.
  3. Validation of diagnosis
     a. Pathological examination reports on tissues and postmortem
     b. Preoperative versus postoperative diagnosis
     c. Admission and discharge diagnoses
  4. Validation or primary diagnostic information. Special studies on accuracy of lab reports, interpretations of x-ray films, etc.
C. Treatment
  1. Preventive management and supervision of certain diseases. Minimal or optimal standards of number of visits or routine follow up in given diseases such as diabetes, hypertension, syphilis, etc.
  2. Patterns of use of drugs, blood and biologicals in general. Examples:
     a. Total prescribed drug utilization per capita and per 1000 physician visits
     b. Use of antibiotics, especially in mixtures
     c. Use of antibiotics without testing for sensitivity of microorganism
     d. Use of "shot-gun" hematinics
     e. Use of multivitamins
     f. Use of tranquilizers

g. Use of blood by amount of blood, age, sex, etc. Incidence of single-unit transfusions
  3. Patterns of use of drugs, blood, and biologicals in specified diagnostic situations
  4. Patterns of surgery
     a. Surgical rates by type of procedure with emphasis on certain operations more open to abuse. Examples: tonsillectomy, appendectomy, hemorrhoidectomy, varicose vein operation; certain gynecological operations including hysterectomy, supracervical hysterectomy, uterine suspension
     b. Patterns of multiple operations including second operations suggestive of possible deficiencies in first operation
     c. Removal of normal tissue at operation
D. Consultation and referral
  1. Patterns of consultation and referral by category of physician making request, type of consultant, disease characteristics, patient characteristics, institutional settings, etc.
  2. Consultations and referrals in specific disease situations, including emotional and psychiatric problems and referral to psychiatrists
E. Coordination and continuity of care
  Number of physicians, hospitals, and other providers involved in the care of a single patient over a period of time or during a single episode of illness or care
F. Use of community agencies and resources
  Volume and patterns of use, in

Exhibit 7-33 Continued

general and for specified conditions or situations

III. Other provider behaviors possibly indicative of strength or weakness in the organization of care
   A. Staff turnover and absenteeism
   B. Illness rates (for example, among nursing students)
   C. Use of health services by providers who are presumably informed about sources of good care

IV. Client behaviors possibly indicative of defects in the organization of care or the client–provider relationship
   A. Complaints: volume and type
   B. Compliance and noncompliance: broken appointments; noncompliance with therapeutic regimen (drugs, diet, rest or exercise, etc.); premature termination of care, discharge against advice
   C. Knowledge
      1. About health and illness in general
      2. About current illness
   D. Changes in knowledge or behavior expected after prior exposure to medical care. For example: knowledge about prenatal and well-baby care resulting from having had a child; appropriate institution of prenatal and well-baby care

V. Characteristics of use of service
   Studies of the utilization of service have important implications for quality. Insufficient care means poor care. Similarly, unnecessary care is not only costly but can also denote poor quality, in surgery for example. It is assumed that adjustments have been made for factors that influence utilization, other than patient care.
   A. Volume of care
      1. Levels of utilization in the general population and population subgroups classified by age, sex, race, income, occupation, education, place of residence, insurance status, etc.
      2. Components of the utilization rates: "initiation": proportion receiving one or more services; "continuation": Number of services for those who receive one or more services
      3. Use by place of care: office, home, hospital, nursing home, etc.
      4. Use by source of care:
         a. Type of health professional
         b. Specialty status

VI. Characteristics of health and other outcomes
   It is assumed that adjustments have been made for factors that influence outcome, other than patient care.
   A. Health outcomes
      1. General mortality, morbidity, and disability rates. The problems of interpretation would be very severe; but one would examine secular trends, geographic variations, etc.
      2. Mortality in special subgroups
         Infant mortality and its components
         Maternal mortality
         Other age- and sex-specific mortalities
      3. Mortality by cause
      4. Longevity
         Life expectancy—general and at given ages
      5. Composite indices of illness or health giving average number of days lost from morbidity and mortality combined or the average number of remaining days after losses have been subtracted
      6. The occurrence of preventible morbidity or disability in

Exhibit 7-33 Continued

the general population. This approach is based on the assumption that given good care, either currently or during years or decades preceeding old age, some of the current morbidity and disability would have been prevented. Examples: prevalence of iron-deficiency anemia; loss of vision due to glaucoma; loss of hearing due to middle-ear disease; rheumatic heart disease; diabetic acidosis; amputations in diabetics and other patients; stage and extent of cancer at time of diagnosis

7. The occurrence of certain complications of, or failures in, therapy. Examples: Decubitus ulcers: cardiac decompensation; incomplete control of diabetics

8. Case fatality rates and operative mortality rates, by type of illness or operation and type of provider, with corrections for demographic and socioeconomic characteristics of patients

9. The occurrence of specified complications during the course of care or following surgery—for example, postoperative infection

10. The restoration of physical function following certain traumatic or neurological diseases. Examples: recovery after fractures; residual disability following strokes

11. Social restoration following mental illness. Examples: ability to remain in the community (as indicated by readmission rates); ability to find and maintain employment

B. Satisfaction
  1. Patient satisfaction is not necessarily, nor even usually, an indicator of the technical quality of care, but attention to patient needs is an important aspect of care and patient satisfaction an important objective in addition to technical performance
  2. Satisfaction of the health professionals providing care. While this is a dimension that is seldom mentioned, it is reasonable to assume that the best technical care cannot be maintained if the persons who provide it are unhappy with the work they do and the conditions under which it is done

Source: A. Donabedian, "Promoting Quality through Evaluating the Process of Patient Care," *Medical Care* 6(May-June 1968): 181. Reprinted with permission. © 1968 J.B. Lippincott Co.

An example of an index has been developed by the U.S. Public Health Service:[46]

$$\text{Index } Q = MDP + \frac{A}{N}(274) + \frac{B}{N}(91) + \frac{C}{N}(274),$$

where

M   = health problem ratio $\dfrac{\text{(Target Group Rate)}}{\text{(Reference Rate)}}$;

D   = crude target group mortality rate per 100,000;
P   = years of life lost due to death;
A   = number of inpatient days;
B   = number of outpatient visits;
C   = days of restricted activity;
N   =target group population;
274 = conversion constant $\dfrac{100,000}{365}$; and
91 = conversion constant $\dfrac{100,000}{365} \times \dfrac{1}{3}$.

The reference group is the comparison group such as U.S. population, or the statewide or local census. The higher the Q value, the greater the impact of the health problem.

Using data from the United States for the period 1963-64, the following data can be plugged into the formula:

Diseases of the Circulatory System

Mortality rate	365.8 per 100,000
Hospital days	34,613 (in thousands)
Physician visits	119,358 (in thousands)
Restricted days	24,392 (in thousands)

Since the target group and the reference group would be the same if the entire U.S. population were used, the value for M becomes 1. The Q value then is arrived at in the following manner:

$$Q = 1 \times 365.8 \times 11.7 + 50.83 + 58.40 + 35.82 = 4{,}425.$$

In the example, this Q value is the highest of the leading disease problems, accurately reflecting the ranking of mortality in the United States and also the impact on the health care delivery system. On all four indicators utilized in this index, diseases of the circulatory system appear to be a top priority problem. For evaluation, the specific indicators could be compared before and after, as well as the Q value, to determine if the activity had an impact on the health care system. Of course, there are other impacting variables that are not included in an index of this type. Until the information can be quantified, indexes will have to rely on reasonably accurate existing statistics.

CLINICAL INDEXES

Although an effort has been made to distinguish between indicators and indexes, the dividing line is not always that clear. Researchers have used indicators and indexes in their assessments, and at times the terms appear to be used on an interchangeable basis. However, in citing examples, the original meanings of the terms used will be used to retain consistency.

D.D. Rutstein and his associates[47] developed a technique that measures the quality of medical care with a clinical method that employs indexes of outcome. These outcomes are classified as unnecessary disease, unnecessary disability, and unnecessary untimely death. Exhibit 7-34 enumerates the clear-cut immediate use of quality of care indexes. In this exhibit, a single case of disease, disability, or untimely death would be enough cause for an immediate evaluation of the health care system. In essence, these indexes are quantitative negative measures that can be used in national evaluation, local assessments, or even individual hospital reviews.

If the user of this clinical index system discovers an unnecessary, untimely death, the investigation should be simple to follow. Thus, the unnecessary case of diphtheria, measles, or polio could be linked to a state legislature that did not appropriate the funds for immunization clinics, to the local health officer who did not implement the immunization program, to the medical society that opposed community clinics, to the physician who did not immunize his patient, or to the mother who neglected to take her child for the immunization. Lung cancer deaths could be due to the patient's reluctance to give up cigarette smoking, the influence of advertising, the lack of an effective health education program in the community, or infrequently, an error in the medical care system.

Certainly, the physician is not solely responsible for the unnecessary disease, disability, or death. However, health care providers usually have the initial contact and the continuing responsibility. Furthermore, health care providers do have the responsibility to provide professional guidance to politicians, administrators, industry, school systems, government services, the community at large, as well as to the individual patient and his family. Examination of the clinical index should provide clues as to which groups should be concerned with the causes of the unnecessary disease, disability, or death. Of course, the advice of health care providers might be disregarded, and the index might not carry much weight with those concerned. Nevertheless, use of the index guarantees that the responsibility has been carried out and that scientific input has entered into the considerations.

Exhibit 7-34 Unnecessary Disease, Disability, and Untimely Death Single Case Indexes*

8TH REV NO.	CONDITION	UNNECESSARY DISEASE	UNNECESSARY DISABILITY	UNNECESSARY UNTIMELY DEATH	NOTES†
000	Cholera	P		P,T	
001	Typhoid fever	P		P,T	
003.0	Other salmonella infections w/food as vehicle of infection	P		P	
005.1	Botulism	P		P	
010-019	Tuberculosis (all forms)			T	
010	Silicotuberculosis	P	P	P,T	P — Occupational
013	Tuberculosis of meninges & central nervous system	P		P,T	Sensitive index
020	Plague			T	
021	Tularemia			T	
022	Anthrax			T	
026	Rat-bite fever			T	
032	Diphtheria	P		P,T	
033	Whooping cough	P		P	
034	Streptococcal sore throat & scarlet fever			T	
037	Tetanus	P		P	Including neonatal tetanus
040-043	Acute poliomyelitis with or without paralysis or other complications (s)	P	P	P	
050	Smallpox	P		P	
055	Measles	P		P	
056	Rubella	P	P	P	Disability in offspring
060	Yellow fever	P		P	
073	Psittacosis	P		P,T	
080	Epidemic louse-borne typhus			T	
081.0	Endemic flea-borne typhus			T	
082.0	Spotted fevers			T	
090	Congenital syphilis	P	P	P,T	
091	Early syphilis, symptomatic			T	
093-094	Major complications of syphilis (s)	P,T	P,T	P,T	
098	Gonococcal infections		T	T	
098.1M	Gonococcal stricture of urethra		T	T	
102	Yaws	P		P,T	
124	Trichiniasis	P		P	
126M	Hookworm disease w/anemia	P		P,T	
127.0	Ascariasis	P		P	
140	Malignant neoplasm of lip	P		P,T	P — Pipe smokers & sun exposure
141.1, 141.2, 141.3, 144&145.0	Malignant neoplasm of dorsal & ventral surfaces, borders & tip (not base) of tongue, floor of mouth, or buccal mucosa (s)	P		P,T	P — Tobacco smokers & cud & betelnut chewers
161	Malignant neoplasm of larynx	P		P,T	P — Cigar & cigarette smokers
162	Malignant neoplasm of trachea, bronchus, & lung	P		P	P — Cigarette smoking, occupational exposure
163.0	Malignant neoplasm of pleura	P		P	P — Asbestos exposure
173	Other malignant neoplasms of skin	P		P,T	Other than melanoma, P — radiation & sun exposure
180	Malignant neoplasm of cervix uteri			T	
188	Malignant neoplasm of bladder	P		P	P — Aniline dyes & cigarette smoking
189.0M	Wilms' tumor			T	Early recognition & treatment
190M	Malignant neoplasm of eye — retinoblastoma		T	T	Genetic — screening & treatment
192.5M	Neuroblastoma			T	Early recognition & treatment (<1 yr of age)
193M	Thyroid carcinoma	P		P	P — Radiation exposure
205	Myeloid leukemia	P		P	P — Radiation exposure
240.0	Endemic goiter	P			Iodine deficiency
242	Thyrotoxicosis with or without goiter			T	
243	Cretinism of congenital origin		T	T	
244	Myxedema		T	T	Thyroid screening test for T4 & TSH
260-269	Avitaminoses & other nutritional deficiencies	P	P,T	P,T	Not associated with neoplasia or malabsorption
268M	Nutritional marasmus (<1 yr of age)	P	P,T	P,T	
274M	Gout — tophaceous	T	T		
278.0	Hypervitaminosis A	P	P	P	
278.2	Hypervitaminosis D	P	P	P	
280	Iron-deficiency anemias	P	P,T	P,T	Good public-health index
281.0	Pernicious anemia		T	T	
281.1	Other vitamin B12 deficiency anemias		P,T	P,T	
281.2	Folic acid deficiency anemia		P,T	P,T	
281.3	Vitamin B6 deficiency anemia		P,T	P,T	
284	Aplastic anemia	P	P	P	P —Benzene exposure, chloramphenicol
320.0, 320.1, 320.8M	Bacterial meningitis (*Haemophilus influenzae* Group B, pneumococcus, streptococcus Group A)			T	Early recognition & prompt treatment

*P denotes prevention, T treatment. M scope not congruent with ICDA definition, & (s) summary statement.

†The symbol "P —" or "T —" in the Notes indicates that the prevention or treatment is limited to the circumstances described by the phrase that follows the symbol.

‡NIC indicates that the condition is not identifiable as such in the ICDA code.

Exhibit 7-34 Continued

8TH REV NO.	CONDITION	UN-NECESSARY DISEASE	UN-NECESSARY DISABILITY	UN-NECESSARY UNTIMELY DEATH	NOTES†
375.1M	Blindness — glaucoma, chronic (primary)		T		
381-383	Otitis media or mastoiditis (or both) (s)		T	T	
390-392	Active rheumatic fever		P	P	P — Prevent recurrences
426	Pulmonary heart disease	P	P	P	P — Occupational & environmental exposure
460-466, 470-474, 480-486, & 490	Acute respiratory infections, influenza, pneumonia, & bronchitis (s)			T	Deaths <age 50 unless associated with immunologic defects or neoplasms
491,492, &519.3	Chronic bronchitis, emphysema, or chronic obstructive lung disease	P	P	P	P — Cigarettes & other environmental risks
493	Asthma			T	T — Self-inhalation therapy deaths <age 50
515-516	All pneumoconioses (s)	P	P	P	
550-553	Inguinal or other hernia of abdominal cavity with or without obstruction (s)			T	Deaths <age 65
574,575	Acute or chronic cholecystitis and/or cholelithiasis (s)			T	Deaths <age 65
680-686	Infections of skin & subcutaneous tissue			T	
692	Other eczema & dermatitis	P	P	P	P — Environmental & occupational exposure to specific agents
710	Acute arthritis due to pyogenic organisms	P	P,T	P,T	P — Secondary to pyogenic infections
712.0M	Blindness — juvenile rheumatoid arthritis		T		Uveitis
720.0	Acute osteomyelitis	P	P,T	P,T	P — Secondary to pyogenic infections
720.1	Chronic osteomyelitis		T	T	
NIC‡	Congenital anomalies associated w/rubella	P	P	P	Including cataract, patent ductus arteriosus, deafness, & mental deficiency
774.0,775.0	Diseases due to Rh incompatibility (s)	P	P,T	P,T	
630-678	All maternal deaths (including abortion) (s)			P	
760-778	Infant mortality, general (s)			P	Plus all other deaths <1 yr of age regardless of cause
310M-315M, 333.0	Mental retardation induced by: Maternal nutritional deficiency Rubella (Maternal) Rh incompatibility Tay-Sachs disease			P	Parent education & genetic counseling (See Table B)
NIC	Man-made (including occupational) diseases induced by (with examples): 1. *Toxic agents,* including direct chemical hazards (carbon tetrachloride); carcinogens (vinyl chloride); mutagens (lead); teratogens (thalidomide); pesticides (cholinesterase inhibitors); contact irritants (occupational dermatoses); dusts (pneumonoconioses); contact sensitizers (nickel); water contaminants (polychlorinated biphenyls); air pollutants (sulfur dioxide). 2. *Physical hazards,* including radiant energy (medical, industrial, & war); noise (rock & roll); & vibration (jack hammers). 3. *Artificial environments,* including space travel, airplanes, caissons, air conditioned sealed buildings, & intensive-care units. 4. *Accidents* (manifold varieties inducing injury). 5. *Biological hazards,* including laboratory accidents, antibiotic-resistant micro-organisms, & contact allergic dermatitis (plants & wood).				
780-793, 795,796	Symptoms & ill-defined conditions				Unless specified as "cause unknown" frequent diagnoses consisting only of symptoms or ill-defined conditions are evidence of poor quality

Source: D.D. Rutstein, W. Berenberg, T.C. Chalmers, C.G. Child, A.P. Fishman, and E.B. Perrin. "Measuring the Quality of Medical Care. A Clinical Method." Reprinted, by permission of *New England Journal of Medicine* 294: (1976): 582. © 1976.

Health planners can utilize this clinical index to evaluate death certificates, admission and discharge records, and follow-up data on the use of community resources.

Conditions listed in the first column are taken from the Eighth Revision, *International Classification of Diseases Adapted for Use in the United States*. The number refers to that classification. Where there is some difference, the letter M, for modified, appears after the number, as in 274M. Most of the conditions listed in the exhibit are single entities. However, the final four—maternal mortality, infant mortality, mental retardation, and man-made diseases—comprise a collection of causation factors rather than a single direct cause. These indexes should still serve as evaluation measures even though the tracing back of some elements might be a complicated process.

INSTRUMENTS AND SCALES FOR VARIOUS ACTIVITIES

Throughout this section on evaluation a number of instruments and scales have already been illustrated. An additional few will be documented here as examples in their totality of an evaluation. This does not mean that other instruments and scales in this book cannot be utilized, adapted, modified, or designed to accomplish an evaluation objective. Health planners can examine the material and come to their own conclusions as to the utility of each method.

Exhibit 7-35 considers employee performance using degrees of performance measured against the performance factors of quality, timeliness, initiative, adaptability, and communication. This particular evaluation scheme has appeared in numerous journals, and the original source has been lost in the transition. Yet, the classification does indicate the possibility of evaluation using five degrees and five factors to construct a table with 25 individual cells. If each cell can be exclusive of each other, then a viable evaluation scheme has evolved.

Although the example relies on humor, the intent is still serious if the health planner can explicitly detail the criteria for placing an institution, an employee, an element of health care, or other factor into that cell—and only that cell.

SELF-ADMINISTERED EVALUATION OF PLANNING

An evaluation of this type chooses the key elements and allows the respondent to measure each of those points. A problem with this type of instrument relates to how fine a distinction the respondent can be expected to make regarding each of the points. Scales have been used with five gradations, one neutral or uncertain and each of the other two on the good or bad side. Respondents do not appear to have too

Exhibit 7-35 Guide to Employee Performance Appraisal

Performance Factors	Far Exceeds Job Requirements	Exceeds Job Requirements	Meets Job Requirements	Needs Some Improvement	Does Not Meet Minimum Requirements
			Performance Degrees		
Quality	Leaps tall buildings with a single bound	Must take running start to leap over tall buildings	Can only leap over a short or medium building with no spires	Crashes into buildings when attempting to jump over them	Cannot recognize buildings at all—much less jump over them
Timeliness	Is faster than a speeding bullet	Is as fast as a speeding bullet	Not quite as fast as a speeding bullet	Would you believe a slow bullet?	Wounds self with bullet when attempting to shoot gun
Initiative	Is stronger than a locomotive	Is stronger than a bull elephant	Is stronger than a bull	Shoots the bull	Smells like a bull
Adaptability	Walks on water consistently	Walks on water in emergencies	Washes with water	Drinks water	Passes water in emergencies
Communication	Talks with God	Talks with his Angel	Talks to himself	Argues with himself	Loses those arguments

Source: Unknown; found in *Health Planning and Public Accountability Seminar Workbook* (Germantown, Md.: Aspen Systems, 1976). Reprinted with permission.

much difficulty choosing the extremes or the middle position. When it comes to the second and fourth positions, the fuzziness arises. Just how much of a distinction does the respondent make between the first and second choice and the fourth and fifth choice? Often, the evaluator combines the responses and ends up with a three-category evaluation: good, neutral, and bad. Therefore, if health planners desire a finer definition in the evaluation, some thought must be given to advising the respondents as to the distinction between the choices. This has been attempted with the agree/slightly agree/uncertain/slightly disagree/disagree categories. Again, the question is whether the respondent can determine the intensity differential between agree and slightly agree. In any event, the health planner should be aware of this problem when constructing an evaluation instrument.

Ten criteria for evaluating your planning are listed in Exhibit 7-36. The respondent is asked to rate each one on a five-point scale from inadequate to adequate. Words in italics emphasize the element in the criterion statement that the respondent is cued to for major consideration. Analysis of the responses should guide the health planner in discovering any self-defined weakpoints in planning. An overall score as well as a score for each of the ten criteria can be compiled for the analysis.

TOTAL COMPARATIVE PROGRAM EVALUATION MODEL

Administrators might wish to compare the total gamut of programs for which their budget is providing the manpower, resources, and supplies. This requires that uniform measures be established for which data are readily available. In addition, the impact of each program should be capable of evaluation as well as across specific variables. Decisions that have to be made can be aided by an evaluation of this type.

In Exhibit 7-37 a paradigm for program impact evaluation of the activities of the Office of Economic Opportunity is given. All the activities are listed across the top and the comparative elements are listed in the left column.

Universe of need is equivalent to the target population identified as requiring the services. Program reach refers to the number of persons actually using the services. Program coverage yields a number that tells the evaluator what proportion of the target population has been serviced. This would be useful as a measure of effectiveness and could be compared across the model among all the activities to determine which activity was most effective. Program cost merely lists all the

Exhibit 7-36 Criteria for Evaluating Your Planning

Criteria	Ratings				
	Inadequate				Excellent
1. Is your plan based on *clearly defined* objectives that are in accord with organization goals?	1	2	3	4	5
2. Is your plan as *clear and simple* as the task will permit?	1	2	3	4	5
3. Does your plan provide for the *involvement* of all *appropriate personnel*?	1	2	3	4	5
4. Is your planning based on *realistic analysis* of forces in the situation?	1	2	3	4	5
5. Does your plan have *stability* and yet provide for flexibility?	1	2	3	4	5
6. Is your planning *economical* in use of human and financial resources needed to implement it?	1	2	3	4	5
7. Can your plan be *divided and delegated* for efficient implementation?	1	2	3	4	5
8. Are the *methods* to be used reliable and up to appropriate standards?	1	2	3	4	5
9. Does your plan provide for adequate *training* of personnel needed for accomplishing the task?	1	2	3	4	5
10. Does your plan provide for continuous *review and reevaluation*?	1	2	3	4	5

Source: Massachusetts Department of Mental Health, *Reference Guide for Area Board Members* (Boston, Massachusetts, 1960), p. 40.

costs for the total activity. Questions can arise here as to whether to include the estimated costs of unpaid volunteers, donated supplies, or other aspects of the activity that might have to be budgeted if these items were not supplied free. Cost per person reached is the measure of efficiency of cost-effectiveness and again can be compared across the model for an evaluation of which activity produces the best per unit cost factor. An activity can be effective but not cost-effective, and planners might wish to consider alternatives that meet the objective at a lower unit cost. Cost of total coverage reveals what budget increase is required to service the total population needing that service. Planners

Exhibit 7-37 Paradigm for OEO Program Impact Evaluation*

Evaluation Data	Job Corps	VISTA	Anti-Poverty Programs[b]							Delegated Programs	Non-OEO Project
			Community Action Programs								
			Organization-Coordination Functions	Legal Services	Service Programs						
					Head Start	Follow Through	Upward Bound	Health Services	Others		
A. Universe of need											
B. Program reach											
C. Program coverage (A/B)											
D. Program cost											
E. Cost per person reached (D/B)											
F. Cost of total coverage (E) x (A)[c]											

G. Measures of program effectiveness:
  1. Immediate objectives
  2. Poverty reduction											

H. Benefit-cost ratio (G/D)											

*John Evans explained the use of the matrix as follows: "Going down the left-hand Evaluation Data column from A through H will indicate how the completed paradigm would be useful in overall agency planning and programming. With extensive and dependable data for each program on universe of need (A) and program reach (B), we can calculate and compare progress on the extent to which they are reaching their target populations (C). A solid figure on program coverage (C) would be very useful in planning and budgeting both within a given program and across the total array of OEO programs. Bringing together for all programs the information on their total costs (D) (on which we have good data) and information on the number of people they reach (B) (on which we don't) would allow us to compute, and compare programs on, the cost per person reached (E). With information on program costs (D), the total universe of need (A), and the present program reach (B), we could determine for each program what the cost of total coverage would be and how much of an increment over present budget outlays this would require (F)" (29, p. 233).

[b] A number of the programs listed have since been delegated to the Departments of Labor and of Health, Education, and Welfare.

[c] A correct computation would not be this simple but would take into account the marginal cost required to expand programs at different levels.

Source: J.S. Wholey, J.W. Scanlon, H.G. Duffy, J.S. Fukumoto, and L.M. Vogt, *Federal Evaluation Policy. Analyzing the Effects of Public Programs* (Washington, D.C.: The Urban Institute, 1970), p. 37.

could use this type of analysis to determine where to place additional increases in funds that an agency might receive. Program coverage and cost per person reached could be powerful influences on the decisions of an administrator with extra money to allocate.

Item G in this model may be difficult to quantify and put into usable numerical form. Poverty reduction can be measured by the numbers of people who no longer earn below the income level established as poverty. Achievement of immediate objectives is more difficult to evaluate, unless the immediate objective is so specified and objective that a measurement can be taken. However, how can the objectives be compared across the various activities. Do all activities have the same objectives? Or can the evaluator just count how many of the first ten objectives of each activity have been met. Some of this quandary has been attacked in the Program Planning Budgeting System (PPBS), wherein the various alternatives are figured on a basis that calculates a numerical cost-benefit ratio. In any event, if this figure can be derived from the data, the health planner will then have three numbers that can be valuable tools for planning: the program coverage ratio, the cost per person reached, and the cost-benefit ratio.

Using this type of evaluative model, health planners can suggest where to spend additional monies, where to cut down, and where to look for alternatives.

A GUIDE TO PROGRAM EVALUATION

Program evaluation must be linked directly back to the description of the program, the grant application, or any other detailed written record about the origin of the activity. Goals, objectives, and targets specified in the descriptive material have to be extracted and compared with what happened during and at the conclusion of the program. Thus, the more specific the objectives and targets are, the easier the program evaluation will be.

Evaluation of a program requires the use of records, interviews, and analysis of operational statistics and special survey data. Again, the data must be linked to the objectives and, it is hoped, be easily acquired and easily measurable.

In the example in Exhibit 7-38, a program to develop a nursing home patient ombudsman service is being evaluated. Direct and individualized services are provided to persons in nursing homes, and efforts are scheduled to organize the community to bring about long term changes in the institution. Concerned citizens—both paid and unpaid—actively help to assume that residents of long term care facilities receive the quality of care and the quality of life to which they are entitled through an ombudsman service. Note that, as the evaluation proceeds, questions are asked and responses are called for in terms

Exhibit 7-38 Evaluation of a Nursing Home Patient Ombudsman
Service

The purpose of evaluation is to learn whether the program is achieving the
desired results; whether the original goals and objectives of the program are
being met; and what changes, adjustments, or legislation are necessary to
enable it to function more effectively.

The evaluation approach recommended in this model would consist of
analysis of operational statistics and records and interviews with volunteers,
agencies, nursing home staff, etc. A more in-depth analysis of problems identified and handled over the period of a few years could test the hypothesis that
such a program of ombudsmen and "back-up" agencies have significantly les-
sened problems confronting patients in nursing homes.

A. Local areas and their "back-up" agencies
   1. How is the program working? Measurement of volunteer recruitment,
      training, placement and on-the-job performance. For example, the
      evaluation would look at:
      a. number of volunteers recruited against the targets set at program
         start-up, number of volunteers still active after a four or six month
         period;
      b. effectiveness of training as determined by on-the-job experiences and
         volunteer perceptions of training;
      c. placement procedures in terms of successful placement of om-
         budsmen in targeted nursing homes and whether volunteers and
         homes have been matched successfully;
      d. on-the-job performance measured against job duties and volunteer
         satisfaction with jobs as compared with original expectations;
      e. cost-benefit analysis of use of volunteers to carry out the program
         objectives; and
      f. number of nursing home residents reached by volunteers.
   2. Measurement of effectiveness of "back-up" agency procedures
      a. Supervision and support services for volunteers.
      b. Relationships with nursing homes.
      c. Communication system and information provided to participating
         agencies and the public.
      d. Relationships and procedures with state ombudsman.

B. The complaint/grievance system
   1. Documentation of grievances; effectiveness and accuracy of procedures.
   2. Number of grievances in a four- or six-month interval; number of pa-
      tients reached.
   3. Number of grievances resolved; quality of resolution.
   4. Problems encountered in operating the grievance system; their origin
      (volunteers, "back-up" agency, nursing home staff, patients and their
      families, regulatory agencies, others).

Exhibit 7-38 Continued

C. State ombudsman program
   1. Statewide statistics on volunteers; number of patients served; number of community agencies and organizations involved; number of nursing homes involved.
   2. Analyses of patient problems identified and resolved at local, regional, or state levels.
   3. Effectiveness in terms of response from state regulatory and policy-making bodies in resolving problems.
   4. Effect on relationships/climate in nursing home; perceptions of patients and their families about the program; awareness of the program; effect on nursing home administrators and staff.

D. Evaluation methodology
   Evaluation should be carried out by independent, experienced professionals not involved in the implementation of the program. A report of the program evaluation should be available to the New York State Office for the Aging, to the program's Advisory Committee, to the federal Administration on Aging, and to the public.

Source: S. Hunter. *A Plan for a New York State Nursing Home Patient Ombudsman Program* (New York: Community Council of Greater New York, 1977), pp. VIII 1-3. Reprinted with permission. © 1977 Community Council of Greater New York.

---

of numbers of people, as well as in terms of their attitudinal and behavioral patterns. Also note that the last item in the program evaluation suggests that the evaluation be carried out by independent, experienced professionals not involved in the program. This aims to reduce bias and assure an objective evaluation.

SELF OR OTHER EVALUATION OF AN OCCUPATIONAL HEALTH PROGRAM WITH A SCORING SYSTEM

Based on published and professionally acceptable guidelines and standards, an objective scoring system has been developed by S.B. Webb, Jr.,[48] to provide a single and flexible method for evaluating occupational health programs. In this system an interdependent relationship is emphasized among the following four components and their relative weights:

- a written guiding philosophy and policy   10%
- organizational structure   10%
- resources   20%
- occupational health services program   60%

This evaluation stresses the long range commitment to occupational health and not only a short term economic payoff for insurance or other reasons. Although the evaluation can be self-administered, outside evaluators should also be able to utilize this format. Furthermore, separate pieces of this evaluation could be used to examine questions about aspects such as employee hospital utilization, laboratory procedures and preplacement examinations.

Exhibit 7-39 reproduces the evaluation model. Note the relative weights attached to the various aspects of the program. For example, under organizational structure, if the health director reports to the president it is worth 3 points, as compared with only .5 point if reporting to a department head.

Problems arise with this type of evaluation in the assignment of numerical weights to the components. Is reporting to the president six times more valuable than reporting to the department head? Health planners can use a panel of experts to arrive at the weights by asking them to make the determinations based on their experience. Research studies might yield data on the statistically significant variables that should be more heavily weighted. Existing standards and guidelines might also indicate a priority order and attach weights to components of programs.

A self-administered evaluation of this type is easy to undertake, score, and analyze. Implementation after the evaluation becomes a critical factor. Health planners might wish to consider the value of having an outside group conduct the evaluation merely for the added impetus toward implementation afterwards.

If the data exist upon which to develop a program evaluation similar to the model in Exhibit 7-39, it would be an appropriate, quick, and relatively inexpensive procedure to undertake for any program.

MEDICAL CARE EVALUATION STUDY ABSTRACT

A report form suggested by the federal government's Bureau of Quality Assurance to document the conduct of a medical care evaluation study is reproduced in Exhibit 7-40. This instrument is a form of a checklist to assure that certain steps are taken as well as a mechanism for keeping records of decisions and expenditure of resources.

Note that starting and completion dates are recorded and the study topic is "management of patients with suspected AMI (active myocardial infarction) within first hour after admission to emergency room." This study was undertaken because this problem was seen as a perceived need with the possibility of preventable mortality/morbidity; the hospital's medical audit committee was assigned the responsibility of meeting the need. Emergency room nurses, respiratory therapists,

Exhibit 7-39 A Model Occupational Health Program and Scoring System for Self-Evaluation

Component 1: A Written Guiding Philosophy and Policy	Weighting
A. Goals	
1. To keep an individual healthy so that he can perform his assigned job with the maximal amount of efficiency.	1.5
2. To match an individual's capacity to perform a specified job with the physical and psychological demands inherent in that job.	0.5
B. Objectives	
1. The maintenance of the health of the worker through specific preventive medicine procedures, frequent checks on employee health status, health education activities, and detection and control of potential health hazards inherent in the work environment.	1.0
2. The provision of emergency medical care for occupational and nonoccupational illnesses or injuries.	0.5
3. The provision of definitive care and rehabilitation for occupational illnesses or injuries in keeping with the medical or surgical skills of the staff.	0.5
C. Medical policy	
1. Preplacement health evaluations for all applicants.	0.35
2. Periodic health evaluations and/or health surveys of all employees or employees in certain age groups regardless of type of work.	0.75
3. Special health evaluations for employees with specific disabilities and new employees transferring to different jobs.	0.35
4. Employee health counseling and health promotion activities.	0.75
5. Treatment of the alcoholic.	0.50
6. Rehabilitation of the ill or injured employee.	0.50
7. Formal liaison with personal family physicians.	0.50
8. Formal liaison with community medical care resources.	0.50
9. Termination health evaluations.	0.35
10. Medical care is rendered by licensed, qualified professionals familiar with the work environment.	0.50
11. Professional consultant services are used for	0.50

Exhibit 7-39 Continued

  examinations and definitive care beyond the
  expertise of the full-time staff.
 12. A record system is maintained that:
   a. Is confidential   0.15
   b. Contains job descriptions   0.15
   c. Is reviewed at regular intervals for up- 0.10
    dating
   d. Is used for purposes of medical investiga- 0.05
    tion

Maximal Score, Component 1:   10.00

Component 2: Organizational Structure	Weighting

 1. Health director reports directly to top management:
   a. President   3.0
   b. Vice president   2.0
   c. Department or section head   0.5
 2. Top management is familiar with manage- 1.0
  rial interpretation of medical policy and assistance can be assured.
 3. Health director is involved directly in advising management regarding company policy
  on:
   a. Employee health insurance benefits   1.0
   b. Retirement program   0.5
   c. Medical department budget and program 1.5
    direction
   d. Industrial relations criteria of efficiency, 1.0
    absenteeism, or labor turnover and effec-
    tive work performance
 4. Formal liaison with company committee
  concerned with:
   a. Safety   0.5
   b. Disaster control   0.5
   c. Health   1.0

Maximal Score, Component 2:   10.0

Component 3: Resources	Weighting

 1. Facilities
   a. Facilities are available for the perform- 1.5
    ance of health evaluations and counsel-
    ing.
   b. Facilities are adequate for dispensing 1.5
    emergency care for occupational and
    nonoccupational illnesses or injuries.
   c. Facilities are attractive, well kept.   1.0
 2. Staff
  (actual number of professional health team 16.0

Exhibit 7-39 Continued

man hours per 100 employees per day ÷
ideal) × maximum points

Maximal Score, Component 3:	20.0

	Weighting
Component 4: Occupational Health Services Program	
1. Preplacement health evaluation	3.0
a. Personal history (0.3)	
b. Family history (0.3)	
c. Occupational history (jobs held, dates, and places) (0.3)	
d. Type of work exposure (0.3)	
e. Organ inventory (0.3)	
f. Functional capacity (0.75)	
g. Psychological evaluation (0.75)	
2. Preplacement laboratory procedures	3.0
a. Chest radiography (0.3)	
b. Audiometry (0.3)	
c. Visual testing (0.3)	
d. Electrocardiography for males over 50 (0.3)	
e. Hematological studies (0.3)	
f. Urinalysis (0.3)	
1. Chemical (0.15)	
2. Microscopic (0.15)	
g. Serodiagnostic test for syphilis (0.3)	
h. Blood typing and Rh factor determination (0.3)	
i. Other radiographic, hematological, or laboratory studies as indicated by previous history, former job-related injury, or illness, or by examination findings (0.3)	
3. Classification system for fitness for employment	2.0
a. Physically fit for any job (0.4)	
b. Physically fit for any job, but has minor remediable defects (0.4)	
c. Physically fit for modified work only in accordance with noted restrictions (0.4)	
d. Physically unqualified for any job applied for (0.4)	
e. Temporarily deferred (0.4)	
4. Immunization program	1.0
5. Personal protective devices as indicated by work environment	3.0
6. Regular health evaluation	5.0
a. All employees (3.0)	

Exhibit 7-39 Continued

b. Management (0.25)	
c. Employees in certain age groups (1.0)	
d. Employees in specific disabilities (0.75)	
7. Periodic occupational health evaluation	2.0
a. Employees exposed to hazards (1.0)	
b. Employees in certain age groups (0.8)	
c. Other illness or absence (0.2)	
8. Job transfer evaluation	2.0
a. All employees (2.0)	
b. Only some employees (0.5)	
9. Specific disability examinations at appropriate intervals for those hired with impairments	2.0
10. Termination physical evaluation	1.0
a. All employees (1.0)	
b. Only some employees (0.2)	
11. Health counseling	5.0
a. Does not include psychological (-2.0)	
12. Special surveys for case finding, according to appropriate age and sex groups and geographic locations	5.0
13. Health education program	5.0
a. Posters, flyers (0.25)	
b. Small group discussion (3.0)	
c. Discussion with supervisors (1.0)	
d. Community seminars (0.75)	
14. Treatment for occupational illness or injury	3.0
15. Emergency treatment for nonoccupational illness or injury	3.0
16. Retiree health program	2.0
17. Regular inspection of plant for potential hazards	3.0
18. Alcohol control program	5.0
19. Rehabilitation program	5.0
Maximal Score, Component 4:	60.0

Source: S.B. Webb, Jr., "Objective Criteria for Evaluating Occupational Health Programs," *American Journal of Public Health,* 65: (1975): 31. Reprinted with permission. © 1975 American Public Health Association.

Exhibit 7-40 Filled In Report Form Documenting a Medical Care Evaluation Study

Bureau of Quality Assurance Health Services Administration	Office of Management and Budget Approval Number	HOSPITAL ID NO.
	PSRO NAME _Rockville PSRO_	PSRO NO. _842_
MEDICAL CARE **EVALUATION STUDY ABSTRACT**	MCE STUDY BEGUN Month _07_ Year _74_	MCE STUDY COMPLETED THROUGH STEPS BELOW Month _09_ Year _74_
	CONDUCTED BY: ☐ PSRO ☑ DELEGATED HOSPITAL	MCE STUDY ID NO. _16_

1. STUDY TOPIC _Management of patients_ (Write In) _with suspected AMI within first hour after adm. to emergency room_

2. METHOD FOR SELECTING STUDY (Check One)
   - ☐ a. PROFILE ANALYSIS
   - ☐ b. CONCURRENT REVIEW
   - ☐ c. OTHER MCE STUDY
   - ☐ d. ANALYSIS OF MEDICAL RECORDS
   - ☑ e. PERCEIVED NEED
   - ☐ f. OTHER (Specify) _____

3. TOPIC CHARACTERISTIC (Check One)
   - ☐ a. INCIDENCE/PREVALENCE
   - ☑ b. PREVENTABLE MORBIDITY/MORTALITY
   - ☐ c. COST OF CARE
   - ☐ d. OTHER (Specify) _____

4. HOSPITAL STUDY RESPONSIBILITY (Check One)
   - ☑ a. MEDICAL AUDIT COMMITTEE
   - ☐ b. UR COMMITTEE
   - ☐ c. SERVICE/DEPT. (Specify) _____
   - ☐ d. OTHER (Specify) _____

5. NON-PHYSICIAN PARTICIPATION (Specify)

   E.R. Nursing

   Respiratory Therapy

   X-ray Technologists

6. DERIVATION OF CRITERIA (Check One)
   - ☑ a. SELF GENERATED
   - ☐ b. NATIONAL ORGANIZATION
   - ☐ c. OTHER PSRO(S)
   - ☐ d. OTHER HOSPITAL(S)
   - ☐ e. OTHER (Specify) _____

7. STUDY SITE (Check One)
   - ☐ a. PSRO-WIDE
   - ☐ b. PSRO SUB-AREA (NO. HOSPITALS _____)
   - ☑ c. INDIVIDUAL HOSPITAL
   - ☐ d. SERVICE /DEPT. OF HOSP. (Specify) _____
   - ☐ e. OTHER (Specify) _____

8. TYPE OF DATA COLLECTION (Check One)
   - ☐ a. RETROSPECTIVE
   - ☐ b. CONCURRENT
   - ☑ c. MIXED

9. SAMPLE CHARACTERISTICS
   - a. NUMBER OF SUBJECTS _50_
   - b. POPULATION _N/A_
   - c. OTHER _all pts. adm. to E.R. with suspected MI in last 3 months_

10. DATA INSTRUMENT (Check One)
    - ☑ a. SPECIAL FORM
    - ☐ b. ROUTINE FORM
    - ☐ c. OTHER (Specify) _____

11. DATA QUALITY CONTROLS (Check all that apply)
    - ☑ a. VERIFIED
    - ☐ b. VERIFIED - SOURCE INADEQUATE
    - ☐ c. VERIFIED - DATA INACCURATE
    - ☐ d. NONE
    - ☐ e. OTHER (Specify) _____

12. DATA PROCESSING (Check One)
    - ☑ a. MANUAL
    - ☐ b. EDP
    - ☐ c. MIXED
    - EDP Cost: $ _____

13. FINDINGS (Check One)
    - ☐ a. COMPLIANCE WITH STANDARDS (Go to item 20)
    - b. VARIATION FROM STANDARDS
      - ☐ (1) VARIATION JUSTIFIED (Go to item 20)
      - ☐ (2) DEFICIENCY IDENTIFIED (Proceed with item 14)
      - ☑ (3) MORE THAN ONE DEFICIENCY (Proceed with item 14, specify number _3_)

Exhibit 7-40 Continued

14.   DEFICIENCY ANALYSIS (Check One)
- [ ] a. KNOWLEDGE
- [x] b PERFORMANCE

- [ ] c. OTHER _____

15.   ATTRIBUTION (Check all that apply)
- [ ] a. ONE HOSPITAL
- [ ] b. MORE THAN ONE HOSPITAL (NO. ____)
- [ ] c. INDIVIDUAL PHYSICIAN
- [x] d. GROUP(S) OF PHYSICIANS
- [x] e. NON-PHYSICIAN(S)
- [x] f. ADMINISTRATIVE
- [ ] g. FURTHER STUDY NEEDED

- [ ] h. OTHER _____

16.   TYPE OF ACTION RECOMMENDED (Check all that apply and describe)

- [ ] a. PRACTITIONER COUNSELLING _____

- b. EDUCATIONAL PROGRAM *efficacy of*
  - [x] (1) SINGLE HOSPITAL *immediate monitor. of*
  - [ ] (2) PSRO SUB-AREA *cardiac rhythm*
  - [ ] (3) PSRO - WIDE _____

- [x] c. ADMINISTRATIVE CHANGE *organize an emergency team for use in ER*
- [ ] d. CHANGE IN CONCURRENT REVIEW

- [ ] e. OTHER REVIEW MODIFICATION _____

- [ ] f. OTHER _____

17.   ESTIMATED RE-STUDY DATE (mo/yr) *Jan. 1975*
18.   IF EDUCATION IS RECOMMENDED, IS THERE LINKAGE WITH EXISTING CONTINUING MEDICAL EDUCATION ACTIVITIES?
- [x] yes   [ ] no

IF YES, PLEASE DESCRIBE: *part of inservice program on value of cardiac monitoring in AMI*

19.   RESPONSIBILITY FOR ACTION (Check all that apply)
- [x] a. MEDICAL STAFF (COMMITTEE)
- [ ] b. HOSPITAL BOARD OF TRUSTEES
- [x] c. HOSPITAL ADMINISTRATION
- [ ] d. SERVICE/DEPT. (Specify) _____

- [ ] e. OTHER (Specify) _____

20.   PERSON HOURS UTILIZED (Round to half hours)

MCE STUDY TASK	PHYSICIAN	OTHER
a. SELECTION AND DESIGN	1	
b. SETTING CRITERIA AND STANDARDS	3	
c. DATA COLLECTION AND DISPLAY		28
d. INTERPRETATION AND ANALYSIS OF FINDINGS	2	2
e. TOTAL	6	31

ADDITIONAL EXPLANATORY REMARKS (USE ADDITIONAL PAPER IF NECESSARY)

16c. (continued): return x-rays to emergency room for review by physician team immediately

RESERVED FOR PROCESSING CONTROL

Source: USDHEW, Bureau of Quality Assurance, *PSRO Management Information System,* p. III-12, undated.

and x-ray technicians were also included in the auditing group. Data collected were a combination of retrospective and concurrent, with 50 patients admitted to the emergency room with suspected myocardial infarction in the last three months as the study group. This study committee probably developed their own instrument for data collection and processed the information manually. They found three deficiencies to be corrected. Recommendations included holding an educational program on the efficiency of immediate monitoring of cardiac rhythm, the organization of an emergency team for use in the emergency room, and the returning of x-rays to the emergency room for review by the physician team immediately. Notice that a remonitoring date has been set, as well as the assignment of responsibility for implementation of the recommendations. Finally, the total staff hours expended in this medical care evaluation are tabulated.

For evaluation purposes, a form of this nature allows for an immediate monitoring of the problem, the responsibilities, and the recommendations, including a follow-up date for rechecking. For more in-depth analysis, the health planner can seek out the departments concerned and gather all the detailed material.

REVIEW AND COMMENT EVALUATION FORM

Federal legislation requires that review and comment procedures be undertaken by a number of agencies. In essence, review and comment is an evaluation of a proposed activity in which the examiners check to determine whether the proposal contains specific information. Furthermore, the examiner decides if the proposal receives approval, or some variation of approval, or is not approved. At times, this type of evaluation form can be compiled individually and then jointly discussed at a committee meeting with a consensus report prepared.

Exhibit 7-41 is a copy of a review and comment form that covers six basic areas for evaluation: the basic plan, economics, environmental relationships, other relationships, community participation, and capabilities. It is possible that additional material will have to be prepared for the evaluators or that training sessions will be appropriate. Many of the subtopics listed under each of the six major areas are open to differing interpretations. Some differences can be resolved in the committee meetings, if these are scheduled. Health planners would do well to try to resolve any vagueness prior to having evaluators apply their time and energy to a review and comment form of this nature.

Exhibit 7-41 Review and Comment Evaluation Form

Name of Proposal:_____ Review Date:_____

Name of Sponsor:_____ Project Number:_____

City and County:_____ Date Application Received For Review:_____

Name of Reviewer: (Individual or Committee)_____

FINDINGS: (check one column for each criteria) *

CRITERIA	Approve without Condition(s)	Approve with Condition(s)	Not Approvable	Not Applicable
1. Basic Plan				
a. Relationship to community need				
b. Projected demand for services				
c. Accessibility for target population				
d. Comprehensiveness of services				
e. Lack of alternatives (present and projected				
f. Effect on health care system development				
g. Appropriate use of present resources				
h. Adequacy of anticipated utilization				
i. Adequacy of plans for evaluation				
j. Avoids duplication				
k. Adequacy of long range plans				
l. Conformity with areawide plans				
2. Economics				
a. Appropriateness of capital expenditures				
b. Adequacy of proposed budget				
c. Comparative unit costs				
d. Consideration of alternative less costly approaches				
e. Increase in per diem rate or charges				
f. Assurance of financial support				
g. Availability of third party payment				
h. Prospects for long-run funding				
i. Impact on underserved and high risk groups				
3. Environmental Relationships				
a. Estimates of noise and measures for control				
b. Transportation access and effect on community				
c. Impact on community and neighborhood character				
d. Effect on housing				
e. Minimize total environmental impact through energy conservation and use of natural resources				
f. Reduction and control of waste effluents				
g. Effect on facility utilization in area				

Exhibit 7-41 Continued

CRITERIA	Approve without Condi- tion(s)	Approve with Condi- tion(s)	Not Approv- able	Not Appli- cable
4. Relationships				
a. CHP involvement in proposal development				
b. Impact on utilization of other resources in area				
c. Conformity to plans of city, county state and regional planning bodies				
d. Extent of cooperation and linkage with provider groups				
5. Community Participation				
a. Community involvement in preparation and design of application				
b. Community response to application				
c. Representation of community interest on governing body				
d. Satisfaction of consumer represen- tation requirements				
6. Capabilities				
a. Ability to comply with legal requirements				
b. Past performance of sponsor in health field				
c. Anticipated ability to meet fiscal and administrative needs				
d. Ability to proceed in timely manner				
e. Ability to generate continuing community support				

* CONDITIONS: (Refer to criteria by number and list conditions placed on project or reasons for disapproval)

Source: Reprinted with permission from *Health Planning and Public Accountability Seminar Workbook* (Germantown, Md.: Aspen Systems Corporation, 1976), pp. 83-84.

The role of the staff in working with the evaluators has to be clearly defined. At times, staff members have gone to extremes in influencing the review and comment decisions. If the review and comment evaluation is designed to allow nonstaff experts to evaluate proposals, then the staff's role should be guidance and not leadership. This appears to be the style for the HSAs and the national review boards. If the review and comment is an internal procedure, then staff evaluation is merely another responsibility.

As already noted, the major drawback of this type of evaluation instrument is the tendency to arrive at varied interpretations of what each item means in the listed examination areas.

CLINICAL EVALUATION USING THE INDICATOR CASE MODEL

B.S. Hulka and her associates[49] have developed the indicator case model to evaluate the quality of health care delivered in practice. This type of evaluation assumes that certain key elements will yield fruitful information relative to an assessment. Eight elements are cited by Hulka, including utilization, cost and convenience, physician performance, communication, compliance, physician awareness of patient concerns about condition, patient satisfaction, and outcome. These are expanded on in Exhibit 7-42. Note that these elements encompass the health care delivery system and not merely the treatment of the patient by the physician. Exhibit 7-43 then proceeds to identify the sources of data for the elements being evaluated. Evaluation data would come from patient interviews, physician's records, institutional records, observations of the patients, and prescriptions. In Exhibit 7-44, the indicator case model is related to the evaluation classification of structure, process, and outcome.

This type of evaluation can be adapted to any situation in which the key elements can be identified and agreed upon by all concerned to be the most appropriate for consideration. However, in addition to the key elements, there must be techniques for collecting data and for a total evaluation. Health planners might have to determine weights for the various elements as some of the other instruments have done. Furthermore, the relationship between the elements sometimes raises questions about the cause and effect of each component. Each component becomes a separate evaluation in itself since the data collection for each one is a task of some magnitude. Yet, the comprehensive Gestalt evaluation is difficult to achieve without consideration of the total picture.

QUICK EVALUATION FOR DRUG ABUSE CENTERS

In this evaluation scheme developed for use by drug abuse centers, five quantitative measures and four qualitative measures are included with data about the cost per client-year. Exhibit 7-45 shows the specific items and explains what they mean. Since the evaluation is oriented toward an operational service, the use of this quick evaluation tends to show how well the program is doing in terms of services to clients. If appropriate comparative data can be supplied to the evaluators, the method can truly yield a quick appraisal of the effectiveness of the services. In addition, any of the specific items that rate low can lead to

Exhibit 7-42 Indicator Case Model: Elements for Assessment

1. Utilization

   Number of ID physician* visits
   Number of different physicians visited: in ID physician's group; outside group
   Hospitalization: number and length of stay
   Referrals: to outside physicians, community agencies, outside laboratories

2. Cost and convenience

   Dollar costs for: physicians, drugs, laboratory, hospital, agencies
   Source of payment: patient, third party
   Time spent by patient: getting to and from doctor's office, waiting in office, waiting between appointment request and appointment
   Transportation: kind and availability

3. Physician performance

   Method of diagnosis
   Management: physical examination, laboratory tests, instructions, medication, other therapy

4. Communication

   Diagnosis
   Medications
   Supportive measures: diet, activity, self-care
   Complications
   Where to get emergency care
   Maintenance of contact and appointment setting

5. Compliance

   Appointments kept
   Drugs taken
   Instructions followed

6. Physician awareness of patient concerns about condition

7. Attitudes toward physicians (patient satisfaction)

8. Outcome
   a. Disease status
   b. Symptomatic status
   c. Functional status

*The "ID physician" is that physician or clinic through which the patient is enrolled into the study. The ID physician is also the patient's usual source of care.

Source: B.S. Hulka, "Evaluation of Primary Medical Care in a Total Community: The Indicator Case Model," in *Evaluation in Health Services Delivery,* edited by R. Yaffe and D. Zalkind (New York: Engineering Foundation, 1974). Reprinted with permission. © 1974 Engineering Foundation. The work resulting in the above was performed under Health Resources Administration Contract HMS 110-73-399.

Exhibit 7-43 Sources of Data for Elements Being Assessed: Indicator Cases

Elements	*Sources of Data*
1. Utilization	Patient interview Physician records Hospital records
2. Cost and convenience	Patient interview Physician records Hospital records Laboratory records
3. Physician performance	Physician records Physician questionnaire
4. Communication	Physician questionnaire Patient interview
5. Compliance	Physician records Patient interview Pharmacy prescription Observation of patient (diabetes)
6. Physician awareness of patient concern	Patient interview Physician questionnaire
7. Attitudes toward physician	Patient interview
8. Outcome	
a. Disease status	Patient interview Physician records Hospital records
b. Symptoms	Patient interview
c. Function	Patient interview

Source: B.S. Hulka, "Evaluation of Primary Medical Care in a Total Community: The Indicator Case Model," in *Evaluation in Health Services Delivery,* edited by R. Yaffe and D. Zalkind (New York: Engineering Foundation, 1974). Reprinted with permission. © 1974 Engineering Foundation. The work resulting in the above was performed under Health Resources Administration Contract HMS 110-73-399.

Exhibit 7-44 Interrelationships Among Variables in the Indicator Case Model

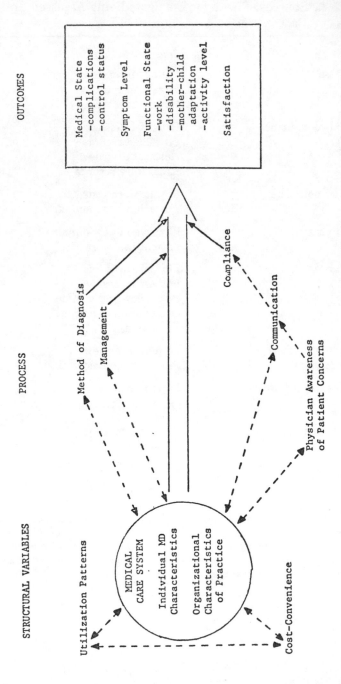

Source: B.S. Hulka, "Evaluation of Primary Medical Care in a Total Community: The Indicator Case Model," in *Evaluation in Health Services Delivery,* edited by R. Yaffe and D. Zalkind (New York: Engineering Foundation, 1974). Reprinted with permission. © 1974 Engineering Foundation. The work resulting in the above was performed under Health Resources Administration Contract HMS 110-73-399.

Exhibit 7-45 Quick Evaluation: Analytical Summary Sheet

A. Cost per client-year:	Outpatient	Residential	Inpatient
(1) Current rate	$ 748		
(2) Current FY through <u>December</u>	$1,252		
(3) Past FY	NA		
B. Other Quantitative Indices:			
1. Ratio of actual to standard budget		0.83	
2. Staff-client ratio		1 to 17	
3. Counselor-client ratio		1 to 37	
4. Staff turnover rate		20%	
5. Percent of positive urinalysis tests		15%	
C. Qualitative Indices:			
1. Level of services provided to clients		low	
2. Scope of record-keeping systems		high	
3. Quality of records		low	
4. Validity of reported data		high	

DEFINITIONS:

A.1: [(Costs for most recent month) X (12)] ÷ (number of clients seen at least twice last week).

A.2: (Costs for current FY to date) ÷ (current FY client-years of treatment to date).

A.3: (Costs for past FY) ÷ (past FY client-years of treatment).

B.1: [Actual budget] ÷ [number of clients seen at least twice last week) X (standard cost per client)]. Standard cost per client is $1,500 for outpatient care, $4,500 for residential care and $30,000 for inpatient care.

B.2: (Number of staff-members) ÷ (number of clients seen at least twice last week).

B.3: (Number of counselors) ÷ (number of clients seen at least twice last week).

B.4: [Number of people employed during past and current FY) − (number of positions filled at least half the time during past and current FY)] ÷ [number of positions filled at least half the time during past and current FY].

B.5:. (Number of positive urinalysis tests) ÷ (total number of urinalysis tests).

C.1: "Medium" consists of individual counseling at least once a week; vocational rehabilitation (i.e., job counseling, training or placement); and two of the following: legal, social or health services. "High" consists of more services and "low" of less.

C.2: "Medium" means the program (a) was able to complete the data forms easily; (b) keeps a formal budget, prepares authorizing documents before disbursing funds, records all expenditures and receipts, and makes periodic financial statements; (c) keeps individual client records, including admission forms and counselors' notes. "High" consists of more records and "low" of less.

C.3: "Medium" means that 70-80% of the records are relatively complete, up-to-date, and consistent. Client records include weekly counselors' notes which seem relevant and useful. "High" indicates that more than 80% meet these conditions and "low" less than 70%.

C.4: "Medium" indicates that data verified by the evaluation team and data reported by the program differ by 10-20%. "High" indicates differences of less than 10% and "low" of more than 20%.

Source: M.A. Toborg, L.I. Dogoloff and M.M. Basen. *Quick Evaluation Methodology* (Washington, D.C.: Special Action Office for Drug Abuse Prevention, Executive Office of the President, Series A, No. 2, 1973), p. A-5.

further examination. A caution in using this type of quick evaluation relates to the availability of accurate data for insertion into the proper boxes. At times, health planners might find that the organization either cannot supply the numbers or might insert the wrong numbers. Item C4 points to tackling that problem.

EVALUATION ALPHABET

Evaluation in health care seems to have developed an extensive "alphabetland." Most of the initials listed and spelled out are self-explanatory. Health planners will see the letters cited and should be aware of their meaning. You will probably add to this list as new methods, techniques, and programs are added (Exhibit 7-46).

EVALUATION PROBLEMS

Health planners must be aware that evaluation efforts do have difficulties with the usual questions regarding reliability and validity. In many health care evaluations involving patients, researchers have discovered that patients want to please the doctor and respond as they think the doctor wishes to hear. Suchman[50] identifies the following major sources of inconsistency:

- subject response can be affected by motivation, fatigue, or mood;
- observer reactions can be affected by the same factors or other personal factors and color the interpretations of the data;
- situations under which the evaluation is made are variable and affect the responses, such as weather, location, and time;
- instruments might be poorly worded, ambiguous, or have double meanings and influence the responses; and
- processing of the data could produce coding and/or mechanical errors, obviously biasing the results.

Evaluation activities should try to reduce the sources of bias or error to a minimum, but without interfering with the evaluation. It should be noted that all measurements do contain some error; there is no absolute level that can be determined without consideration of the variables in the appraisal. How much error is acceptable is also a difficult question; its answer depends on the purpose of the evaluation. Reliability can be controlled by attention to those factors indicated above that induce variable change in the collection of data. Reliability results when the probability of obtaining the same results with the repeated use of the same measuring instrument yields a high level of agreement.

Although a health planner can achieve high reliability, he might not have high validity. On the other hand, there can be no validity without reliability. Validity means the degree to which any measure actually

Exhibit 7-46 Evaluation Alphabet

CHAMP	Certified Hospital Admissions Monitoring Program
CME	Continuing Medical Education
CON	Certificate of Need
DUR	Drug Utilization Review
EMCRO	Experimental Medical Care Review Organization
HAPP	Hospital Admissions Pre-Certification Program
HASP	Hospital Admission and Surveillance Program
JCAH	Joint Commission on Accreditation of Hospitals
LOS	Length of Stay
MAC	Maximum Allowable Cost
MAP	Medical Audit Program
MCE	Medical Care Evaluation
MIIS	Medical Interpretive Information System
NHDS	National Hospital Discharge Survey
NHS	National Health Survey
OSCHUR	On-Site Concurrent Hospital Utilization Review
PACE	Physicians Ambulatory Care Evaluation Program
PAIS	Patient Activity Information System
PAS-MAP	Professional Activity Study–Medical Audit Program
PCA	Patient Care Appraisal
PDUR	Pre-Discharge Utilization Review
PEP	Performance Evaluation Procedure
PMR	Periodic Medical Review
POMR	Problem Oriented Medical Records
PPI	Physician Performance Index
PROMIS	Problem Oriented Medical Information System
PSRO	Professional Standards Review Organization
QAP	Quality Assurance Program
QUEST	Quality, Utilization, Effectiveness Statistically Tabulated
SOAP	Subjective Data, Objective Data, Assessment, and Plans
UHDD	Uniform Hospital Discharge Data
UR	Utilization Review

succeeds in measuring what it was supposed to measure. An evaluation instrument might be reliable—that is, the device can be considered stable. However, the same instrument can be valid in one situation and invalid in another. Thus, validity is a broader problem than reliability. The factors affecting validity have also been detailed by Suchman:[51]

- Propositional validity wherein the basic assumptions of the study are "wrong." Objectives may derive from invalid theories, or there may be invalid conclusions from valid theories.
- Instrument validity wherein inappropriate or irrelevant indices are used.

- Sampling validity wherein the sample of the population might not be representative, and the no responses might also skew the sample.
- Observer or evaluator validity wherein a consistent bias is introduced and sways the respondents in a particular direction, lowering the validity of the responses.
- Subject validity wherein deliberate misinformation is given by the subjects to impress the observer, to conceal data, or to create a favorable impression with the invalid data.
- Administration validity wherein the actual operation of the evaluation can make the results invalid, such as weather conditions, season of the year, training of the researchers, and the auspices of the study.
- Analysis validity wherein the person analyzing the data may have invalid rationales for interpreting the data to prove preconceived viewpoints of personal vested interests.

A comparison of the factors affecting reliability and validity clearly indicate the relationship between the two considerations.

Validity can be determined in several ways; and health planners must realize that, at times, validity can be so because someone merely said it was so. Following are some methods for determining validity.

- Face validity. A measure is valid because it is obviously significant, and the evaluator may decide this by himself.
- Consensual validity. This is the same as face validity, but a panel of experts comes to an agreement instead of only one person.
- Correlational validity. A measure is highly correlated to a known, valid measure of the same area of concern.
- Predictive validity. A correlation of present measures with events to take place in the future.

For example, an evaluation of medical schools assumes that students with high IQs will go to medical school (face validity). Admission committees at the schools confirm this assumption (consensual validity). Preadmission test scores correlate to the high IQ theory (correlational validity). It is predicted that medical schools will continue to receive students with high IQs in the future (predictive validity).

Health planners should easily see the problems with validity that are determined by a single vote, a group vote, or a future crystal ball. When the method can be correlated and tied to other valid measures, the validity stands a better chance of avoiding criticism. This is not to say that the other techniques are not used and, in some instances, highly respected because of the individual or individuals involved in the determination of the valid measures.

In an article on evaluation and measurement, L.W. Green[52] pinpointed some dilemmas that are worth consideration. The dilemmas are cited as extremes as follows:

rigor vs. significance,
internal vs. external validity,
experimental vs. placebo effects,
effectiveness vs. economy of scale,
risk vs. payoff,
long vs. short term evaluation, and
spending enough vs. spending too much.

In carrying out a rigorous evaluation, the planner might concentrate too much effort on maintaining a tight protocol; the results could be trivial. At times, the changes in the evaluation can produce significant results and still keep the design within reasonable bounds. Thus, it is important that health planners work to develop adequate designs, utilize solid statistical analyses, assure detailed documentation and reporting, and ensure replication.

Internal validity means that the evaluation showed that the activity caused some change. External validity refers to the ability to generalize from the evaluation of the project. If planners concentrate on internal validity, the conclusions cannot be generalized, and vice versa. This calls for attention to the objectives as well as to the political aspects of the activity.

Placebo effects are always a problem in evaluations. Health planners could find it difficult to pinpoint the experimental aspects of the activity as opposed to those that accounted for any change. A "Hawthorne effect" can occur, where the subjects express their desire to please the investigators by producing more or by giving responses that they know the researchers want to hear.

Effectiveness and economy are two words often heard in evaluation. Is it appropriate to use fewer people, or will the results be biased? If the numbers of personnel involved in the activity are increased, there might be some loss of effectiveness since the staff has to do more. However, this results in a lower per unit cost, and administrators appreciate that fact. Some possible ways around this dilemma involve the technique of aggregating people into groups for the activity; the use of trained aides to reduce professional manpower costs; the utilization of technological advances such as cable television, programmed instruction, and computer-assisted instruction; and the inclusion of a variety of approaches within the activity.

Risk versus payoff considerations might suggest to the health planner that it would be appropriate to choose the optimum time to initiate activities to maximize the payoff and minimize the risk. A maxim for health planners dictates that an activity should be started when the opportunity for success is greatest. Certainly, if this rule is followed, the evaluation will also stand the greatest chance for success. Not only does this type of risk/payoff consideration offer some protection for the health planner's job, but it also bolsters those who have committed themselves to the activities.

Long or short term evaluation problems naturally relate to a funding capability. But they should also consider the true effects of the activity under review. Sometimes observations are made too early, and the impact is delayed, with a sleeper effect occuring after the evaluation is concluded. On the other hand, the early measured impact might disappear after a short time and revert back to prior status. Evaluation might take place during an historical upward trend. If not enough time is allocated for the evaluation, the change could be falsely attributed to the activity, when in truth the change was taking place anyhow. Another backlash situation occurs when the activity is prematurely terminated, and the evaluation shows a downward curve in value. A portion of the consideration of long or short term evaluation must be directly related to the objectives of the program. If permanent changes are anticipated, the evaluation should plan for long term monitoring. Immediate changes can be measured with short term evaluation.

How much to spend on evaluation can be answered with the statement that the planner should only spend what is needed to get the job done. However, the concepts of cost-benefit analysis and cost-effectiveness enter into these decisions. Threshold spending means allocating only enough money to achieve the goal, with extraneous matters omitted from the evaluation. On the other end, saturation spending would put enough money into the review to squeeze out every last drop of worthwhile data and conclusions to the point of vanishing returns. Booster spending would be picking the best points at which to inject funds into an evaluation (similar to a booster vaccination that results in an increase in protective antibodies). Generally, health planners should try to resolve the money problems early enough that the evaluation can be integrated into the planning cycle without having to change techniques or methods late in the game. That move gains relatively little for the evaluation effort.

Low Utilization of Evaluations

Considerable evaluation does take place, and a considerable number of reports with recommendations end up gathering dust on shelves. Four basic reasons have been cited for the low utilization of evaluations:[53]

- Organizational inertia. Organizations tend to maintain the status quo and to resist change. Evaluation usually implies that changes are needed.
- Methodological weakness. Poorly conducted studies produce poorly respected conclusions. Decision makers tend to trust their own instincts or experiences rather than the results of poorly done studies.
- Design irrelevance. Critical programs and vital policy issues often are unrelated to the evaluation undertaken.
- Lack of dissemination. Concerned policy and decision makers might never see or hear about the conclusions of the evaluations. Sometimes the evaluation is deliberately buried to keep the information from being communicated to relevant individuals and organizations.

Although organizational inertia probably will always exist, the other three roadblocks can be broken through with some effort. Certainly, there are enough methods existing to assure a strong methodology for evaluation. Critical issues should be a prime consideration of planners who do not wish to spin their wheels. Dissemination will certainly take place if the planning process includes those who are to be involved in the implementation and those to be affected by any changes. Part of the process should be devoted to the publication and the spreading of information. In fact, a number of federal legislative mandates in recent laws specifically call for health planning information to be open to all and for public hearings that share the information with all concerned individuals and agencies.

There also appears to be a growing trend toward abstract evaluation studies, which make the summaries widely available. This allows interested parties to have the basic data and to request the original material if additional data are required.

REFERENCES

1. E.A. Codman, "The Product of a Hospital," *Surgery, Gynecology and Obstetrics* 18 (April 1914): 491.

2. S.R. Garfield, M.F. Collen, R. Feldman, K. Soghikian and R. Richart, "Evaluation of an Ambulatory Medical Care Delivery System," *New England Journal of Medicine* 294, no. 8 (February 19, 1976): 426.

3. C.H. Weiss, "The Politicization of Evaluation Research," *Journal of Social Issues* 26, no. 4 (1970): 57.

4. V.E. Weckwerth, *On Evaluation: A Tool or a Tyranny* (Minneapolis, Minn.: Systems Development Project, University of Minnesota, 1969), p. 1.

5. E.A. Suchman, Evaluation Research. *Principles and Practice in Public Service and Social Action Programs* (New York: Russel Sage Foundation, 1967), p. 91.

6. *Ibid.*, p. 31.

7. G. James, "Outline for the Evaluation of Tuberculosis Programs" (Akron, Ohio: Department of Health, undated) mimeographed.

8. R.H. Brook, *Quality of Care Assessment: A Comparison of Five Methods for Peer Review* (Washington, D.C.: U.S. Government Printing Office, 1973), pp. 1-3.

9. J.S. Wholey, J.W. Scanlon, H.G. Duffy, J.S. Fukumoto and L.M. Vogt, *Federal Evaluation Policy. Analyzing the Effects of Public Programs* (Washington, D.C.: The Urban Institute, 1970), p. 23.

10. B.A. Meyers, *A Guide to Medical Care Administration, Volume 1* (Washington, D.C.: American Public Health Association, 1970), p. 62.

11. E. Herzog, *Some Guidelines for Evaluative Research* (Washington, D.C.: HEW Children's Bureau, 1959), p. 23.

12. J. Elinson. Lecture at Columbia University School of Public Health and Administrative Medicine - Course title: Evaluation in Public Health, 1959.

13. Suchman, *op. cit.*, p. 141.

14. Suchman, *op. cit.*, p. 143.

15. National Institute of Mental Health, *Program Evaluation in the State Mental Health Agency. Activities, Functions, and Management Uses* (Washington, D.C.: Government Printing Office, 1976), pp. 3-7.

16. S. Levey and N.P. Loomba, *Health Care Administration. A Managerial Perspective* (Philadelphia: J.B. Lippincott Company, 1973), p. 424.

17. D.F. Bergwall, P.N. Reeves and N.B. Woodside, *Introduction to Health Planning* (Washington, D.C.: Information Resources Press, 1974), pp. 204-206.

18. Herzog, *op. cit.*, pp. 81-88.

19. Suchman, *op. cit.*, pp. 60-68.

20. Wholey *et al.*, *op. cit.*, pp. 24-26.

21. Task Force Report. *Quality Control and Evaluation of Preventive Health Services* (New York: Prodist, 1976), p. 106.

22. James, *op. cit.*

23. O.L. Deniston, I.M. Rosenstock, W. Welch and V.A. Getting, "Evaluation of Program Efficiency," *Public Health Reports* 85 (1970): 835.

24. Weckwerth, *op. cit.*, pp. 15-16.

25. A. Ciocco, "On Indices for the Appraisal of Health Department Activities," *Journal of Chronic Diseases* 11 (May 1960): 509.

26. J. Elinson, "Methods of Sociomedical Research," in *Handbook of Medical Sociology*, edited by H.E. Freeman, S. Levine, and L.G. Reeder (Englewood Cliffs, N.J.: Prentice Hall, 1972), pp. 488-489.

27. H.L. Blum, "Evaluating Health Care," *Medical Care* 12 (December 1974): 999.

28. A. Donabedian, "Evaluating the Quality of Medical Care," *Milbank Memorial Fund Quarterly, Part 2,* 44 (July 1966) 104.

29. R. Greene, *Assuring Quality in Medical Care. The State of the Art* (Cambridge, Mass.: Ballinger, 1976), p. 45.

30. L.L. Weed, *Medical Records, Medical Education and Patient Care* (Cleveland: Case Western Reserve Press, 1969).

31. M.I. Roemer, "Evaluation of Health Service Programs and Levels of Measurement," *Public Health Reports* 82 (July 1968).

32. R.M. Grimes and S.K. Mosely, "An Approach to an Index of Hospital Performance," *Health Services Research* 2, no. 3 (Fall 1976): 288.

33. S. Shindell, "The Elements of Professional Standards Review," *Journal of Legal Medicine* 1 (September-October 1973): 34.

34. B. Backhaut, *Factors Affecting the Cost of Health Care;* J.S. Gonnella, *Factors Affecting the Continuity of Health Care;* J. Lebow, *Factors Affecting the Availability of Health Care;* R. Penchansky, *The Concept of Access;* A.D. Spiegel, *Factors Affecting the Acceptability of Health Care;* A.D. Spiegel and B. Backhaut, *Factors Affecting the Quality of Health Care* (Springfield, Va.: National Technical Information Service, 1977).

35. A. Harwood, "The Hot-Cold Theory of Disease. Implications for the Treatment of Puerto Rican Patients," *Journal of the American Medical Association* 216, no. 5 (May 17, 1971): 1153.

36. Wholey *et al., op. cit.*

37. M.E. Shaw and J.M. Wright, *Scales for the Measurement of Attitudes* (New York: McGraw-Hill, 1967).

38. L.G. Reeder, L. Ramacher and S. Gorelnik, *Handbook of Scales and Indices of Health Behavior* (Pacific Palasades, Calif.: Goodyear Publishing Company, 1976).

39. P.A. Lembcke, "Medical Auditing by Scientific Methods. Illustrated by Major Female Pelvic Surgery," *Journal of the American Medical Association* 162 (October 13 1956): 646.

40. R.I. Lee and L.W. Jones, *The Fundamentals of Good Medical Care.* Publication no. 22 of the Committee on the Costs of Medical Care (Chicago: University of Chicago Press, 1933).

41. A. Donabedian, "Promoting Quality Through Evaluating the Process of Patient Care," *Medical Care* 6 (May-June 1968): 181.

42. J.A. Solon, "Measurement of Health Status," in Evaluation of Health Services Delivery, edited by R. Yaffe and D. Zalkind (New York Engineering Foundation, 1974), pp. 263-267.

43. Health Resources Administration, *Selected Bibliographic References on Methodologies for Community Health Status Assessment* (Washington, D.C.: U.S. Government Printing Office, 1976).

44. National Center for Health Statistics, *Clearinghouse on Health Indexes. Cumulated Annotations, 1975* (Washington, D.C.: U.S. Government Printing Office, 1977), p. 1.

45. Donabedian, "Promoting Quality Through Evaluating the Process of Patient Care," *op. cit.*

46. Public Health Service. *Health Planning. A Programmed Instruction Course* (Washington, D.C.: U.S. Government Printing Office, 1968), p. 141.

47. D.D. Rutstein, W. Berenberg, T.C. Chalmers, C.G. Child, A.P. Fishman and E.B.

Perrin, "Measuring the Quality of Medical Care. A Clinical Method," *New England Journal of Medicine* 294, no. 11 (March 11, 1976): 582.

48. S.B. Webb, Jr., "Objective Criteria for Evaluating Occupational Health Programs,"*American Journal of Public Health* 65 (January 1975): 31.

49. B.S. Hulka, "Evaluation of Primary Medical Care in a Total Community: The Indicator Case Model," in *Evaluation in Health Services Delivery,* edited by R. Yaffe and D. Zalkind (New York: Engineering Foundation, 1974), pp. 163-170.

50. Suchman, *op. cit.,* pp. 118-119.

51. *Ibid.,* pp. 120-126.

52. L.W. Green, "Evaluation and Measurement: Some Dilemmas for Health Education," *American Journal of Public Health* 67 (1977): 155.

53. Wholey *et al., op. cit.,* p. 50.

An Example of the Planning Process in Family Planning*

HOW TO PLAN

Planning is the process through which decisions are transformed into action. The elements of planning, which are the same regardless of the field, are identifying the problem, setting objectives, assessing resources, considering solutions, planning action, implementing the plan, and evaluating the outcomes. This process may seem more difficult to use in the educational field where the steps and processes are more abstract than they are in direct services.

Exhibit A-1 illustrates the steps in planning the educational component of a family planning program. While identifying the problem (Step A), setting program objectives (Step B), and assessing resources (Step C) are responsibilities that belong primarily to program administrators, they are included in the chart so one can see how the educational component fits into the entire planning process. The educational perspective, moreover, should be included in each of the first three planning steps—although it may be provided by staff members other than educators.

AN EXAMPLE OF THE PLANNING PROCESS

The Hightown Family Planning Agency serves one million residents; 450,000 reside in Hightown and the remaining 550,000 in the suburban and surrounding rural area. The agency has been in operation for two years and reflects the realistic initial planning of the staff and board. The development of services and the recruitment of family planning patients is proceeding close to schedule.

---

*The material and exhibit in this Appendix come from S.G. Deeds, *A Guidebook for Family Planning Education* (Columbia, Md.: Westinghouse Population Center, 1973).

Exhibit A-1 Planning Process for the Educational Component

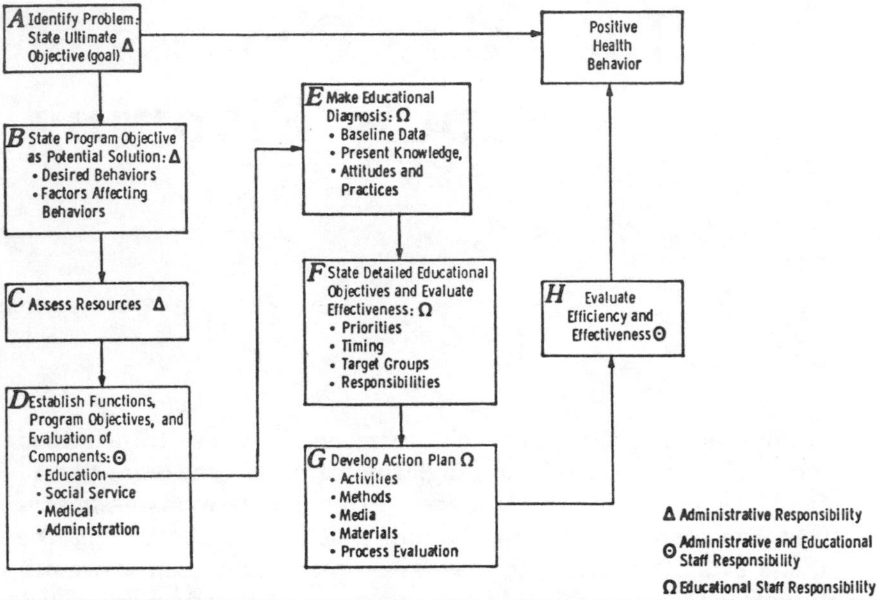

The agency's strategy was to provide basic contraceptive services to 40 percent of the estimated couples in need during the first 18 months of operation. Services would be provided at two major clinics and, occasionally, at loaned facilities. The development of other services such as sterilization and fertility testing, as well as the addition of new locations as a result of postpartum programs in hospitals, subsidized services in private doctors' offices, and prenatal clinics began in the latter part of the second year. Utilization and coordination of these existing resources are to be given full-scale attention during the third year to determine the extent of additional clinic sessions and locations required in the last two years of the program to reach the estimated number needing services.

In the original planning the defining of educational objectives resulted in identifying staff skills needed in the educational division: administrative, planning, and supervisory; public relations; community organization; training; small-group discussion; audiovisual production.

As you join the staff you find an educational director, a trainer with group discussion skills, a public relations program run by a community organizer and an executive staff, and a budget for purchasing audiovisual materials on contract. Your job is to plan a program for young adults and teenagers. Steps A to D will already have been taken before you arrived. However, your activities must be planned in the context of established goals and must be based on the data already collected. Hence you will need to know what action your agency has taken in these areas.

A: Identify the Problem and Set Ultimate Objectives

The ultimate objective of the Hightown Family Planning Agency is to improve the health of the residents of the county by providing family planning services and maximizing access to other available health services. This goal was based on an analysis of health problems which included:

- an infant mortality rate higher than the national average,
- a high maternal death rate,
- evidence of malnutrition and morbidity among preschool children, and
- drop-outs from high school attributed to unplanned pregnancies.

The long term objective stated by the planners is to:

- reduce high infant and maternal death rates and unplanned pregnancies by providing family planning services to 25,000 couples in need in five years, and
- coordinate related health services for families of the couples in need to reduce morbidity and malnutrition among children.

B: Propose Behavioral Objectives as Solutions to the Problem

Modes of behavior and practices that would help solve the problem noted include:

- increasing the time span between pregnancies,
- delaying a woman's first pregnancy to age 20,
- planning pregnancies and therefore reducing the number of women seeking abortions,
- reducing the number of pregnancies for high-risk mothers,
- avoiding pregnancy after a female is 35 years old,
- using prenatal care in the first trimester of pregnancy,
- raising the dietary level of mothers and children,
- improving the level of personal hygiene of mothers and babies,
- using preventive health services for babies and preschoolers.

The reasons these practices are not being adopted to the extent desired include: services are unavailable or inaccessible due to cost, distance, or time; family income is insufficient for proper diet; prospective clients are unaware of available services, reasons for planning families, and methods for planning families; the community does not believe young mothers, over-35 mothers, and their babies are at high risk; the community does not believe that large families sometimes lack psychological and emotional as well as physical support; and community customs support early marriage and job-seeking and large families.

The factors favoring the desired changes in behavior include: resources for services are available through federal grants; underutilized health resources in the community are available; a communications network of television, radio, and newspapers reaches 85 percent of the population; churches working with ethnic groups are disposed to family planning; the medical community is concerned about high mortality rates and public health; political officials support family planning and health grants; and some of the school officials view family planning favorably.

Assess Resources

An assessment of resources would involve compiling a list of available sources of funding, space, and equipment. It would also involve tabulating the resources of other related agencies that have personnel training facilities, funds, related programs, etc. Agencies to be considered include: governmental and intergovernmental agencies (community planning, information, education, labor); voluntary agencies such as the Cancer Society, Red Cross, religious groups, unions, and women's or youth groups; medical and allied health training institutions; libraries; and commercial institutions.

Available manpower was assessed with the following type of chart:

Agencies That May Supply Workers	Main Duties	Duties in Health Education	Health Education Training	Supervisor's Responsibility in Health Education	Difficulty in Involving Workers in Health Education Program
Family planning agency					
Health agencies					
Social service agencies					
Welfare agencies					
Educational programs Community colleges Schools					
Other groups YWCA YMHA County extension Homemakers 4-H					

D: Establish Functions and Program Objectives

The agency's program objectives are:

- confine pregnancy to women between 20 to 35—the most healthful age for both the mother and the child,
- avoid procreation when a woman is over 35,
- postpone pregnancy until a woman is 20 years old,
- practice child spacing by allowing two years to elapse between pregnancies,
- limit the number of children according to the physical and emotional needs of the family, as defined by the client, and
- ensure that couples successfully use effective and safe fertility control methods.

The following are examples of objectives defined in terms of the knowledge and attitudes (subobjectives) of the specific target couples, their close contacts, medical and health personnel, other related agency personnel, the general community, and the family planning agency staff:

- Both young people and adults know and believe that the preferred age for females to bear children is between 20 and 35.
- Both young people and adults in the fertile age group know about family planning methods and where services can be obtained. They can select and use safe, effective, and suitable methods successfully.
- Youth and adults make decisions to plan a pregnancy at the preferred age and use measures to postpone pregnancy.
- Medical and allied health professionals are convinced of the safe age range, use professional influence to foster awareness, and provide family planning services and/or referral to help clients limit childbearing to that age.
- Health workers, educators, group workers, and welfare staff incorporate health aspects of human reproduction in their educational efforts; they encourage their contacts to limit pregnancy to the preferred age range.
- Opinion leaders in the community provide psychological and social support for encouraging childbearing at the optimum age.
- Providers of family planning counseling and service know the biological and emotional factors which make 20 to 35 the optimum age for pregnancy, are aware of all fertility control options, and are able to communicate that information effectively to their patients.

The first year of the educational plan, which involved generating large-scale community support for family planning and providing information on the availability of services, was judged successful. This judgment was based on the expressions of support from numerous agencies, a favorable press, continuous funding support from the governmental bodies, and community surveys showing that 40 percent of the general public could identify sources for provision of family planning information and that 67 percent of the population between 20 and 45 knew of the need for and the availability of services.

Staff training in communication and listening skills is proceeding on schedule. Patient education in the clinics is provided through a combination of methods including individual instruction, group discussion, and presentation of factual information by audiovisuals and pamphlets. Word-of-mouth referrals are on the increase.

The general success of the program thus far does not extend to the youth population. The knowledge of contraception and availability of services revealed in the community survey is not reflected in the attendance of that age group in the clinic. In addition, other behavior described below indicates the need for an intensive effort with that group.

After orientation and consultation with the educational staff, your assignment becomes additional community exploration and diagnosis.

E: Make Educational Diagnosis

Research produced the following information:

- Existing baseline data indicate that 425 babies were born to women under 20 in the county in 1972.
- School personnel are concerned because the drop-out rate is high at three high schools. A study shows that a major reason for dropouts during the last two years of high school is unplanned pregnancy. The study shows additionally that the high risk group is characterized by close steady dating, low scholastic and career motivation for females, and diffuse career motivation for males.
- Health personnel identify problems of early pregnancy such as prematurity, poor nutrition, the need for mothering skills, and economic problems affecting both mothers and children.
- Students state that access to family planning clinics depends upon parental consent. Queries on other methods of contraception reveal gaps in knowledge and understanding.

- Parents' attitudes regarding family planning information programs range from permissive to strict. Parents feel a need for such programs for students but are unwilling to take a public stand. Many seem unsure and uncomfortable about their ability to present information to their children.

F: State Detailed Objectives and Evaluate Effectiveness

Your long term objective, it is agreed, is to reduce the number of babies born to women under age 20 by 20 percent in the next two years. Your educational strategy might shape up the following way:

- make fertility control services accessible to young people who are ready and willing to accept and use them;
- encourage the teenagers who are sexually active but unwilling to use fertility control services to consider such services to be to their advantage; and
- in the process of generating the community and social acceptance necessary for young people to gain accessibility to services and information, begin to effect changes in attitude that will bring about longer range community change. This would be support for later marriage, alternatives to marriage for females such as careers and advanced education, smaller families, realistic vocational counseling and careers for young men, increased youth employment opportunities, and greater promotion of hobbies and recreation, which may discourage early pairing and steady dating.

The educational strategy was based on the following planning assumptions:

- direct access to fertility control services by young adults and teenagers would reduce the rate of pregnancy in that group;
- direct access to medical methods of fertility control would require that young persons perceive their ability to gain parental permission;
- direct access to medical methods of fertility control would also increase if the law requiring parental consent were modified;
- access to nonmedical fertility control services would increase if youth and vendors knew about and approved their use;
- knowledge of fertility control methods would increase if educational programs were provided in schools
- sexually active teenagers, uncommited to pregnancy avoidance,

will not use available methods unless a change in knowledge and attitude occurred;

- some commitment and attitude change in the above group would result from the first five changes listed above;
- identification of the hazards and risks of early and multiple pregnancies must be presented to uncommitted groups by using group-specific methods; and
- the present community climate must change to support the desired attitudes and practices.

To carry out the educational strategy, the following short term objectives and evaluation mechanisms were established:

- Make a factual presentation of the local family planning problem and its health aspects via mass media using a new format each week for 26 weeks. This objective may be evaluated by documenting public opinion as it is expressed in editorials, letters to the editor, newspaper features, and local talk show.
- Gain support for community leaders, service clubs, religious groups, neighborhood associations, and youth groups. Criteria for evaluation include written statements, letters of support, speeches, letters to lawmakers, discussions, and reviews in local television and radio programs.
- Encourage health and welfare agencies to change any policy, service, or procedure which does not support the family planning program. How well this objective is achieved may be measured by comparing agency records, policy statements, referral patterns, and counseling and education contacts both before the educational program and after its implementation.
- Get 50 percent of the parents of teenagers who believe young people should have access to birth control services to support their viewpoint publicly and to support adult education classes for parents to assist them in communicating with and educating their children. The criteria for evaluation include signed petitions for such classes initiated by PTA efforts and the establishment of classes based on requests and enrollment.

G: Develop Action Plan

An action plan detailing activities, responsibilities, and methods might be set up in the following fashion:

Short Term Objective	Activity	Responsibility	Purpose	Methods & Media
Gain support of community leaders	Interviews, conferences, written documents and articles	Health leaders, social scientists	Bring facts to attention; enlist support in solving problems	Kit of materials with statistical evidence, case histories, examples
Gain support of service groups	Talks, discussions, programs	Educators, health professionals, youth leaders, agency-based members	Bring facts to attention, involve service groups in the study & solution of problems, enlist support	Talks reinforced with written materials, audio-visuals, newsletters
Help health and welfare agencies to anticipate change & begin planning change	Seminars, workshops study groups, & staff conferences	Administrators, experts, policy-level board & staff	Discuss data, study present practices & needed change, enlist community for change	Wide variety of media: face-to-face & small group discussions audio-visuals, printed materials.

H: Evaluate Efficiency and Effectiveness

Three types of program assessment will be made: process, effectiveness, and efficiency evaluations.

- *Process evaluation.* A process evaluation will involve answering the following types of questions: Are conditions conducive to reaching the subobjective of support from community leaders and groups? Have the health leaders who will make contacts been recruited and trained? Are they contacting and interviewing the community leaders? What is the response to the materials that have been developed? Are they effective? This kind of analysis makes it possible to revamp activities and assumptions to use available resources most effectively.
- *Effectiveness evaluation.* Did the contacts, talks, and background materials accomplish the subobjective of developing support? Did the subobjectives collectively accomplish the educational objective—to change legislation, to gain certain actions from youth, from parents, from school, etc.? What evidence has been collected, positive and negative, showing change? Has the birth rate shifted?

- *Efficiency evaluation.* Was the accomplishment (output and benefit) worth the expenditure of resources? The outcome (accomplishments) of an information communication effort would be patient knowledge and the benefit resulting would be the desired practices (compliance). In the case of communication with relatives, the educational output would be social support for the patient and the benefit resulting would be compliance and public support.

Some costs that might be used to analyze benefits quantitatively include an estimate of the social and dependency costs of young parents, the costs of school drop-outs and low career achievement, and the costs related to maternal and infant mortality and morbidity. This estimate would provide baseline data. At the end of two years, or whatever period you have projected, the number of events avoided, in this case pregnancies of mothers under age 20, could be calculated. The existing rate could then be compared with the rate projected to have occurred without the program. Assuming that your objective has been successfully reached, the amount saved could then be compared with the resources expended in your particular educational program. Such efforts can sometimes be useful in generating support for educational efforts with administrators and consumer boards. This is just one example of an efficiency evaluation. Similar approaches may be used to evaluate portions of the program at shorter time intervals.

Illustrative Material from Community At the Crossroads: A Drug Education Simulation Game. The Social Seminar.*

Community at the Crossroads is a two- to five-hour game simulation of a community response to the problem of drug abuse. It is intended for use primarily by teachers, other school personnel, and students. However, it may also be played by community groups interested in encouraging discussion of drug abuse prevention and education.

Simulation materials include 32 player's cards, a director's guide, a film discussion guide, 32 role cards, 32 copies of the police report, 32 copies of the clergyman's report, and 32 copies of the budget report. All this material is packaged in a box for handy storage.

The material duplicated below is taken from the Player's Guide that is distributed to each participant.

DESCRIPTION OF THE SIMULATION AND ITS OBJECTIVES

Cummington, U.S.A., can be and is anywhere in America. Its specific characteristics may be more or less like those of the town in which you live or work, but the problems it faces are typical of all communities today. The residents of Cummington have just been forced to realize that they have "a drug problem."

For the next few hours you will be intimately and emotionally involved in trying to define what direction the community will take in response to this problem. You will participate in a simulation—a simplification or representation of reality in which participants assume a variety of roles. In a series of scheduled and structured meet-

---

*Created by the National Institute of Mental Health, HEW, 1971.

ings, you will attempt to define the nature and extent of Cummington's drug problem and community strategies for dealing with that problem.

There are no simplistic solutions to the problems of drug abuse in America, nor will you find any in Cummington. Communities must search their own resources—both institutional and human—to determine what they have and what they need. The basic nature of the community must be explored for possible answers to the question, "Why here?" You will hear responses from all members of the community. You will discover that parents, children, teachers, community officials, law enforcement agencies, and social agencies must work together in a cooperative spirit if Cummington is to achieve anything more than an argumentative stalemate.

Some Background

About six months ago, based on his reading of the national press, the mayor of Cummington suggested that a Drug Abuse Advisory Council (DAAC) be established. At that time, however, there was little concern in the community about drugs, and therefore, the suggestion received little attention and less support. The past two weeks, however, have seen the citizens of Cummington sit up and take notice. Where they might once have thought that Cummington was a model community immune to the social problems striking the rest of the country, they now know that such immunity does not exist. Recent events have established that drugs are being used by young people in Cummington. These events, which you will find detailed in the scenario, have forced the residents of Cummington to begin to come to grips with the situation.

Many residents have been hounding the mayor and the city council to "do something!" In answer to this pressure, the mayor again put forth his idea and last week appointed an eight-member Drug Abuse Advisory Council. Its function, he said, is to act as a sounding board so that the total community will voice opinions as to steps that might be taken to curb the use and abuse of drugs. The council's function, however, is to be more than advisory. The mayor, the community council, and the school committee have agreed to put the DAAC's recommendations into action.

Tonight the DAAC has scheduled a meeting with a representative sample of Cummington's population. Besides the eight members of the Council, there will be students, parents, and teachers present. Each of these people has expressed an interest in the problem and has agreed to volunteer time to the DAAC.

You are one of these people. As such, you will be given a confidential role profile as a citizen of Cummington. These individuals hold the wide variety of opinions found in any community. In the course of the simulation, several alternative courses of action will undoubtedly be offered. Individual participants may support or oppose these proposals for entirely different reasons. It is important to seek out these reasons so that true understanding will develop.

A Word About Your Role

Different role profiles are provided to assure that certain attitudes will be voiced during the coming meetings. Although you may not personally agree with or even like the role you play, the game has been so designed that there will be ample opportunity both during the actual simulation and afterward, in a critique session, to explore all points of view.

Try to imagine how the person you are portraying would react to various arguments and what counterarguments he would make. Also be aware of nonverbal methods of communication such as facial expressions and hand and body gestures. These techniques will help to validate your role. Remember, however, that in real life people do change their minds. Be prepared to accept arguments that you think are valid and to change the position of your role as you see fit.

Obviously, the role profile can only be a guide to an individual's behavior. You must take it from there and make it into a real person. As the simulation progresses, you will find yourself relying less on the role and more on your own instincts of human behavior.

The material below is taken from the Director's Guidebook.

DESCRIPTION OF THE SIMULATION AND ITS OBJECTIVES

"A Community at the Crossroads" is a role-playing simulation dealing with a community's response to a complex social problem—drug abuse. This simulation is a simplification or representation of reality in which participants assume the roles of teachers, students, parents, and city or town leaders. Through a series of scheduled and structured meetings the participants define the nature and extent of the drug problem and then determine strategies and programs for dealing with that problem.

Cummington, U.S.A., is a fictitious community, but it could be any community in America. Its citizens have very recently been forced to realize that they have a "drug problem." However, the citizens are confused, alarmed, disorganized on what course of action the community must take to solve its problem.

"A Community at the Crossroads" has been designed to help that community (and especially yours) in formulating a plan of action. The simulation recreates the various attitudes that people hold about drug abuse, and how these attitudes can help or hinder efforts for solution. The roles of the police, medical profession, and schools are examined so understanding develops on how they can assist in coping with the problem.

By playing in the simulation, the participants will be exposed to various points of view, many of which will differ from their own. Indeed, some participants may play roles involving attitudes antithetical to their own, and, in tests of the simulation, the mere playing of such a role is, in itself, a valuable learning experience for the participant.

No simulation is intended to be the solution to a community's drug problem. Rather, it provides a forum for people to come together in a simulated real-life situation to begin to solve their problem. "A Community at the Crossroads," therefore, is not based on any particular city or town. The game's reality arises from the topic presented—drug abuse—and from the more general subject of human behavior when individuals are confronted with a possibly unifying, yet potentially divisive, issue.

The simulation teaches primarily through communication among participants. When teachers and students with community members examine what the role of the school should be in dealing with the problem, they and parents, members of the professions, and city officials will better understand what their roles should be.

Finally, "A Community at the Crossroads" is a vehicle for showing that drug abuse *is* a community problem, a complex problem that does not lend itself to simplistic solutions and a communitywide issue that requires the support and cooperation of all community members and· social institutions.

DESCRIPTION OF MEETINGS

Meeting One: Orientation (15-20 minutes)

The simulation director will distribute the clergyman's report before the start of the meeting.

All participants will be introduced to and welcomed by the Drug Abuse Advisory Council, chaired by the clergyman. The clergyman will make a few brief remarks based on his report. He will then open to the floor a general discussion of the incidents which have occurred in Cummington, the nature and extent of the drug problem in Cummington, and the purpose of the DAAC.

At the close of the meeting, the clergyman will direct the participants to divide into four role groups: (1) parents, (2) teachers, (3) students, and (4) the DAAC. The groups will discuss what specific steps the community might take in responding to its drug problem.

Simulation Director's Notes for Meeting One

1. Before starting the game, you should take several participants aside and inform them that when the clergyman opens the discussion to the floor, they should voice their viewpoints. We suggest you prompt the individuals playing roles #10, 12, 19, 23, 30, 21. By prompting certain roles all participants will then "open up," and you preclude a period of waiting before discussion begins.

2. Before starting, remind the clergyman that he should *not* read his report to the group. Also, his remarks should be brief.

3. The meeting should be brief (approximately 15-20 minutes). It is intended to get disparate viewpoints and attitudes "out in the open."

4. Remind participants before the start of play that they should refer to the Sequence and Nature of Meetings section of the Player's Manual before each session begins.

Break

Approximately five minutes will be allowed between meetings. Participants should spend this time reviewing the proposals for a school disciplinary policy, a drug treatment and counseling center, and a drug education program.

Meeting Two: Role Groups (30-45 minutes)

The overall purpose of this meeting is for each role group to discuss the goals of the community in responding to its drug problem and to develop tentative recommendations regarding acceptance or rejection of the three proposed plans.

Each person should introduce himself briefly and tell about his background. These introductions need not include everything in the role profile.

Each group should choose a discussion chairman and a secretary. It will be the secretary's responsibility to report the groups recommendations at the next DAAC meeting.

The chairman should then direct the discussion to the three proposals that have been put before the community. Participants should give their general reactions to these plans and discuss what the specific goal and long range implication of each plan is. This should lead into a discussion of the validity of these goals for the city of Cummington. Based on this discussion, the secretary should prepare a report giving the group's tentative recommendations for acceptance or rejection of the proposed plans, based on the community's goals.

Simulation Director's Notes for Meeting Two

1. The role groups should meet in separate rooms.

2. You should go to each role group and remind them that the purpose of the meeting is to discuss the situation in Cummington and to come up with only *tentative* recommendations concerning the proposed plans of action.

3. You will probably discover that most if not all role groups will find it difficult to advance even tentative recommendations because of the polarity of viewpoints within their respective groups. This is good and is intended. Meeting two is not a planning session (although it seems so). It is intended to allow participants to vent their feelings and to begin to understand that compromise will be necessary if positive drug problems are to be initiated.

Meeting Three: Drug Abuse Advisory Council Open Meeting (20-30 minutes)

At the start of this meeting, the simulation director will distribute copies of (1) the police chief's report and (2) the budget.

The clergyman will call for reports of the four role groups. Following the reports, the chairman will open the floor to discussion on the police chief's report and how it relates to the goals of the community. The group should also discuss how the budget relates to the proposed plans.

At the close of this meeting, the clergyman will divide the participants into smaller groups. This time, however, they will be task force committees. Each committee will represent a cross section of the community's roles (parents, teachers, students, and the DAAC).

Simulation Director's Notes for Meeting Three

1. Be sure to distribute police and budget reports before meeting begins.

2. Allow participants five minutes to review the reports before starting the meeting.

3. Clergyman again chairs this meeting.

Break:

There will be a five-minute break between meetings. Participants should study the four proposed plans (school disciplinary policy, drug treatment and counseling center, drug education, and police recommendations) and the budget.

Meeting Four: Task Force Committees (45-60 minutes)

Each committee should choose a discussion chairman and a secretary. It will be the secretary's responsibility to make the group's final report to the DAAC. Each individual should briefly introduce himself in his role. The overall purpose of this meeting is to determine the priorities of the community in light of budgetary restrictions. Each group should discuss and answer the following questions:

1. Should the school disciplinary policy be implemented as is? Should it be modified; and, if so, in what way? How much money should be allocated to the program? Should the policy be rejected?

2. Should the community establish a drug treatment counseling center as outlined by Mr. Leonard? Should some sort of facility be established? If so, what kind? How much money should be allocated to the program? Should no new facility be added?

3. Should the community implement the police chief's recommendations? Should they modify his plan? If so, in what way? How much money should be allocated to the police department? Should the police chief's plan be rejected?

4. Should the community establish a drug education program? If so, what kind, for whom, administered by whom, and with what viewpoint (e.g., factual, legal, attitudinal)? How much money should be allocated to such a program?

5. Participants may propose any alternative plan of action not listed above.

Note: The total amount of money allocated among these four programs cannot exceed the total figure given in the budget.

Simulation Director's Notes for Meeting Four

1. This is the key meeting of the game. Participants will meet in the heterogeneous task force committees.

2. Each task force must make *final* recommendations regarding proposed programs.

Meeting Five: Drug Abuse Advisory Council Open Meeting
(20–30 minutes)

The clergyman will call for reports from the four task force committees. He will open the floor to general discussions regarding the recommendations of the task force committees.

Simulation Director's Notes for Meeting Five

1. Each task force presents recommendations.

2. There will be no general discussion until all task forces have presented recommendations.

3. The open discussion should be brief, and the clergyman should terminate the meeting and the game by telling the participants that the DAAC will weigh the recommendations and report to the community in the near future.

Meeting Six: Critique (30 minutes)

Participants will reassume their real identities. The simulation director will open discussion on the following questions:

1. How do you think the DAAC will vote and why?
2. What did you learn from the simulation?
3. Where does the community go from here?

The critique session is especially important for the participants. The simulation director should direct the discussion to an examination of the issues in the game as they relate to the community's own drug problem. The simulation director should also emphasize the need for follow-up discussions and planning.

ROLE 4: PSYCHIATRIST

You are 40 years old and have been a doctor in Cummington for ten years. You are respected in the medical community for being a good

Simulation Sequence Diagram

Nature of Meeting	Players	Tasks	Time
Orientation	All participants together	1. Discuss recent events in Cummington 2. Discuss nature and extent of problem 3. Discuss purpose of DAAC 4. Clergyman's report	15–20 minutes
Break		Review sections of Player's Manual dealing with school policy, treatment center, and drug education	5 minutes

Role Groups	1. Parents
	2. Students
	3. Teachers
	4. DAAC
		1. Discuss goals and implications of
		  (a) school disciplinary policy
		  (b) drug treatment and counseling center
		  (c) drug education program
		2. Develop tentative recommendations for acceptance or rejection of three plans
			30–45 minutes

DAAC Open Meeting	All participants together	1. Role group reports 2. Discuss police report 3. Discuss budget	20–30 minutes
Break		Review sections of Player's Manual dealing with school policy, treatment center, and drug education, as well as police report and budget	5 minutes
Task Force	Four heterogeneous Task Force groups. Task Force A: 1, 8, 9, 10, 17, 24, 25, 27 B: 6, 7, 11, 16, 18, 21, 26, 29 C: 2, 5, 12, 14, 20 23, 30, 31 D: 3, 4, 13, 15, 19, 22, 28, 32	1. Determine priorities of community in implementing drug abuse programs based on budgetary restrictions. 2. Develop specific recommendations regarding acceptance, modificiation, cost, or rejection of four proposed plans, based on budgetary restrictions.	45–60 minutes

Simulation Sequence Diagram continued

Nature of Meeting	Players	Tasks	Time
DAAC Open Meeting	All participants together	1. Task force reports 2. General discussion of recommendations	20–30 minutes
Critique	All participants assume real identity	Discussion of 1. How the DAAC will probably vote and why? 2. What was learned from the simulation? 3. Where does community go from here?	20–30 minutes

therapist and the author of two perceptive and innovative books on psychiatric counseling. You have been connected with the Community Health Center for five years, and in that time have talked with many youngsters involved in drugs. You have learned to see things through their eyes as well as your own, and you realize that the problem is more than kids just wanting to break the law or rebel. You see the use of drugs—what it means legally and morally—as the beginning of a new value system. Yet, many kids are being treated as misfits and freaks by adults just for smoking pot. You don't condone the use of hard drugs, feeling that many kids who get involved with hard drugs *are* sick. However, you feel they are turning to drugs because of what the society has done to them, the same way that an alcoholic turns to liquor. Furthermore, you don't lump marijuana in the category of hard drugs.

You agree with many of the kids to whom you've spoken that Cummington needs a center for drug users or potential drug users that is not connected with the local or federal government and that is completely nonpunitive. You've found out from the kids who *do* come to the Community Health Center that many kids don't come because they don't want to be judged, and because they are afraid they'll be turned over to the authorities. You feel that if the proposed treatment and counseling center were run the way you think it should be, it could really help a lot of kids who otherwise wouldn't be helped. "The Community Health Center is just not big enough or structured properly to deal with the kind or size of the drug problem that we have."

You also favor intelligent and objective drug education programs for the schools and the community. You've found out by talking with kids that "nothing turns them off so much as a moralistic sermon on drugs, and when governmental pamphlets are given to them, they think the government is trying scare tactics on them." One kid said, "If they lie about the dangers of pot, and they *have* lied, why should we (kids) believe the government when they talk about the dangers of other drugs?" You know the kids are also well aware of the hypocrisy of adults who tell them not to smoke pot or use drugs when they smoke cigarettes, take pills, and drink.

Scenario

Front Page News, Cummington Courier

Police Raids in Cummington; Drugged Girl Falls From Building

Fleeing the scene of a "pot party," a Cummington teenager fell in an attempt to climb down a series of balconies at the rear of an apartment building. She was seriously injured and is receiving treatment at Cummington City Hospital. Doctors say that she was under the influence of a hallucinogenic drug, probably LSD. The incident followed drug raids by State and local police.

At 10 p.m. last night, four members of the Cummington police force joined a five-man State police unit to conduct three simultaneous raids. They acted on information from an as yet unknown source.

At the new Fairfax Building in the west end, five local high school students were caught at a "pot party" in a third floor apartment. Six young adults were apprehended at a similar party in a first floor apartment. They were William and Dorothy Sears, both 27, John Dorsett, age 29, and Carol Dorsett, age 26, Peter Mathews, age 29, and Ruth Mathews, age 28.

On Parker Street, on the East Side, six teenagers were arrested at a "salad bowl" party, The six individuals were arrested on charges of the possession and use of illegal drugs and for being in the presence of illegal drugs. Police found a plentiful supply of amphetamines, barbiturates, general stimulants, and marijuana.

All the startled participants were taken, without protest, to the local police station. Chief Kramer questioned the students and contacted all of their parents. At about midnight, 10 of the students were released on $50 bail each, in the custody of their parents.

One boy, who was charged with possession of 3 ounces of marijuana, was released on $1,000 bail. Juvenile hearings for all the students are scheduled in about 3 weeks.

All the teenagers are students at Cummington High School and live in Cummington. Names are being withheld in accordance with the State's juvenile crime regulations.

The six adults were charged on several counts—possession, use, and being in the presence of illegal drugs. They were released the following morning on bail of $1,000 each and will be represented by their lawyer at a court hearing, also scheduled in about 3 weeks.

The judge concluded this brief session by admonishing the young couples. "I've levied a high bail on you," he said, "because you ought to know better. This case is going to be an example for people to think about."

Police Chief Kramer had these comments this morning: "We've been aware that drugs have been coming into Cummington during the past few months. The State police have asked us to keep an informal record on the situation here, and they will cooperate with us when action is necessary. Yes, this was the first action taken in Cummington, but I wouldn't say that it'll be the last."

Questioned as to the parents' reactions, Chief Kramer said, "Sure, they were shocked. These are kids who've never been in trouble before. One parent told me it was the worst disgrace in the history of their family. There may be some more disgraced families," Kramer concluded.

Cummington Courier Editorial

Wisdom of the Elders

We've had a little more than a week now to get used to the idea that we've got a drug problem here in Cummington.

Our shock and disbelief really showed how innocent we were. Of course, we all knew of a drug problem in the country, but here in our fair city? Never!

And we don't even have a good scapegoat. Had outsiders been involved, we could have maintained our community pride and rallied our forces against them.

But the facts are that drugs are here and the users are some of our very finest youths. The shock has worn off a bit, but we're rather confused. We're asking one another, "What's going wrong with society? Have we been too permissive with our children?"

We can't solve all of society's problems or intellectually analyze all of our values. But, what we can do is to take charge—act confidently and swiftly to solve this problem.

Let's use the rather dusty value called "wisdom of the elders" to bolster our confidence and stir us to action.

Let's put a drug education program in the schools. Let's teach the teenagers about the existing narcotics laws that were made by concerned legislators and are used by honorable judges. Let's teach them about the dangers of drugs that have been documented by dedicated scientists. Why not have the enforcers of the law, the respected men in blue, be the teachers of this drug education?

When the results are in, we'll undoubtedly conclude that when "the elders" are inactive or not visible, by choice or by pressure, problems do develop in a community. But, when experienced adults act, problems are solved.

Director's Guide

Description of the simulation and its objectives	1st P—representation of reality with the actors identified. 3rd P—formulate a plan of action with cooperation from all concerned. Last P—Need for interaction to solve problems.
Description of meetings	What to do for each six meetings scheduled. Read the simulation director's notes for each meeting. For meeting one, the director is told to prompt people playing specific roles to motivate others to "open up" at the session. Clergyman is told not to read his report and make remarks brief. For meeting two, the director tells groups to come up with tentative recommendations. Separate rooms for meetings are indicated. For meeting four, director is told this is key meeting and each task force must make final recommendations. For meeting six, the director asks for responses to given questions with participants. Reassuming their real identities. This gives the director a critique of the feasibility of implementing the recommendations.
Simulation sequence diagram	This diagram presents visually the meetings—who participates, the tasks, and the time limitation. This is a condensation of the real life action over a much longer period of time.

Role profile for psychiatrist

Illustrates the type of information that the player needs to fulfill the representation. Gives attitudes held by psychiatrist as well as a basis for interactions with other players.

Players Manual

Description of the simulation and its objectives

Similar to the director's guide with the addition of the scenario information in the background. Note the call for action. Players are told how to act out their role and to be aware of nonverbal techniques.

Scenario

This sets the scene and puts the players into a situation where they must move forward and plan to meet the crisis. This is the same situation the health planner is in regarding implementation. The policy decision has been made and he must proceed.

Bibliography

Adizes, I., and Zukin, P. "A Management Approach to Health Planning in Developing Countries." *Health Care Management Review* 2 (Winter 1977): 19.

Ahmed, B.M., Levine, J., and Rosen, B. "Assessment of Program and Priorities." *Psychiatric Quarterly* 49 (Fall 1977): 163.

Altman, S. "Rationalizing the American Health Care Delivery System: A Summary of the Health Planning and Resources Development Act of 1974." *World Hospital* 12, no. 1 (1976): 94.

Anderson, J.S., Smoyer, C.S., and Willshier, J.J. "Local Health Planning Advances Under Consumer-Provider Direction." *Hospitals* 51 (April 6, 1977): 63.

Andrews, G., Nield, L., and McDonell, G. "A Note on the Objectives For Regional Hospital Planning." *National Hospital Health Care* 2 (May 1976): 19.

Annas, G.J. "Allocation of Artificial Hearts in the Year 2002: Minerva V. National Health Agency." *American Journal of Law and Medicine* 3 (Spring 1977): 59.

Ardell, D.B. "From Omnibus Tinkering to High-Level Wellness: The Movement Toward Holistic Health Planning." *American Journal of Health Planning* 1 (October 1976): 15.

Atkisson, A.A., and Grimes, R.M. "Health Planning in the United States: An Old Idea With a New Significance." *Journal of Health Politics, Policy and Law* 1 (Fall 1976): 295.

Ball, A.E. "State and Local Regulation Will Prove Most Effective." *Hospitals* 50 (March 1, 1976): 89.

Bauer, K.G. "Hospital Rate Setting—This Way to Salvation." *Milbank Memorial Fund Quarterly: Health & Society* 55 (Winter 1977): 117.

Bauman, P., and Banta, H.D. "The Congress and Policymaking for Prevention." *Preventive Medicine* 6 (June 1977): 227.

Beech, R.P., Fiester, A.R., and Silverman, W.H. "Demographic Data and Mental Health Planning." *Administration in Mental Health* 3 (Spring 1976): 166.

Bengoa, J.M., and Beaton, G.H. "Some Concepts and Practical Considerations in Planning and Evaluation." *WHO Monograph Series* 62 (1976): 213.

Berg, R.L. "Refine Political Strategies in HSAs." *Hospital Progress* 58 (September 1977): 64.

Berki, S.E., and Kobashigawa, B. "Socioeconomic and Need Determinants of Ambulatory Care Use: Path Analysis of the 1970 Health Interview Survey Data." *Medical Care* 14 (May 1976): 405.

473

Bice, T.W., and Salkever, D.S. "Certificate-of-Need Programs: Cure or Cause of Inflated Costs." *Hospital Progress* 58 (July 1977): 65.

Blockstein, W.L. "Current Concerns in Health and Their Relationship to the Planning Process." *American Journal of Pharmacy* 149 (March-April 1977): 37.

Bloom, A. "The Right of Public Access to Information Submitted Under the Requirements of the Health Planning Act." *Public Health Reports* 92 (September-October 1977): 411.

Blum, H.L. "From a Concept of Health to a National Health Policy." *American Journal of Health Planning* 1 (July 1976): 3.

Boeh, J.H. "Public Utility Regulation of Hospitals May Fall Short of Goals in Actual Operation." *Hospitals* 51 (November 1, 1977): 51.

Boog, P.E. "HSAs and Their Effect on Student Health Services." *Journal of the American College Health Association* 25 (June 1977): 287.

Bosch, S.J., and Deuschle, K.W. "The Role of a Medical School in the Organization of Health-Care Services." *Bulletin of New York Academy of Medicine* 53 (June 1977): 448.

Braun, H., Kugelman, R.F., and Massey, M.M. "An Evaluation of the Agency Assessment Program—Implications for the Health Systems Agency Community." *American Journal of Health Planning* 1 (July 1976): 52.

Bricknell, J.G. "The Health Service: Reappraisal of Priorities." *Nursing Mirror* 143 (July 1976): 69.

Bryant, J.H. "Principles of Justice as a Basis for Conceptualizing a Health Care System." *International Journal of Health Services* 7, no. 4 (1977): 707.

Cardus, D., and Thrall, R.M. "Overview: Health and the Planning of Health Care Systems." *Preventive Medicine* 6 (March 1977): 134.

Cleverley, W.O. "Cost Containment in the Health Care Industry." *Topics and Health Care Finances* 3 (Spring 1977): 1.

Cloe, L.E. "Health Planning for Computed Tomography: Perspectives and Problems." *American Journal of Roentgenology* 127 (July 1976): 187.

Cochran, W.G., "The Role of Statistics in National Health Policy Decisions." *American Journal of Epidemiology* 104 (October 1976): 370.

Coleman, J.R., and Kaminsky, F.C. "A Financial Planning Model for Evaluating the Economic Viability of Health Maintenance Organizations." *Inquiry* 14 (June 1977): 176.

Connor, G.R. "State Government Financing of Health Planning." *American Journal of Health Planning* 1 (October 1976): 48.

Cooper, B.S., and Rice, D.P. "The Economic Cost of Illness Revisited." *Social Security Bulletin* (February 1976).

Cummings, K.W. "Psychiatrists and Legislative Issues: Making Their Voices Heard." *Health Service Manager* 9 (February 1976): 1.

Dallas, J.L. "The HSA and the PSRO: Toward a Linkage." *Public Health Reports* 91 (January-February 1976): 46.

Danielson, J.M. "Health Consortium Response to Total Health Care Needs." *Hospitals* 51 (March 1, 1976): 69.

DePozo-Olano, J., and Holland, T. "The Application of New Technological Concepts in the Delivery of Health Services." *Ethics in Science & Medicine* 4, no. 1-2 (1977): 67.

Dittman, D.A., and Peters, J.A. "A Foundation for Health Care Regulations: P.L. 92-603 and P.L. 93-641." *Inquiry* 14 (March 1977): 32.

DuFlorey, C., Weddell, J.M., and Leeder, S.R. "The Epidemiologist's Contribution to Medical Care Planning and Evaluation." *Australian-New Zealand Journal of Medicine* 6 (February 1976): 74.

Earle, P.W. "AHA Plan Preserves Pluralistic System." *Hospital Progress* 58 (February 1977): 61.

Eisdorfer, C., "Issues in Health Planning for the Aged." *Gerontologist* 16 (February 1976): 12.

Elchlepp, J.G., and Henning, W.K. "Medical Center Plans Future By Analyzing Alternatives." *Hospitals* 50 (September 1976): 65.

Elinson, J. "Insensitive Health Statistics and the Dilemma of the HSAs." *American Journal of Public Health* 67 (May 1977): 417.

Endicott, K.M. "A Federal Perspective on the Role of the Journal and Planning to Enhance Health and Well-Being." *American Journal of Health Planning* 1 (July 1976): 1.

Erhardt, C.L. "The Underutilization of Vital Statistics." *American Journal of Public Health* 67 (April 1977): 325.

Ermann, M.D. "The Social Control of Organizations in the Health Care Area." *Milbank Memorial Fund Quarterly* 54 (Spring 1976): 167.

Ferrell, C.R., and Wincenciak, S.L. "A Model of Statewide Planning for the Vocational Rehabilitation of Deaf Persons." *Journal of Rehabilitation* 43 (May-June 1977): 36.

Fink, D.L. "Holistic Health: Implications for Health Planning." *American Journal of Health Planning* 1 (July 1976): 23.

Finney, R.D., Pessin, R.P., and Matheis, L.P. "Prospects for Social Workers in Health Planning." *Health and Social Work* 1 (August 1976): 7.

Fisher, L. and Freeman, S.J. "Community Resources Consultants: An Experimental Approach to Aftercare." *Canadian Mental Health* 24 (March 1976): 33.

Geller, N.L., and Yochmowitz, M.G. "Regional Planning of Maternity Services." *Health Services Research* 10 (Spring 1975): 63.

Gemmell, M.K. "Local Government and Health Systems Agencies." *National League for Nursing* Pub. No. 52-1647 (1976).

Gibson, G. "Measures of Emergency Ambulance Effectiveness: Unmet Need and Inappropriate Use." *Journal of the American College of Emergency Physicians and the University Association for Emergency Medical Services* 6 (September 1977): 389.

Gibson, G., Pickar, E.R., and Wagner, J.L. "Evaluative Measures and Data Collection Methods for Emergency Medical Services Systems." *Public Health Reports* 92 (July-August 1977): 315.

Ginzberg, E. "Paradoxes and Trends: An Economist Looks at Health Care," *New England Journal of Medicine* 296 (April 7, 1977): 814.

Goss, M.E., Battistella, R.M., Colombotos, J., Freidson, E., and Riedel, D.C. "Social Organization and Control in Medical Work: A Call for Research." *Medical Care* 15 (May 1977): 1.

Greene, J.C. "HSA's And All That. A Solution." *Journal of the Michigan Dental Association* 59 (September 1977): 494.

Greer, A.L. "Training Board Members for Health Planning Agencies. A Review of the Literature." *Public Health Reports* 91 (January-February 1976): 56.

Griffith, J.R., and Chernow, R.A. "Cost Effective Acute Care Facilities Planning in

Michigan." *Inquiry* 14 (September 1977): 229.

Gutierrez, J.L. "Health Planning in Latin America." *American Journal of Public Health* 65 (October 1975): 1047.

Hargreaves, W.A., Atkisson, C.C., and Sorenson, J.E. *Resource Materials for Community Mental Health Program Evaluation.* DHEW Pub. No. (ADM) 77-328 (1977).

Harmon, G.J. "Start Planning By Defining the Community, Its Future Needs." *Hospitals* 50 (June 16, 1976): 105.

Harrington, M.B. "Forecasting Areawide Demand for Health Care Services: A Critical Review of Major Techniques and Their Application." *Inquiry* 14 (September 1977): 254.

Hartgerink, M.J. "Health Surveillance and Planning for Health Care in the Netherlands." *International Journal of Epidemiology* 5 (March 1976): 87.

Hertzman, M., and Montague, B. "Cost-Benefit Analysis and Alcoholism." *Journal of Studies on Alcohol* 38 (July 1977): 1371.

Herzlinger, R. "Why Data Systems in Nonprofit Organizations Fail." *Harvard Business Review* 55 (January-February 1977): 81.

Hester, P. "Evaluation and Accountability in a Parent-Implemented Early Intervention Service." *Community Mental Health Journal* 13 (Fall 1977): 261.

Heyssel, R.M. "Countdown to 1984: Health Care Priorities." *Hospital Progress* 58 (October 1977): 60.

Heyssel, R.M. "External Constraints Necessary to Control Hospital Bed Surplus." *Hospital Progress* 58 (April 1977): 6.

Hill, D.B. "Identification of Hospital Cost Determinants: A Health Planning Perspective." *Inquiry* 13 (March 1976): 61.

Hope, W., Jr. "Consumers and PL 93-641." *Journal of the National Association of Private Psychiatry Hospital* 8 (Summer 1976): 24.

Human, J. "Normative Planning for a Better Long Term Care System." *American Journal of Health Planning* 1 (October 1976): 43.

Hungerford, G.D., and Ross, P. "Computed Tomography: Some Clinical, Technical and Health Planning Considerations." *Journal of the School of Medicine Association* 73 (August 1977): 357.

Hutchins, V.L. "New Policies in School Health." *Journal of School Health* 47 (September 1977): 428.

Iglehart, J.K. "The Cost and Regulation of Medical Technology: Future Policy Directions." *Milbank Memorial Fund Quarterly: Health & Society* 55 (Winter 1977): 25.

Jones, W.J. "Hospitals Should Exercise Role in Shaping Health Policies." *Hospitals* 50 (June 16, 1976): 119.

Johnson, E.A. "Puzzlement for Hospital Planners." *Hospital Health Service Administration* 21 (Spring 1976): 64.

Johnson, O.G., Neuman, A.K., and Ofosu-Amaah, S. "Health Information System Installation: Principles and Problems." *Medical Care* 14 (March 1976): 210.

Kaplan, J.M., and Smith, W.G. "The Use of Attainment Scaling in the Evaluation of a Regional Mental Health Program." *Community Mental Health Journal* 13 (Summer 1977): 188.

Kaplis, N.A., and Silberman, S.L. "A Teaching Program in the Sociopolitical Determinants of Health Care." *Journal of Dental Education* 41 (August 1977): 511.

Kendig, H.L., Jr., and Warren, R. "The Adequacy of Census Data in Planning and

Advocacy for the Elderly." *Gerontologist* 16 (October 1976): 391.

Kirklin, J.W., Bridgers, W.F., and Hearn, T.K., Jr. Panel Discussion: "The Allocation of Medical Resources: Who Should Decide and How." *Alabama Journal of Medical Science* 14 (July 1977): 316.

Klarman, H.E. "National Policies and Local Planning for Health Services." *Milbank Memorial Fund Quarterly* 54 (Winter 1976): 1.

Kleinman, J.C. "Age-Adjusted Mortality Indexes for Small Areas: Applications to Health Planning." *American Journal of Public Health* 67 (September 1977): 834.

Lander, L. "Health Systems Agencies." *Health PAC Bulletin* 70 (May-June 1976): 1.

Lane, D.S., and Mazzola, G. "The Community Hospital As a Focus for Health Planning." *American Journal of Public Health* 66 (March 1976): 465.

Lave, J.R., Lave, L.B., and Leinhardt, S. "Medical Manpower Models: Need, Demand and Supply." *Inquiry* 12 (June 1975): 97.

Lee, P.R. "The Frontiers of Health Planning." *American Journal of Health Planning* 1 (October 1976): 1.

Lee, P.R. "Switzer Memorial Lecture: A New Perspective un Health, Health Planning, and Health Policy." *Journal of Allied Health* 6 (Winter 1977): 8.

Lipsky, M., and Lounds, M. "Citizen Participation and Health Care: Problems of Government Induced Participation." *Journal of Health Politics, Policy and Law* 1 (Spring 1976): 85.

Litsios, S. "Developing a Cost and Outcome Evaluation System." *International Journal of Health Services* 6, no. 2 (1976): 345.

Loflin, B. "PL-93-64: National, State and Regional Health Planning." *Journal of the Tennessee Medical Association* 56 (April 1976): 42.

Maatsch, J.L., Hoban, J.D., Sprafka, S.A., Hendershot, N.A., and Messick, J.R. *A Study of Simulation Technology in Medical Education. Appendix D: An Annotated Bibliography.* Ann Arbor: Michigan State University, 1976.

MacStravic, R.E. "Planning System/Hospital Relations: Phases and Fallacies." Hospital Progress 57 (March 1976): 58.

MacStravic, R.E. "Size and Performance of Planning Agencies." *Health Services Research* 12 (Summer 1977): 163.

Mandel, M.D. "New Opportunities for the Public to Shape the Nation's Institutional Health Care Services." *American Journal of Law and Medicine* 3 (Spring 1977): 49.

Marmor, T.R., Wittman, D.A., and Heagy, T.C. "The Politics of Medical Inflation." *Journal of Health Politics and Policy Law* 1 (Spring 1976): 69.

Mason, H.R. "Academic Preparation for Professionals Engaged in Comprehensive Health Planning." *Journal of Community Health* 1 (Spring 1976): 226.

Meredith, G. "Perspectives on Occupational Therapy's Role in Health Systems Agency Activities." *American Journal of Occupational Therapy* 31 (August 1977): 454.

Meredith, J. "Program Evaluation Techniques in the Health Services." *American Journal of Public Health.* 66 (November 1976): 1069.

Mittenthal, S.D. "A System Approach to Human Services Integration." *Evaluation* 3, no. 1-2 (1976): 142.

Mooney, A. "The Great Society and Health: Policies for Narrowing the Gaps in Health Status Between the Poor and the Non-poor." *Medical Care* 15 (August 1977): 611.

Morrone, F. "The National Health Planning Information Center." *Public Health Reports* 91 (January-February 1976): 19.

Muszynski, S. "Mental Health Care and Treatment: Will Health Planning Make a Difference." *Hospital and Community Psychiatry* 27 (June 1976): 398.

Nechasek, J.E. "Health Systems Agencies: Implications and Prospects for the Allied Health Professions." *Journal of Allied Health* 5 (Fall 1976): 55.

Norris, E.L., and Larsen, J.K. "Critical Issues in Mental Health Service Delivery: What Are the Priorities?" *Hospital and Community Psychiatry* 27 (August 1976): 561.

North, A.J., Jr., Wilkinson, P., and Oliver, T.K., Jr. "Regional Planning of Hospital Facilities for Children." *American Journal of Diseases of Children* 131 (April 1977): 400.

Nutt, P.C. "The Merits of Using Experts or Consumers as Members of Planning Groups: A Field Experiment in Health Planning." *Academy of Management Journal* 19 (September 1976): 378.

Parker, B.R., and Srinivasan, V.A. "Consumer Preference Approach to the Planning of Rural Primary Health Care Facilities." *Operations Research* 24 (September-October 1976): 991.

Petus, J. "Hospital Characteristics Influence Planning Approaches, Practices." *Hospitals* 50 (September 1, 1976): 83.

Phillips, D.F. "Regulations and Data Systems: Questions of Demands Versus Needs." *Hospitals* 51 (October 1977): 85.

Pierce, C.F. "Partnerships in Planning: Getting Everyone Into the Act." *Hospitals* 50 (June 16, 1976): 113.

Portnoy, S. "Planning Must Exist At All Levels of the System." *Hospitals.* 50 (June 16, 1976): 65.

Prothro, G.W., and Schlezinger, I.H. "Health Systems Agencies—Just Another Hurdle." *Journal of the Oklahoma State Medical Association* 69 (February 1976): 38.

Prussin, J.A. "Applications of Operational Research to Health Care Delivery Systems and Facilities Planning." *World Hospital* 12, no. 3 (1976): 185.

Reeves, P.N. "Issues in Health Plan Development: A Critique of the Guidelines for Plan Development Under PL 93-641." *American Journal of Health Planning* 1 (1977): 27.

Reider, A.E., Mason, J.R., and Glantz, L.H. "Certificate of Need: The Massachusetts Experience." *American Journal of Law and Medicine* 1 (March 1975): 13.

Reinke, W.A. "Alternative Methods for Determining Resource Requirements: The Chile Example." *International Journal of Health Services* 6, no. 1 (1976): 123.

Revelle, C., Bigman, D., Schilling, D., Cohon, J., and Church, R. "Facility Location: A Review of Context-Free and EMS Models." *Health Services Research* 12 (Summer 1977): 129.

Rice, D.P., and Wilson, D. "The American Medical Economy: Problems and Perspectives." *Journal of Health Politics, Policy and Law* 1 (Summer 1976): 151.

Robbins, A. "Who Should Make Public Policy for Health." *American Journal of Public Health* 66 (May 1976): 431.

Romeder, J.M., and McWhinnie, J.R. "Potential Years of Life Lost Between Ages 1 and 70: An Indicator of Premature Mortality for Health Planning." *International Journal of Epidemiology* 6 (June 1977): 143.

Rosenfeld, L.S., and Rosenfeld, I. "National Health Planning in the United States: Prospects and Portents." *Internation Journal of Health Services* 5, no. 3 (1975): 441.

Ross, J. "Putting it All Together." *American Journal of Health Planning* 1 (January 1977): 8.

Rubel, E.J. "Implementing the National Health Planning and Resources Development Act of 1974." *Public Health Reports* 91 (January-February 1976): 3.

Rubenstein, L., Mates, S., and Sidel, V.W. "Quality of Care Assessment by Process and Outcome Scoring. Use of Weighted Algorithimic Assessment Criteria for Evaluation of Emergency Room Care of Women with Symptoms of UTI." *Annals of Internal Medicine* 86 (May 1977): 617.

Salkever, D.S., and Bice, T.W. "The Impact of Certificate-of-Need Controls on Hospital Investment." *Milbank Memorial Fund Quarterly* 54 (Spring 1976): 185.

Sauber, S.R. "State Planning of Mental Health Services." *American Journal of Community Psychology* 4 (March 1976): 35.

Schneer, E.C., and Fielding, J.E. "Quantifying the Need for Hospital Beds." *New England Journal of Medicine* 297 (November 10, 1977): 1065.

Schneider, D.P., and Foley, W.J. "A Systems Analysis of the Impact of Physician Extenders on Medical Cost and Manpower Requirements." *Medical Care.* 15 (April 1977): 277.

Schoeman, M.E., and Mahajan, V. "Using the Delphi Method to Assess Community Health Needs." *Technological Forecasting and Social Change* 10 (1977): 203.

Scutchfield, F.D. "Alternate Methods for Priority Assessment." *Journal of Community Health* 1 (Fall 1975): 29.

Siegmann, A.E. "A Classification of Sociomedical Indicators: Perspectives for Health Administrators and Health Planners." *International Journal of Health Services* 6, no. 3 (1976): 521.

Sieverts, S. "Is P.L. 93-641 Concerned With Long Term Care? It's Up To You." *Hospitals* 49 (October 16, 1975): 69.

Sieverts, S. "Putting P.L. 93-641 Into Proper Perspective," *Hospitals* 50 (June 16, 1976): 125.

Silver, G.A. "Medical Politics, Health Policy. Party Platforms, Promise and Performance." *International Journal of Health Services* 6, no. 2 (1976): 33.

Simler, S.L. "Health Systems Agencies are Seeking More Power Over Capital Expenditures." *Modern Health Care* 7 (August 1977): 35.

Skerry, W. "P.L. 93-641: Beyond Planning Toward Control." *Hospital Progress* 57 (March 1976): 10.

Skrinjar, B. "A Health Information System for the Management of an Integrated Health Service." *World Hospital* 12, no. 1 (1976): 27.

Skuza, B.H. "Health Planning and Resources Development: An Opportunity for Optometry." *Journal of American Optometric Association* 47 (February 1976): 143.

Smith, V.S. "A Statewide Cooperative Approach to Health Manpower Planning." *Journal of Allied Health* 5 (Spring 1976): 52.

Snoke, A.W., and Snoke, P.S. "Linking Private, Public Energies in Health and Welfare Planning." *Hospitals* 50 (August 16, 1976): 53.

Solomon, M.A. "Implementation of Legislative Requirements for Emergency Medical Services in Prepaid Group Practice Organizations." *Public Health Reports* 92 (July-August 1977): 307.

Somers, A.R., and Somers, H.M. "A Proposed Framework for Health and Health Care Policies." *Inquiry* 14 (June 1977): 115.

Stiles, S.V., and Johnson, K.A. "Regulatory and Review Functions of Agencies Created by the Act." *Public Health Reports* 91 (January-February 1976): 24.

Stone, D. "Professionalism and Accountability. Controlling Health Services in the United States and West Germany." *Journal of Health Politics, Policy and Law* 2 (Spring 1977): 32.

Strauss, M.D., Marten, C.J., and Kempner, M.A. "Toward An Invisible College: Training of Personnel for Local and State Health Agencies." *Public Health Reports* 91 (January-February 1976): 51.

Strosberg, M.A. "Technology and the Governance of the Health Care Industry: The Dilemma of Reform." *Journal of Health Politics, Policy and Law* 2 (Summer 1977): 212.

Stuehler, G. "The Hospital-Based Planner 'In His Time Plays Many Parts.'" *Hospitals* 50 (June 16, 1976): 75.

Tekolste, E. "Health Care: The Clash Between Resources and Limitations." *Hospital Progress* 58 (May 1977): 74.

Terenzio, J.V. "The National Health Planning and Resources Act of 1974." *Bulletin of the New York Academy of Medicine* 52 (December 1976): 1236.

Thompson, T. "Working With P.L. 93-641: The Health Occupation Educator's Viewpoint." *Journal of the National Medical Association* 69 (February 1977): 122.

USDHEW, Health Resources Administration. *Public Health Reports* (January/February 1976 issue with a special section on health planning).

USDHEW, Health Resources Administration. *The Priorities of Section 1502. Papers on the National Health Guidelines*. Pub. No. (HRA) 77-641 (1977).

USDHEW, Health Resources Administration. *Baselines for Setting Health Goals and Standards. Papers on the National Health Guidelines*. Pub. No. (HRA) 76-640 (1976).

USDHEW, Health Resources Administration. *Proceedings of The Public Health Conference on Records and Statistics*. Pub. No. (HRA) 77-1214 (1977).

USDHEW, Health Resources Administration. *Board and Staff Composition of Health Planning Agencies*. Pub. No. (HRA) 78-609 (1978).

Walker, G., and Gish, O. "Mobile Health Services: A Study in Cost-Effectiveness." *Medical Care* 15 (April 1977): 267.

Walsh, D.C., and Bicknell, W.J. "Forecasting the Need for Hospital Beds: A Quantitative Methodology." *Public Health Reports* 92 (May-June 1977): 199.

Wang, V.L., Fonaroff, A., and Dawson, J. "Problem Solving for Common Goals in Two Types of Community Agencies." *American Journal of Public Health* 65 (August 1975): 809.

Weatherford, R.P. "Hospital Planning at HSA." *American Journal of Health Planning* 1 (October 1976): 35.

Werlin, S.H., Walcott, A., and Joroff, M. "Implementing Formative Health Planning Under P.L. 93-641." *New England Journal of Medicine* 295 (September 23, 1976): 698.

West, J.P., and Stevens, M.D. "Comparative Analysis of Community Health Planning: Transition From CHPs to HSAs." *Journal of Health Politics, Policy and Law* 1 (Summer 1976): 173.

Whiting, R., and Casaday, W.L. "Associations Are Source of Planning Assistance," *Hospitals* 50 (September 1, 1976): 68.

Wildavsky, A. "Doing Better and Feeling Worse: The Political Pathology of Health Policy." *Daedalus* 105 (Winter 1977).

Wolf, R.M. "The Use of Evaluation Data in Planning." *National League for Nursing* Pub. No. 21-1637 (1976).

Youngerman, R.A. "Implementing P.L. 93-641: Progress of the North Central Georgia

Health Systems Agency." *Journal of the Medical Association of Georgia* 66 (March 1977): 141.

Zhuk, A.P. *Public Health Planning in the U.S.S.R.* DHEW Pub. No. (NIH) 76-999 (1976).

Zimmerman, J.P. "Service Areas and Their Needs Must Be Reassessed." *Hospitals* 49 (September 1, 1975): 46.

Zwick, D.I. "Health Policy Guidelines and Holistic Care." *American Journal of Health Planning* 1 (January 1976): 49.

Index

of drug abuse centers (quick), 435, 439, 440
of effectiveness in planning, 455-456, 457-458
of efficiency in planning, 457-458
errors in, 440
five A's of, 339
five D's in, 340-341
framework of, 346-348
guide to program, 422-424
guidelines for, 353-354, 375-376, 379-382
health status index and, 408, 414
of hospitals, 317-318, 348-351
impact and process, 331, 332
indexes for, 400, 403-405
indicators for, 400, 403-408, 409-412
instruments for, 417, 418
matrix for, in preventive health, 333-339
measurement instruments for, 369-372
measurement typologies in, 340-343, 344
medical care, studies, 354-357
medical care, study abstract of, 425, 430-432
model screening criteria for PSRO, 398-403
of occupational health program, 424-429
Office of Economic Opportunity and, 331-333
patient care, 358-366
PL 93-641 and, 355-358
placebo effect and, 443
of planning process, 457
problems of, 440-444
program impact, 331-332
program strategy, 332-333
project, 333
project rating, 333
psuedo-, 324-325
of PSROs, 351-354
purpose of, 323-325
reliability in, 440-443
research designs for, 366-369
review and comment form for, 432-434
risk/payoffs considerations in, 444

rules for, 327
scales for, 417, 418
self-administered, of planning, 417-419
standards for, 333, 386
steps in process of, 321-322, 325-327
study example of, 337-339
subversion of, 325
total comparative program model of, 419-422
utilization of, 445
validity and, 440-443
words used in classification categories in, 334-335, 336, 339
See also Health planning
Exceptional children, directory for, 85

F

Facilities. *See* Clinics; Hospitals; Medical facilities
Family planning clinics
  health resources for, 94
  hospitals and, 246-247
Family Planning Programs, evaluation study example for, 337-339
Federal government
  evaluation policy of, 320, 331-333
  health planning guidelines of, 386-396
  involvement of, in health planning, 9-10, 11, 23-24, 241, 250, 331, 386-396
  report form for medical care evaluation, 425, 430-431
  See also Federal legislation
Federal legislation
  evaluation of health care and, 323, 341, 351, 432, 445
  Hill-Burton Act, 9, 52
  influence of, on health planning, 9-10, 11, 23-24
  PL 93-641, 9, 24, 136-143, 179-181
  PL 94-63, 179
  PSROs and, 13
  Social Security, 9, 180
  See also Federal government
Feedback evaluation techniques, cost-benefit analysis and, 166

About the Authors

Allen D. Spiegel, Ph.D., is an Associate Professor of Preventive Medicine and Community Health for the State University of New York, Downstate Medical Center, College of Medicine. In public health since 1951, Dr. Spiegel's experiences include a wide range of activities in medical and health care services, comprehensive health planning, public health education and health and medical communications. Formerly, Dr. Spiegel was with the New York City Health Department, the Medical Foundation, Inc. of Boston, was a U.S. Public Health Service Special Research Fellow at Brandeis University, and a consultant on numerous health and welfare projects. He has authored and co-authored more than 100 articles, reports and pamphlets on health care and edited and contributed to a number of books on community and mental health including a leading reference work, *Perspectives in Community Mental Health*. He is also co-author of *Medicaid: Lessons for National Health Insurance* and the author of *The Medicaid Experience*.

Herbert Harvey Hyman, Ph.D., is a Professor in the Graduate Program on Urban Affairs, Hunter College, City University of New York. He has served as a consultant to HEW for the implementation of PL 93-641, and has been active for a number of years as an executive, project director, and consultant in health planning and community health programs. He is the editor of *Health Regulation: Certificate of Need and 1122,* published in 1977, and the author of *Health Planning: A Systematic Approach,* published in 1975, and *The Politics of Health Planning,* published in 1973. Dr. Hyman received his Ph.D. from Brandeis University. He holds a B.A. degree from Ohio University and a Master's Degree in Social Work from the University of Connecticut.